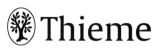

Complementary Oncology

Adjunctive Methods in the Treatment of Cancer

Josef Beuth, M.D.
Professor
Director, Institute of Scientific Evaluation
of Naturopathic Methods
University of Cologne
Cologne, Germany

Ralph W. Moss, Ph.D.
Research Scientist
Brooksville, ME, USA

With contributions by:
Ulrich Abel, Arndt Büssing, E. Dieter Hager,
Heide Jenik, Karl Friedrich Klippel, Hagen Knaf,
Patrick Lang, Ilse Ledvina, Rudolf van Leendert,
Kedar N. Prasad, Volker Rusch, Dieter Prätzel-
Wolters, Volker Schirrmacher, Berthold Schneider,
G.N. Schrauzer, Jörg Sigle, Gerhard Uhlenbruck,
Kurt S. Zänker

47 illustrations

Thieme
Stuttgart · New York

Library of Congress Cataloging-in-Publication Data

Grundlagen der Komplementäronkologie. English.
Complementary oncology : adjunctive methods
in the treatment of cancer / [edited by] Josef Beuth,
Ralph W. Moss ; with contributions by Ulrich Abel ...
[et al.].
p. ; cm.
Revised translation of the German ed.,
published in 2002.
Includes bibliographical references.
ISBN 3-13-137451-9 (alk. paper) –
ISBN 1-58890-323-0 (alk. paper)
1. Cancer – Adjuvant treatment. 2. Cancer – Alternative
treatment.
  [DNLM: 1. Neoplasms--therapy. 2. Complementary
Therapies. QZ 266 G889 2005a] I. Beuth, J. II. Moss,
Ralph W. III. Abel, Ulrich, 1952- IV. Title.
RC271.A35G7813 2005
616.99'406–dc22
2005008532

This book is an authorized and completely revised
translation of the German edition published and copy-
righted 2002 by Hippokrates Verlag, Stuttgart, Germany. Title of the German edition: Grundlagen der
Komplementäronkologie: Theorie und Praxis.

Translator: Ursula Vielkind, Ph. D., C. Tran., Ontario,
Canada.

Cover Images
Tabár L, Tot T, Dean PB. Breast Cancer—The Art and
Science of Early Detection with Mammography,
Thieme 2005.
We would like to thank the authors for their kind per-
mission to use these images.

© 2006 Georg Thieme Verlag,
Rüdigerstrasse 14, 70469 Stuttgart, Germany
http://www.thieme.de
Thieme New York, 333 Seventh Avenue,
New York, NY 10001 USA
http://www.thieme.com

Typesetting by Satzpunkt Ewert GmbH, Bayreuth
Printed in Germany by Druckhaus Götz, Ludwigsburg

ISBN 3-13-137451-9 (GTV)
ISBN 1-58890-323-0 (TNY)   1 2 3 4 5 6

Important note: Medicine is an ever-changing science
undergoing continual development. Research and clinical experience are continually expanding our knowledge, in particular our knowledge of proper treatment
and drug therapy. Insofar as this book mentions any
dosage or application, readers may rest assured that the
authors, editors, and publishers have made every effort
to ensure that such references are in accordance with
**the state of knowledge at the time of production of
the book.**
  Nevertheless, this does not involve, imply, or express any guarantee or responsibility on the part of the
publishers in respect to any dosage instructions and
forms of applications stated in the book. **Every user is
requested to examine carefully** the manufacturers'
leaflets accompanying each drug and to check, if necessary in consultation with a physician or specialist,
whether the dosage schedules mentioned therein or the
contraindications stated by the manufacturers differ
from the statements made in the present book. Such examination is particularly important with drugs that are
either rarely used or have been newly released on the
market. Every dosage schedule or every form of application used is entirely at the user's own risk and responsibility. The authors and publishers request every user to
report to the publishers any discrepancies or inaccura-
cies noticed. If errors in this work are found after publication, errata will be posted at www.thieme.com on the
product description page.

Preface

New approaches to curative cancer therapy are being explored and evaluated around the world. For example, great hopes have been placed in the Human Genome Project as well as in advances in the fields of molecular biology, molecular genetics, and immunology.

Searching for new substances of therapeutic importance (e. g., in rain forests and oceans, or by developing new technologies) also seems promising. However, this is a time-consuming and expensive process because it is an indispensable prerequisite that such treatments be scientifically evaluated before they are clinically applied. Currently, the optimization of curative cancer therapy seems to be most possible through the development of interdisciplinary concepts of oncological therapies.

In the United States, the use of tumor-destructive standard therapies (surgery, radiation, and chemotherapy) did not significantly lower cancer mortality over the last 30 years. Despite expensive efforts in both research and therapy in response to President Nixon's declaration of war against cancer in 1971, the age-adjusted cancer mortality has even increased by about 6%. Good therapeutic results were achieved only for relatively rare types of tumors (such as lymphoma, leukemia, and testicular tumors). This failure to achieve positive results in the statistically major forms of cancer has spurred the demand for new concepts of treatment and has ushered in the scientific, experimental, and clinical efficacy testing of therapeutic measures used in complementary oncology.

In the United States, as many as 91% of all cancer patients now use complementary measures, often without the knowledge of the attending oncologist. Their main motives are:
- to actively participate in fighting their disease or promoting their recovery
- to activate the immune system
- to optimize the standard therapy.

These understandable wishes need to be addressed with critical (though favorable) open-mindedness, and therapists should get it straight in their minds that active patients in fact profit from the activation of their psychoneuroimmunological system.

As per their definition, therapeutic measures in complementary oncology are not intended to replace approved standard therapies. Hence, they are not "alternative therapies." Measures in complementary oncology that prove to be important additions to the tumor-destructive therapies simply claim to optimize these standard therapies.

Preliminary data from scientifically based clinical studies have demonstrated the importance of various measures. The benefits to the patients included improvement in their quality of life, reduction of their symptoms and side effects due to standard therapy, and improvement of their immunological state.

In the present book, efficacy-tested measures of complementary medicine are integrated for the first time in a scientific manner into an oncological treatment plan. Due to the organization of the book and its clearly arranged tables it is not only suitable as a handy reference for the practicing oncologist, but it provides an extensive and critical insight into the relevant test results for the scientifically minded oncologist.

Chapters 1 to 7 offer a critical analysis of the current situation in oncology and introduce the reader to tumor immunology. Other chapters deal with study designs and the problems arising when evaluating oncological studies. This part ends with the presentation of the QoL-Recorder, a tool designed to assist in determining the quality of life—a secret aspect behind therapeutic results, which has been neglected until recently.

Chapters 8 to 20 are competent introductions to complementary therapies for which scientifically based data are available from clinical studies (evidence-based medicine [EBM] level 1 [randomized controlled studies] and level 2 [cohort studies]).

In Chapter 21 the integration of these measures into the standard therapy of solid tumors is presented in the form of tables. Here, the duration and the intensity of the treatments are listed for various types of cancer.

Chapter 22 presents many promising concepts of treatment, but it is still too early to integrate them into the treatment plan.

Our thanks go to Angelika M. Findgott for her charming but straight initiation and accomplishment of this project; Ursula Vielkind for her excellent translation; Stefanie Langner and the staff at Thieme International for the opportunity to realize this project. Finally, we wish to thank all authors of this book for their critical stocktaking of complementary oncology.

Josef Beuth, M. D., Cologne, Germany
Ralph W. Moss, Ph. D., Lemont, Pennsylvania

List of Contributors

Ulrich Abel, Ph. D.
Professor
University of Heidelberg
Heidelberg, Germany

Arndt Büssing, M. D.
University of Witten/Herdecke
Department of Applied Immunology
Herdecke, Germany

E. Dieter Hager, M. D., Ph. D.
Director of BioMed-Clinic
for Complementary Oncology
Bad Bergzabern, Germany

Heide Jenik
Rudolf van Leendert
Institute of Scientific Evaluation of
Naturopathic Methods
University of Cologne,
Cologne, Germany

Karl Friedrich Klippel, M. D.
Professor
General Hospital Celle,
Celle, Germany

Kedar N. Prasad, Ph. D.
Antioxidant Research Institute
Premier Micronutrient Corporation
Novato, CA, USA

Dieter Prätzel-Wolters, Professor
Hagen Knaf, Ph. D.
Patrick Lang, Ph. D.
Fraunhofer-Institute for Techno-
and Business Arithmetics
Kaiserslautern, Germany

Volker Rusch, Ph. D.
Institute of Integrative Biology
Herborn, Germany

Volker Schirrmacher, Ph. D.
Professor
German Cancer Research Centre Heidelberg
Tumorimmunology
Heidelberg, Germany

Berthold Schneider, Dr. phil. Nat.
Professor
Medical University Hanover
Institute of Biometrics
Hanover, Germany

G. N. Schrauzer, M. D.
Professor
Biological Trace Element
Research Institute
Chula Vista, CA, USA

Jörg Sigle, M. D.
Private Practice
Freudenstein, Germany
Department of General Medicine
University of Göttingen
Göttingen, Germany

Gerhard Uhlenbruck, M. D.
Professor
Ilse Ledvina
Institute of Immunobiology
University of Cologne
Cologne, Germany

Kurt S. Zänker, M. D.
Professor
University of Witten/Herdecke
Institute of Immunobiology
Herdecke, Germany

List of Abbreviations

α-TS	α-tocopherol succinate
ADCC	antibody-dependent cellular cytotoxicity
AJCC	American Joint Committee on Cancer
APC	antigen-presenting cell
ASCO	American Society of Clinical Oncology
ASI	active specific immunotherapy (for cancer)
ATBC	α-tocopherol plus β-carotene
ATRA	all-*trans* retinoic acid
ATV	autologous tumor vaccine
AVI	autovaccine for intestinal tract
AWB	Anwendungsbeobachtungen (specific observational studies; a German variant of postmarketing surveillance studies)
BALT	bronchus-associated lymphoid tissue
BCG	bacillus of Calmette-Guerrin
BfArM	Federal Institute for Drugs and Medical Devices
BSC	best supportive care
CALGB	Cancer and Leukemia Group B
CAM	complementary and alternative medicine
CAP	catabolite activation protein
CARET	β-Carotene and Retinol Efficacy Trial
CDC	complement-dependent cytotoxicity
CHART	continuous hyperfractionated accelerated radiotherapy
CMF	cyclophosphamide, methotrexate, fluorouracil (chemotherapy)
CML	chronic myeloid leukemia
CR	complete remission
CRF	case report forms
CTL	cytotoxic lymphocyte
DACH	German, Austrian, and Swiss Societies of Nutrition
DC	dendritic cells
DGE	German Society of Nutrition
DHA	dehydroascorbic acid
DHT	deep hyperthermia
DNA	deoxyribonucleic acid
DRI	dietary reference intake
DTH	delayed-type hypersensitivity
DTIC	5-(3,3-dimethyl-1-triazeno)-imidazol-4-carboximide (dacarbazine)
EBM	evidence-based medicine
EBV	Epstein–Barr virus
ECOG	Eastern Collaborative Oncology Group
EGCG	epigallocatechin gallate
EGF	epidermal growth factor
EGFR	epidermal growth factor receptor
EMEA	European Agency for the Evaluation of Medicinal Products
FDA	Food and Drug Administration
FGF	fibroblast growth factor
FKJ	fine-needle catheter jejunostomy
GAC	germ-free animal characteristics
Gal	galactose
GalNAc	N-acetyl-D-galactosamine
GCP	good clinical practices (placebo controlled, prospective randomized, double-blind multicenter study)
GEP	good epidemiological practices
GM-CSF	granulocyte–macrophage colony-stimulating factor
GSH-Px	glutathione peroxidase
HAA	heterocyclic aromatic amines
HADS	Hospital Anxiety and Depression Scale
HAMA	human antimouse antibody
HBP	hepatic binding protein
HL	hepatic lectin
HLA	human lymphocyte antigen
HRQOL	health-related quality of life
HSP	heat shock protein
ICH	International Conference on Harmonization of Technical Requirements for Registration of Pharmaceuticals for Human Use
ICHP	intracavitary hyperthermic perfusion (perfusion hyperthermia)
IHT	interstitial hyperthermia
IL	interleukin
IMS	Institute for Medical Statistics

iNO	inducible nitric oxide synthetase
IOM	Institute of Medicine
IPHP	intraperitoneal hyperthermic perfusion
IplHP	intrapleural hyperthermic perfusion
IRA	infrared-A radiation
IRB	Institutional Review Board
ISGNAS	International Study Group of New Antimicrobial Strategies
ITT	intention-to-treat analysis
IVHP	intravesicular hyperthermic perfusion
JNCI	Journal of the National Cancer Institute
LAK	lymphokine-activated killer cell
LCL	lymphoblastoid cell line
LHT	local hyperthermia
LPS	lipopolysaccharide
MAC	microflora-associated characteristics
Mab	monoclonal antibody
MALT	mucosa-associated lymphoid tissue
MCP-1	monocyte chemotactic protein 1
MFH	magnetic fluid hyperthermia
MHC	major histocompatibility complex
Mn-SOD	manganese superoxide dismutase
MSKCC	Memorial Sloan-Kettering Cancer Center
NAC	N-acetylcysteine
NANA	N-acetylneuraminic acid
NB	neuroblastoma
NCI	National Cancer Institute
NCS	national consumption study
NDV	Newcastle disease virus
NK	natural killer cell
NOD/SCID	onobese diabetic/severe combined immunodeficiency disorder (mice)
NSCLC	non-small cell lung carcinoma
OS	overall survival
PAC	polycyclic aromatic carbohydrates
PBL	peripheral blood lymphocytes
PDGF	platelet-derived growth factor
PDQ	Physician's Data Query
PDTC	pyrrolidine dithiocarbamate
PEG	percutaneous endoscopic gastrostomy
PEJ	percutaneous endoscopic jejunostomy
PH–GSH–Px	phospholipid–hydroperoxide–glutathione peroxidase

PHS	Physicians Health Study
PHT	perfusion hyperthermia
PLAP	placental alkaline phosphatase
PR	partial remission
PSA	prostate-specific antigen
PSMA	prostate-specific membrane antigen
PUG	percutaneous ultrasonographic gastrostomy
QALYs	quality-adjusted life years
QLQ	Quality of Life Questionnaire
QoL	quality of life
RCT	randomized controlled trial
RDA	recommended dietary (or daily) allowance
RHT	regional hyperthermia
RSV	respiratory syncytial virus
SAQLI	Calgary Sleep Apnea Quality of Life Index
SCLC	small-cell lung cancer
SD	stable disease
SEREX	serological analysis of antigens by recombinant expression cloning
SHT	superficial hyperthermia
SHBG	sex hormone-binding protein
SOP	standard operating procedure
STH	somatotrophic hormone (somatotropin)
TA	tumor antigen
TAA	tumor-associated antigen
TATA	tumor-associated transplantation antigen
TCA	tumor cell activity
TCR	T-cell receptor
TGF-β	transforming growth factor β
TIMP	tissue inhibitor of metalloproteinase
TLR	Toll-like receptor
TNF-α	tumor necrosis factor α
UICC	International Union Against Cancer
VEGF	vascular endothelial growth factor
VIL	vaccine infiltrating lymphocyte
VLP	viruslike particles
WBHT	whole-body hyperthermia
wIRA	water-filtered infrared A radiation

Contents

8 Cancer and Nutrition 91

9 Exercise in Cancer Prevention and Follow-up 116

10 Psycho-oncology 130

11 Biological Basis for Using High Dose Multiple Antioxidants as an Adjunct to Radiotherapy, Chemotherapy, and Experimental Cancer Therapies 151

12 Selenium in Oncology 171

13 Proteolytic Enzymes 183

14 Lectin-Standardized Mistletoe Extracts 189

15 Mistletoe Extracts from the Anthroposophical Point of View 197

16 Thymic Peptides 207

17 Probiotic Therapy 212

Current Issues in the Treatment of Cancer

Since the main causes of death were first considered in medicine, cardiovascular disease has proven to be the leading cause, with cancer in second place. Each year since these statistics have been taken, the number of deaths from cancer has remained the same, while the number of deaths resulting from cardiovascular disease has decreased. In 2001 over half a million people died of cancer in the U.S. (see Fig. 1). It is estimated today that in just a few years from now the death toll from cancer will exceed that from cardiovascular disease.

The dramatic decline in deaths from heart disease can easily be attributed to modern technological and social improvements made to our lives in the past century: the availability of hospital services with intensive care units, roads and transportation allowing rapid response to cardiac attacks, communication systems, and, indeed, better understanding and medical surgical and pharmacological care for heart conditions.

The situation is very different where cancer is concerned. Although we have all these improvements, the number of cancer incidences has exceeded the anticipated growth and age of the population. The number of deaths has remained the same, which means that many people who have cancer may not necessarily die as a result. However, this does not represent an improvement

US Mortality, 2001

Rank	Cause of Death	No. of deaths	% of all deaths
1.	Heart Diseases	700,142	29.0
2.	**Cancer**	**553,768**	**22.9**
3.	Cerebrovascular diseases	163,538	6.8
4.	Chronic lower respiratory diseases	123,013	5.1
5.	Accidents (Unintentional injuries)	101,537	4.2
6.	Diabetes mellitus	71,372	3.0
7.	Influenza and Pneumonia	62,034	2.6
8.	Alzheimer's disease	53,852	2.2
9.	Nephritis	39,480	1.6
10.	Septicemia	32,238	1.3

Source: US Mortality Public Use Data Tape 2001, National Center for Health Statistics, Centers for Disease Control and Prevention, 2003.

Fig. 1

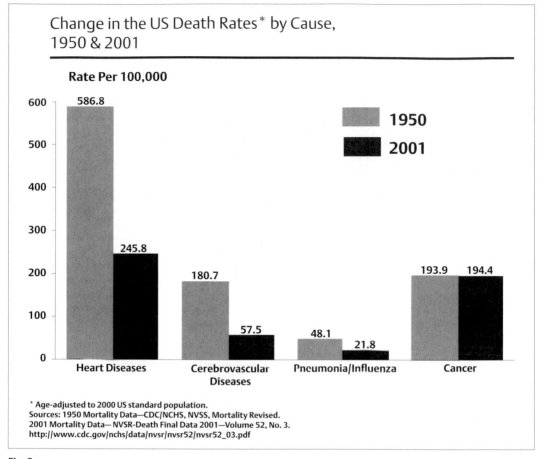

Change in the US Death Rates* by Cause, 1950 & 2001

Rate Per 100,000

- 1950
- 2001

Heart Diseases	Cerebrovascular Diseases	Pneumonia/Influenza	Cancer
586.8	180.7	48.1	193.9
245.8	57.5	21.8	194.4

* Age-adjusted to 2000 US standard population.
Sources: 1950 Mortality Data—CDC/NCHS, NVSS, Mortality Revised.
2001 Mortality Data— NVSR-Death Final Data 2001—Volume 52, No. 3.
http://www.cdc.gov/nchs/data/nvsr/nvsr52/nvsr52_03.pdf

Fig. 2

in cancer cure rates, though we have succeeded in some cases such as with childhood leukemia and lymphoma. People do not die from cancer because we have improved their treatments in order to allow a delay in recurrence. In addition, most people facing cancer are older and have other complicating conditions that may result in their death. For estimated cancer deaths by specific sites refer to Figure 2.

The probability of men who live to be 80 years of age getting cancer is 1 in 2, while for women it is 1 in 3, with mainly prostate cancer increasing the probability for men. The overall risk of death resulting from cancer varies significantly according to cancer sites and ethnicity. Overall, African Americans have an 11 % higher risk of dying from cancer than Whites.

A further interesting observation is that cancer rates are much higher in the developed countries than in developing or third-world countries. A particularly confusing case is that of breast cancer. Breast cancer rates in Western countries are up to 15 times higher than in Africa and up to 5 times higher than in China and Japan. It has been observed that breast cancer incidence rates of second generation daughters of East Asian immigrants to the U.S. equals that of the general population. This observation suggests that it is not the genetic make up of the East Asians that provide protective benefit to breast cancer but rather environmental factors or life style. It has been suspected that the Asian diet is associated with the reduced risk. Since industrialization has rapidly taken place in China the breast cancer rates in the cities have increased dramatically.

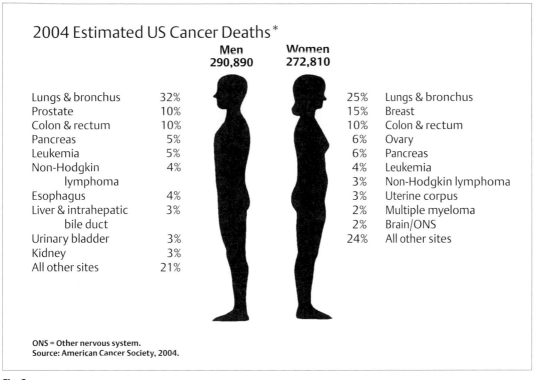

2004 Estimated US Cancer Deaths*

Men
290,890

Women
272,810

Lungs & bronchus	32%	25%	Lungs & bronchus
Prostate	10%	15%	Breast
Colon & rectum	10%	10%	Colon & rectum
Pancreas	5%	6%	Ovary
Leukemia	5%	6%	Pancreas
Non-Hodgkin lymphoma	4%	4%	Leukemia
		3%	Non-Hodgkin lymphoma
Esophagus	4%	3%	Uterine corpus
Liver & intrahepatic bile duct	3%	2%	Multiple myeloma
		2%	Brain/ONS
Urinary bladder	3%	24%	All other sites
Kidney	3%		
All other sites	21%		

ONS = Other nervous system.
Source: American Cancer Society, 2004.

Fig. 3

This may lead us to the conclusion that industrial pollution is the primary cause of breast cancer. However, this is an oversimplified conclusion, and studies attempting to determine industrial pollutants (such as petrochemicals, pesticides and herbicides, electromagnetic fields, microwave emissions, etc.) as a cause were unsuccessful in showing them to be a conclusive cause of the initiation or promotion of breast cancer. Two examples of industrialization have been implicated. As cancer is a disease mostly encountered as we age, the fact that we live much longer than people did just a century ago increases our risk. In addition, for the first time in history in the developed world we have too much food. A significant increase in overall body mass index has been observed in almost all countries. In Japan protein consumption has increased 6 times over since the 1970's, which resulted in an average 6 in (25 cm) increase in height over the previous generation. Similar trends occurred in the U.S. and Europe earlier in the 20th century.

So why would the good things that come with industrialization result in an increase in cancer incidence and death? Cancer is a disease of uncontrolled cell growth. Cell growth is mediated by a complex signaling system mediated by many innate processes. Cell growth is needed for growth, development, procreation, and repair. The cells are therefore susceptible to messages that regulate all these processes. As a result of evolution, the body has adapted to respond to a variety of both internal and external signals. For example, the amount and type of nutrients made available through ingestion facilitates the growth and development of an individual. After the body reaches a certain level of maturity and size, an internal system of hormones regulates the growth and maturity of reproductive ability. Both examples indicate how cell growth may be mediated but in fact set a complex coordinated signaling inside each individual cell that results in its replication (the mitotic process). Cancer occurs when the controls on the processes that regulate the growth and death of cells within the cell are damaged. The cell can lose control in one of four main ways; growth is either promoted or simply not halted, or death is inhibited or simply not initiated. There are genes and proteins within the cell that are responsible for each of these processes. They can change their behavior unexpectedly. This is called mutation. It is currently thought that for a cell to become cancerous it needs to acquire at least four different hits, or particular mutations. Many controls involved in the regulation of growth have to become damaged for the cell to become out of control.

Following this process of initiation or carcinogenesis there must be a way for these cells to continue growing. A supportive environment is required to promote growth; also, ways for the cells to expand, infiltrate surrounding areas, and then break free from their original location to move, lodge, and grow elsewhere. This is a process we call metastasis.

Unfortunately, when we try to isolate the potential genes and proteins involved in the process there are too many of them. They are not easy to target with therapy and, when mutated, they cannot easily be repaired. In addition, each cancer case is different. Despite much effort to understand and target therapies, the pharmaceutical and biotechnology industry has failed to produce more than a handful of useful therapies. Most of the successful targeted therapies are only applicable to specific cases, yet they provide great hope for people. As an example of this, we have been aware of the association between estrogen inhibition and breast cancer recurrence for more than a century. Until the late 1980's, when the estrogen antagonist, tamoxifen, became available, all we could offer to women with breast cancer was oopherectomy, and this only to pre-menopausal women, who represent only a small proportion of women with breast cancer. Later we learned that the efficacy of tamoxifen was further subject to the expression level of the estrogen receptor in the woman's tumor, and only 60% have sufficient expression of this protein. This highlights the fact that not all breast cancers are alike and that not all breast can-

cers require a similar mechanism to promote their growth.

This leads us to the current issue in hand. When and why should patients use a complimentary therapy for the treatment of their cancer? The definition that authors use for this book is that complementary treatment is used to aid or help the current existing therapies employed by standard oncology practice and should not attempt to cure or be used as alternatives to accepted therapies. There are very few cancers where chemotherapy, radiation, hormonal therapy, and immunotherapy such as cytokines or monoclonal antibodies are not used to compliment surgery and so are not viable independent treatments for cancer. They are most commonly used as adjuvants or as palliative treatment in the case of advanced disease. Therefore, the purpose of the suggested treatments is to enhance the effect of the standard therapies, reduce their side effects and toxicities, and potentially improve functions that can improve clinical and survival outcomes. The following question then arises: What is the burden of proof required in order to use any such therapy to be accepted by the general medical community? Another question raised by the contributors is aimed at challenging the current definition of treatment efficacy for any particular cancer: Are the standards employed by clinical trials for the treatment of cancer relevant for a patient's life, survival, or the disease? I think the reader will find the chapters in this book informative and detailed. I also think the challenge is real and we may have to rethink our standards for both the treatment and for future evaluation of the treatment of cancer.

Isaac Cohen, O. M. D., L. Ac.
Chief Scientific Officer
Bionovo, Inc., Emeryville, California
Guest Scientist
University of California, San Francisco
Mt. Zion, Comprehensive Cancer Center and
Department of Ob/Gyn, Center for Reproductive
Endocrinology

— 1 Introduction to Complementary Medicine in Oncology
Joseph Beuth

— Introduction

New developments of complementary medicine in oncology have emerged out of a general disappointment with the results of more traditional treatment options. Despite innovative approaches toward tumor destruction, including surgery, chemotherapy, or radiotherapy, cancer mortality rates have not been reduced in the United States or other industrialized countries in the past twenty years. The age-adjusted mortality rates have even increased by about 6 %. Notable treatment success has only been achieved in rare cancers (such as leukemia, lymphomas, and testicular carcinoma) (3).

Global analyses conducted independently by Abel (1) and Moss (16) dampened the optimism associated with chemotherapy for advanced carcinomas, especially when "responses" (temporary tumor shrinkages) are used as a measure of therapeutic success.

These authors urged the medical establishment to think about new therapeutic strategies. While conventional oncology still promoted the application of high-dose chemotherapy, which can only be survived through measures of intensive clinical care, some less toxic complementary approaches underwent scientific and clinical trials.

The effectiveness of high-dose chemotherapy of epithelial tumors (e. g., breast cancer) still remains to be proved (15). The use of chemotherapy for advanced tumors does not result in significant survival outcomes (1, 16). A statement made by the drug administration in Germany, about unconventional alternatives with respect to aggressive tumor treatment, should be mentioned: "The practice of drug therapy as the main pillar of treatment offered in medicine by all industrialized nations is based on the scientific acknowledgement of certain laws (drug–receptor interactions, dose–response relationships, demonstrated effects on the disturbed regulation of biochemical and psycho–physiological processes) and on the testing of these medicines according to internationally accepted clinical–pharmacological and biometric methods." (7)

The consistent application of this statement should result in an ethical consensus and lead to the following set of requirements:
- Scientific study and evaluation (proof of efficacy) of *all* therapeutic concepts
- Limitation to diagnostics and therapeutics with proved efficacy and their inclusion into health insurance plans
- Development of a comprehensive plan for adequate prevention, prophylaxis, diagnosis, therapy, and follow-up of cancer

While the importance of tumor prevention has moved into the forefront of public consciousness, due to intense awareness campaigns by the cancer societies of various nations, the areas that include diagnosis, therapy, and follow-up need to catch up. Widespread passive follow-up ought to be replaced with an active treatment plan tailored to the respective indications of the patient's disease. In order to reach this goal, oncologists should aim to expand on proved complementary medicinal approaches and optimize the timing of therapy. Particularly the induction of immune suppression (11, 13), the surgery-induced spread of metastases (10), as well as the impairment of quality of life (9, 13) due to the use of traditional therapies can be compensated by a timely combination with complementary medicinal approaches.

— Overview of Methods

Complementary medicine should primarily be seen as an addition or enhancement of current standard treatment options in oncology. It is to be differentiated from "alternative medicine," which seeks to find replacements for conventional toxic approaches. Although complementary and alternative medicines are grouped together in the popular acronym "CAM," they are in fact quite different in their aims. Since many alternative treatments are still poorly documented, equating the two could lead to a misguided and undeserved rejection of all complementary medicine.

That many of the methods discussed in this book can complement standard treatment has been proved in clinical trials that have shown an increase in the quality of life, as well as in total survival time. Biometrically secured and prospectively randomized data are presented for these approaches, for the most part from placebo-controlled clinical trials and cohort trials according to Good Epidemiological Practice (GEP), which will be described shortly (Table 1.1).

Nutrition Advice

The National Cancer Institute of the United States attributes about 35% of all types of cancer to malnutrition (5, 17). The potential for prevention of cancer is thus large, and general nutrition guidelines for primary and secondary prevention are of much value (according to the German Society of Nutrition [DGE] and the American Institute for Cancer Research).

Once cancer becomes apparent, success of therapy, or the healing process, is decisively determined by the patient's nutritional state. Fundamentally, a specific advisory for the patient's optimized nutrition is of great importance at this point, since malnutrition and cachexia can have a significant effect on the quality and duration of life. Malnutrition increases cancer mortality by about 30% (17), and cachexia worsens the prognosis of disease significantly, since it is associated with reduced response to treatment, more complications, and therefore prolonged hospitalization.

Table 1.1 Scientifically proved complementary methods in oncology

		Recommended procedures	Expanded procedures	Demonstrated effects
Nutrition advice		×		QoL ↑
Exercise		×		IM, QoL ↑
Psycho-oncologic guidance		×		QoL ↑, ST ↑
Vitamin substitution	Vitamins A, C, E		×	QoL ↑
	Balanced mixture		×	QoL ↑
Mineral substitution	Sodium selenite	×		IM, QoL ↑
Enzyme therapy			×	QoL ↑, R ↓, MET ↓, ST ↑
Indication-specific measures	Mistletoe therapy	×		IM, QoL ↑
	Thymus peptide extracts		×	IM, QoL ↑
(activation/restoration of immune cells)	Microbiology therapy		×	IM
Tumor-specific/ antiproliferative measures	Blockage of adhesion molecules		×	MET ↓, ST ↑
	Hemocyanin therapy	×		R ↓
	Hyperthermia		×	IM
	Monoclonal antibodies		×	R ↓, MET ↓, ST ↑
	Differential induction	×		ST ↑
	Hormonal therapy	×		R ↓, ST ↑

↑ prolonged/improved; ↓ reduced; IM, immune modulation; QoL, quality of life; MET, metastases; R, relapse; ST, survival time.

Exercise, Physical Activity

Focused gymnastics, moderate exercise (of longer duration), or physical activity has proved beneficial in the prevention and follow-up of cancer (2, 21). This has led to:
- Improvement in bodily functions, including regeneration of previous abilities (for example, restitution of shoulder–arm–joint mobility after cancer-destructive therapy for breast cancer).
- Activation/modulation of hormones and immune system responses and positive influence on mood, sensitivity to pain and quality of life through the release of neuropeptides (e.g., β-endorphins).
- Result in psychological stabilization through social contacts (sense of belonging to a team or group).

Psycho-Oncological Support

Psychotherapeutic measures should be an integral part of any immediate treatment or rehabilitation of today's cancer patient. It is widely known that handicaps may lead to psychosomatic diseases and that these can be relieved or even cured with appropriate psychological aid or therapeutic modalities.

In addition, psychotherapeutic measures are indicated for dealing with disease in the following types of problems and symptoms:
- Emotional disturbances, such as fear and depression
- Conflicts within a relationship or family
- Impairment in social behavior
- Social withdrawal tendencies
- Psychological impairment with physical decline and deterioration
- Problems in accepting the disease
- Discrepancies between therapeutic expectancy and actual treatment options
- Inadequate behavior toward disease

Psychotherapy is an integral part of acute and rehabilitative treatment in oncology.

Substitution of Essential Minerals and Vitamins

The cancer patient has an increased requirement for essential micronutrients that are rarely adequately supplied even through a wholesome and balanced diet. This especially holds true before or during tumor-destructive therapy, since the need for micronutrients in these phases is increased due to side effects such as reduced appetite, nausea, vomiting, diarrhea, and perspiration.

It has been demonstrated that a deficit in micronutrients (vitamins and minerals) results in a reduced tolerance of current standard cancer therapy.

The role of micronutrients in the primary and secondary prevention of cancer is multifunctional. Vitamins and minerals inhibit the activation of cancer-causing substances as well as inflammatory processes. Other micronutrients can prevent the reuptake of cancer-inducing substances into the cell and protect cellular DNA by disabling the adhesion of cancerous compounds (2, 17).

The indication-specific substitution with essential micronutrients (combination of balanced vitamins and minerals) as a prevention of cancer as well as a compensation of therapy-induced nutritive deficits has proved beneficial in intervention studies and controlled clinical trials.

Enzyme Substitution

A standard combination of proteolytic enzymes (papain, trypsin, chymotrypsin) resulted in a reduction of disease and therapy-induced symptoms, depending on the stage of disease progression as well as the type of cancer (results were noticeable in patients with plasmacytoma, colorectal cancer, and breast cancer). Additionally, an increase in quality of life, survival time and regression intervals, or metastasis-free intervals was noticed (4). Treatment with proteolytic enzymes that are adapted to the respective stage and type of cancer, may enhance standard therapy and now qualifies as evidence-based medicine.

Phytotherapy

Treatment with mistletoe extract as the prototype of phytotherapy is the most common complementary procedure in Central European oncology. According to a questionnaire, more than 80 % of all German cancer patients use some form of complementary therapy (62 % use mistletoe extracts) (20). Patients give the following reasons for complementary use of mistletoe extracts:

- Involvement of patients themselves in the process of cure and coping with disease
- Optimization of standard therapy
- Reduction in side effects of standard therapy
- Augmentation of patient's immune system
- Desire for a holistic approach of therapy
- Wish to not leave any option untried

Current medical therapy with mistletoe extracts is performed using standardized lectin extracts. Preclinical research using mistletoe extracts or its defined components (lectins, viscotoxins, polysaccharides, vesicles) are far advanced. The following results have been noticed:

- Immune modulation
- Cytotoxicity
- Induction of apoptosis
- Stabilization of DNA
- Antitumor effect
- Anti-infectious effect

Initial controlled trials showed stage-specific effects in certain cancers (breast carcinoma, colorectal carcinoma, glioblastoma): reduction in side effects with simultaneous improvement in quality of life and reproducible immune system regeneration using mistletoe extract therapy (8, 9, 12, 13). Also, an effect on survival was noticed using standardized mistletoe therapy in an intervention trial.

Mistletoe therapy has proved useful in controlled clinical trials performed by the author and others. One should keep in mind the stage and type of cancer, since clinical trials have shown that mistletoe therapy has no advantage, for example, in patients with epithelial cancer of the throat (19). Systemic diseases (leukemia, lymphoma) are a contraindication for immunotherapies with mistletoe extracts.

Thymic Peptide Therapy

Standardized thymic peptide preparations (i.e., biochemically defined fractions of thymic peptides, such as thymosin α-1, thymopentin, thymic humoral factor) are applied to stimulate the immune system (e.g., in the event of immune suppression following standard therapy). Experimental and preclinical effects have been demonstrated for these substances (including the modulation, stimulation, or restoration of immune cells, and antitumor, antimetastasic, or antiviral activity). In addition following application, there are well-documented observations that demonstrate a positive influence on the immune system and the quality of life (such as the reduction in the side effects of tumor-aggressive therapeutic measures) (14).

At this point, it should be mentioned, however, that mere observational studies do not result in definitive proof of efficacy.

Despite many clinical studies, it yet remains to be proved whether treatment with thymic peptides can effectively prevent relapse and metastasis and thereby prolong survival time. All trials showed certain weaknesses and deficits and have not met the criteria of scientific standards. The initial trials that were non-GCP-compliant were promising (14) and still need to demonstrate proof of efficacy in current GCP-compliant multicenter studies.

Probiotic Therapy

The secretory immune system of the gastrointestinal tract is considered part of the humoral immune system (MALT – mucosa-associated lymphoid tissue). Also part of this system are the mucosa of the respiratory tract (BALT – bronchial-associated lymphoid tissue), the mucosa of the urogenital tract, and the mammary glands. It has been proved experimentally that the physiological function of the immune system is closely related to the mucosal microflora. This is the underlying principle upon which the outcome of microbiological (probiotic) therapy rests.

Probiotics (e. g., *Propionobacterium* species, *Lactobacillus* species, *Enterococcus* species, *Bifidobacterium* species) belong to the physiological microflora of the body and have shown to be efficient immune modulators in clinical and experimental trials (11).

Blockade of Adhesion Molecules

A specific adhesion mechanism of hepatocytes and tumor cells has been observed through clinical studies of tissue and tumor cells. Experimental in-vitro trials, as well as in-vivo studies (using murine tumor models), have proved that metastasis in the liver is initiated through galactoside-specific binding of hepatic lectins to the terminal galactose on tumor cell receptors.

The blockade of liver lectins resulted in a numerically significant reduction of liver metastases in two experimental murine models. This well-documented fundamental mechanism presents the opportunity of blocking liver lectins through galactoglycoconjugates during the perioperative time period, when the tumor cells reach the circulation.

Three controlled clinical trials have shown that by blocking liver lectins through perioperative galactose infusions, the adhesion of tumor cells and the development of liver metastases have significantly been reduced in patients with colorectal or gastric cancer (10). A validation study has to further prove the value of this promising complementary therapeutic strategy.

Hyperthermia

Hyperthermia is based on external physical heat application and can be categorized according to its focus and extent of expansion into:
- **Whole body hyperthermia:** treatment of advanced-stage cancer
- **Deep hyperthermia:** treatment of localized cancer, for example, of internal organs or bones
- **Superficial hyperthermia:** treatment of skin cancer/metastases
- **Perfusion hyperthermia:** treatment of cancerous/metastatic invasion of hollow organs
- **Interstitial thermography/hyperthermia:** treatment of regional cancer

A combination of hyperthermia with standard or immune therapies is expected to result in additive and synergistic effects. Hyperthermia (in combination with chemotherapy/radiotherapy) is currently being subjected to scientific testing worldwide. It is absolutely vital to perform evaluations of this therapeutic measure without preconceived notions. Hyperthermia has been used for many centuries as a tumor-reductive therapy. Although there are many clinical trials (PubMed cites 400 references to randomized controlled trials), there is still a lack of definitive clinical results. The first controlled clinical studies have been promising and all seem to point to hyperthermia as a complementary treatment measure that enhances standard tumor-destructive therapies.

All of the aforementioned therapeutic approaches are currently being evaluated further, and exaggerated claims are unwarranted. Since proof of efficacy for specific tumor types and stages is measured separately, additional studies must be completed so that defined complementary medicinal concepts may be integrated into evidence-based oncology.

Occasional discrediting of complementary procedures as scientifically unfounded is the result of inappropriate equation with unsound fringe methods. Relevant complementary oncology procedures are currently being studied in standardized GCP/GEP-compliant trials for efficacy, which serves to safeguard the patient. The studies are, in addition, visibly positioned in the guidelines of specialty groups to improve quality assurance.

Fringe Methods

It is imperative to beware of unsound therapeutic and diagnostic measures that have not undergone any scientific testing for efficacy, but are sometimes erroneously associated with scientifically proved complementary medicine. These procedures are being intensely advertised (internet, television, tabloids) and wrongly suggest the following after application:
- Reduction in tumor growth and mass
- Slowing of growth of metastases
- Prolongation of survival time
- They are the sole beneficial treatment modality after all other options have failed
- Delay of the necessity of chemotherapy
- Intensified chemotherapy and radiotherapy effectiveness

Although we should always remain open to new concepts, such procedures are usually not based on sound scientific principles and may ultimately prove life-threatening for the patient (if he or she delays possibly curative measures).

Table 1.2   Examples of diagnostic and therapeutic procedures that have not been sufficiently evaluated

Nonevaluated diagnostic procedures	Nonevaluated therapeutic procedures
• Redox-serum analysis	• Galavit
• Darkfield microscopy	• Ukrain
• Enderlein diagnosis/biophotonic diagnosis	• Megamin
• Tumor-cell detection in peripheral blood	• Essiac Tea
• Irrelevant molecular biological or immunological parameters	• Recancostat
	• PC-SPES
	• SPES
	• Noni juice
	• Thymus extracts/total organ extracts
	• Dr. Rath's vitamins

Promotion can take the shape of directly advertising a doctor's practice to the public. Since this is still looked at with considerable suspicion, there is also a strong undercurrent of indirect and masked promotion, with the worrisome result that doctors are guided less and less by conscientious check on the quality of their actions according to an ethical standpoint. It is not surprising that self-proclaimed expertise and financial remuneration of ambitious individuals, as well as irresponsible and exaggerated advertisement of scientifically unsound and insufficiently evaluated (and usually costly) therapeutic and diagnostic procedures are more and more commonly seen in medical practice.

In addition, this especially holds true for all specialties in which chronically diseased and fearful patients must be managed just as well as they are in the field of oncology. It has become common for self-proclaimed "specialists" in their area of expertise to abuse public health organizations and self-help groups by giving presentations and slide shows in an attempt to acquire patients. One has also seen the growth of disreputable clinics, practices, laboratories, and unproved diagnostic and therapeutic procedures with promises of a cure.

The chronically ill cancer patient is often ridden with survival fears in addition to sacrificing quality of life. Although many such patients have become self-educated "experts" on their own disease, others are at the mercy of their attending doctors. This leaves the door open for considerable abuse with recommendations for diagnostics and medications with no proven effectiveness or safety.

Conclusion

Complementary procedures in medicine are currently widely debated by the scientific community, because the required scientific proof of effectiveness for most of the therapeutic approaches has not yet been met with definite results. In the past years, basic research and clinical evaluation of defined complementary therapeutic concepts in oncology have been intensified in an attempt to integrate these procedures into evidence-based medicine.

According to definition, scientifically based therapies of complementary medicine cannot replace the much studied conventional tumor-destructive therapies (operation, chemotherapy, and radiotherapy) and are thus not to be seen as "alternative therapy." Complementary approaches in oncology that are advised as additional therapy to standard tumor-destructive therapy claim to optimize this therapy. The first data emerging from scientifically sound clinical trials prove that defined complementary procedures are beneficial for the patient.

References

1. Abel U: Chemotherapie fortgeschrittener Karzinome. Stuttgart, Germany: Hippokrates Verlag; 1995.
2. Arnold von Versen B: Der Einsatz von Mikronährstoffen bei Tumorerkrankungen und zur Tumorprävention. Dtsch Z Onkol. 2001; 33:19–29.
3. Bailar JC, Gornik HL: Cancer undefeated. N Engl J Med. 1997; 336:1569–1574.
4. Beuth J, Ost B, Pakdaman A, et al.: Impact of complementary oral enzyme application on the postoperative treatment results of breast cancer patients—results of an epidemiological mulitcentre retrolective cohort study. Cancer Chemother Pharmacol. 2001; 47:53–62.
5. Doll R, Peto R: The causes of cancer. Quantitative estimates of avoidable risks of cancer in the United States today. J Natl Cancer Inst. 1981; 66:1193–1208.
6. Grossarth-Maticek R, Kiene H, Baumgartner SM, et al.: Use of Iscador, an extract of European mistletoe (*Viscum album*), in cancer treatment: prospective nonrandomized and randomized matched-pair studies nested within a cohort study. Alternative Therapies. 2001; 7:57–78.
7. Haustein KO, Höffler D, Lasek R, et al.: Außerhalb der wissenschaftlichen Medizin stehende Methoden der Arzneitherapie. Dtsch Ärztebl. 1998; 95:800–805.
8. Heiny BM, Albrecht V, Beuth J: Lebensqualitätsstabilisierung durch Mistellektin-1 normierten Extrakt beim fortgeschrittenen kolorektalen Karzinom. Onkologe (Suppl. 1). 1998; 4:35–39.
9. Heiny BM, Beuth J: Mistletoe extract standardized for the galactoside-specific lectin (ML-1) induces β-endorphin release and immunopotentiation in breast cancer patients. Anticancer Res. 1994; 14:1339–1342.
10. Isenberg J, Stoffel B, Stuetzer H, et al.: Liver lectin blocking with D-galactose to prevent hepatic metastases in colorectal carcinoma patients. Anticancer Res. 1998; 17:3767–3772.
11. Isenberg J, Stoffel B, Wolters U, et al.: Immunostimulation by propionibacteria: Effects on immune status and antineoplastic treatment. Anticancer Res. 1995; 15:2363–2368.
12. Lenartz D, Dott U, Menzel J, et al.: Survival of glioma patients after complementary treatment with galactoside-specific lectin from mistletoe. Anticancer Res. 2001; 20:2073–2076.
13. Lenartz D, Stoffel B, Menzel J, et al.: Immunoprotective activity of the galactoside-specific lectin from mistletoe after tumor destructive therapy in glioma patients. Anticancer Res. 1996; 16:3799–3802.
14. Maurer HR, Goldstein AL, Hager ED: Thymic Peptides in Preclinical and Clinical Medicine. Munich, Germany: Zuckschwerdt Verlag; 1997.
15. Minckwitz G, Dan Costa S, Kaufmann M: Hochdosis-Chemotherapie beim Mammakarzinom. Dtsch. Ärzteblatt. 1997; 94:2835–2837.
16. Moss R: Questioning Chemotherapy. Equinox Press NY. 1995. German edition: Fragwürdige Chemotherapie. Heidelberg, Germany: Haug; 1997.
17. Prasad KN, Cole WC: Cancer and Nutrition. Amsterdam, Netherlands: IOS Press; 1998.
18. Schüle K: Bewegung und Sport in der Krebsnachsorge. Forum DKG. 2001; 2:39–41.
19. Steuer-Vogt MK, Bonkowsky V, Ambrosch P. et al.: The effect of an adjuvant mistletoe treatment programme in resected head and neck cancer patients: a randomized controlled clinical trial. Eur J Cancer. 2001; 37:23–31.
20. Stoll G: Die Misteltherapie in der Onkologie. Z. Onkol/J Oncol. 1999: 31:31–34.
21. Uhlenbruck G: Bewegungstraining in der Krebsnachsorge: Einfluss auf immunologische und psychologische Parameter. Forum DKG. 2001; 2:34–36.

2 The Conventional Treatment of Cancer: The Case of Non-Small Cell Lung Cancer

Ralph W. Moss Ph. D.

Introduction

The purpose of this chapter is to review critically the three main conventional treatments for cancer: surgery, radiotherapy, and chemotherapy. I will illustrate problems involved in assessing their effectiveness by focusing on one kind of malignancy, non-small cell lung cancer (NSCLC). I have chosen lung cancer because it is among the most prevalent causes of cancer death worldwide and NSCLC is overwhelmingly the most common type of cancer at this anatomical site. I shall discuss the effectiveness of the standard methods in the treatment of various stages and substages of the disease.

The central question is whether conventional treatments, singly or in combination, have been proved to be effective and reasonably safe. There are many definitions of effectiveness, which leads to widespread confusion. Some people think effectiveness should be measured by the complete removal en bloc of a growth and its surrounding tissue; by the prevention of local, regional, or distant recurrences; or by the shrinkage of measurable tumor for a prescribed length of time.

> My definition of **effectiveness**, however, hinges on an increase in the **median overall survival** (OS) of all the patients who are given the treatment.

Ideally, a description of effectiveness involves a comparison with patients who do not receive the treatment in question but receive a placebo or "sham" treatment. The effectiveness of any treatment must also be studied in the context of its long-term impact on the patient's quality of life (QOL).

The best way of attaining such evidence is through prospective, randomized controlled trials (RCTs). According to the Institute of Medicine (IOM) of the US Academy of Sciences, an RCT is:

"... a formal study carried out according to a prospectively defined protocol. It is intended to discover or verify the safety and effectiveness in human beings of interventions to promote well-being, or to prevent, diagnose, or treat illness ... Properly conducted clinical trials are a necessity in health care because very few interventions produce such large or striking results that they can be evaluated by observation alone" (1).

What Are the Characteristics of a Successful Clinical Trial?

According to the IOM:

"To generate the most reliable information, clinical trials require certain design characteristics (particularly assignment of participants to interventions by 'randomization') and they must include enough participants to exclude the play of chance as a likely explanation for results. ... Regardless of the sophistication and complexity of the design and analysis, the question of whether 'a' is better than 'b' is the essence of the clinical trial" (1).

Since the end of World War II, clinical trials have been widely used throughout the industrialized world for the testing of new drugs and vaccines. After the well-known thalidomide disaster, and the consequent enhancement of the powers of the US Food and Drug Administration (FDA) in 1962, the US government has required clinical trials before it will allow any new diagnostic procedures or therapeutic agents onto the marketplace. (As I shall explain below, this standard has been eroded in recent years.)

RCTs should be large enough to yield a meaningful result (be adequately powered) and should hopefully involve more than one medical center. The **RCT** is the "gold standard" of testing. There is a perception among both medical professionals and the lay public that the conventional treatments for cancer (primarily surgery, radiation, and chemotherapy), which are in use worldwide, have been proved through this rigorous scientific process. In fact, the presence or absence of RCTs is supposed to form the boundary line between conventionally proved treatments and those nonconventional treatments that are collectively referred to as conventional and alternative medicine (CAM). Any claims of effectiveness for CAM is routinely met with the rejoinder: "Where are the RCTs to support such approaches?"

The question implies that conventional cancer treatments rest on a solid foundation of successful RCTs and that such trials are the basis for declaring these treatments proved and effective. The purpose of this chapter is to determine whether such claims for conventional cancer treatments can in fact be documented through reference to the standard medical database, Medline.

We immediately confront a problem: the focus of FDA reform in the 1960s was pharmacological agents. But two of these three main anticancer modalities, surgery and radiation, were excluded from the stringent 1962 FDA regulations. In legal parlance, they were grandfathered into US law (i. e. accepted based solely on their prior widescale use). Essentially, no formal approval process was deemed necessary before surgery or radiation therapy was employed as treatments for cancer patients. This exemption covered not just past treatments but future ones as well: cancer surgeons and radiation oncologists were essentially given carte blanche from the US government to introduce new or modified techniques for treating cancer. Other governments followed suit.

Perhaps for that reason, clinical trials of these two older modalities are more limited in number and scope than they are for drug-based therapies. In fact, on a percentage basis, there are approximately three times as many RCTs of cancer chemotherapy as there are for cancer surgery (Table 2.1).

However, despite this *legal* carte blanche, the *scientific* requirements of proof obviously remain the same for surgery or radiation as for any other treatment. No treatment can be considered effec-

tive until and unless it has been subjected to the highest possible standards of proof. Whenever feasible and ethical, this is the RCT. A World Health Organization publication addresses this question. "Radiotherapy must justify its place in the armamentarium of cancer-fighting technologies. Not only must it constantly be subject to clinical trials evaluating its role, it must also be reviewed in terms of its cost–benefit and utility in the circumstances in which it is used" (61). The same should be said of cancer surgery and chemotherapy.

▄ History of Clinical Trials

The idea of comparing one regimen or treatment directly with another is very old (5, 15). There is even reference to an early "clinical trial" in the Old Testament. Daniel and his companions were resolved to eat and drink a purely vegetarian diet. But Babylon's chief palace official feared that "if you eat something else and end up looking worse than the other young men" the King might be angry. And so Daniel proposed the following test: "For the next ten days," he said, "let us have only vegetables and water at mealtime. When the ten days are up, compare how we look with the other young men, and decide what to do with us. . . . Ten days later, Daniel and his friends looked healthier and better than the young men who had been served food from the royal palace" (12).

The foundations of the modern RCT were laid in the nineteenth century. A great French physician, Pierre Charles Alexandre Louis (1787–1872), wrote that "the edifice of medicine reposes entirely upon facts, and that truth cannot be elicited, but from those that have been well and completely observed" (45). Through a statistically driven study, Louis showed that bloodletting (the cornerstone of the conventional medicine of his day) was much less effective for inflammations than had previous-

Table 2.1 Research database on cancer treatment			
	Surgery	**Radiotherapy**	**Chemotherapy**
Total no. of articles	442 419	128 491	274 449
No. RCTs	7 221	3 920	12 737
RCT as % of whole	1.6 %	3.0 %	4.6 %

(Source: PubMed, http://www.ncbi.nlm.nih.gov/entrez/query/fcgi, search carried out on 12 April 2005).
RCT = randomized controlled trial

ly been supposed. Louis declared that the rate of death of different patient populations "can only be attributed to the employment, or omission, of bloodletting" (44).

But the development of RCTs primarily came from Great Britain before and after World War Two: Major Greenwood (1880–1949) was an early biostatistician who deplored the sloppy substantiation of the claims of most clinicians. One of his students was Austin Bradford Hill (1897–1991). In 1937, the editors of *The Lancet* asked Hill to write a series of articles on the proper method of applying statistics to medical questions. These articles were later published as the classic work *Principles of Medical Statistics.* In their preface, the editors prophetically declared:

"In clinical medicine today there is a growing demand for adequate proof of the efficacy of this or that form of treatment. Often proof can come only by means of a collection of records of clinical trials devised on such a scale and in such a form that statistically reliable conclusions can be drawn from them. However great may be our aversion to figures, we cannot escape the conclusion that the solution of most of the problems of clinical or preventive medicine must ultimately depend on them" (30).

After World War II "it was no longer possible for the clinician, however distinguished, to discuss the prognosis and treatment of disease unless his words were supported by figures," wrote L.J. Witts, Nuffield Professor of Clinical Medicine at Oxford University. "The accelerating pace of discovery entailed the constant trial of new remedies, whose value could not be left to be determined by the slow processes of time and fashion as in the past" (85).

Hill's first clinical trial, completed in 1946:

- defined in advance the characteristics of who would, and would not, be treated
- objectively documented the response to treatments
- established a neutral committee to define the ethical issues posed by the trial.

One commentator noted at the time: "A notable feature of this trial was the frank realization by all concerned of the fallibility of human judgment in general and of clinical and radiological judgment in particular. … *The principle of the elimination of personal bias is fundamental in all experiment,* but it is of particular importance in clinical research.

Thus, in the selection of patients for inclusion in either treated or control groups, the final decision was made purely on a chance basis" (63).

In the last few decades, RCTs have emerged as the universally acknowledged gold standard of medical research (48). Almost a quarter of a million controlled trials have been carried out around the world (9). There are presently at least 2200 ongoing clinical trials available to cancer patients, publicized through US government websites such as www.cancer.gov and www.clinicaltrials.gov.

▬ Surgery as a Cancer Therapy

Surgery has been called "the mainstay of therapy for malignant neoplasia" and "the most effective curative and palliative treatment for most solid tumors" (47). Its first uses actually predate recorded history. Yet it is only within the last century or so that surgery has become a respected profession. According to a standard textbook, "Throughout most of recorded history, surgeons have been the objects of societal opprobrium because of the unspeakable perioperative suffering endured by their patients" (49).

Before the late nineteenth century, extensive surgery more frequently resulted in death than in the cure of the patient. It was the discovery of anesthesia that led to a dramatic improvement in cancer surgery and its growing acceptance. For example, in the decade before the introduction of anesthesia the Massachusetts General Hospital in Boston performed just 400 operations. But from 1894 to 1904, over 24000 operations were performed there.

The greatest innovations in cancer surgery were associated with Central European doctors, such as Theodor Billroth (1829–1894) and his student Emil Theodor Kocher (1841–1917). In America, William Stewart Halsted (1852–1922) transplanted the German model of organized postgraduate surgical education to America. In 1890, he described the radical mastectomy that bears his name. This Halsted operation was so extensive that it undeniably caused a great deal of suffering for many of the patients who survived. But, presumably, it was dramatically more effective at saving or prolonging patients' lives. This operation became the prototype for radical cancer surgery at every anatomical site.

The use of the "**Halsted radical**" was based on a theory that was itself not subjected to experimental testing. This theory was that cancer spread in a stepwise fashion through the tissues and then through the lymphatic system, and that essentially cancer was a local or regional, not a systemic, disease. Halsted said that breast cancer spread through first and second order regional lymph nodes. In a famous lecture, he spoke of how breast cancer "in spreading centrifugally, preserves in the main continuity with the original growth, and before involving the viscera may become widely diffused along surface planes" (49).

This theory turned out to be unsupportable. Yet enormous numbers of patients were subjected to drastic operations without adequate experiments to test this underlying hypothesis. Since breast cancer was considered a "local affection," surgeons were exhorted to apply "greater endeavor with the cognition that the metastases to bone, to pleura, to liver are probably parts of the whole ..." (27). Here was the rationale for radical resection en bloc of the fascia of the major muscles, and for wide resection of the skin of the breast ... and eventually to the "extended radical mastectomy," in which excision en bloc was extended to include the internal mammary and supraclavicular lymph nodes and even portions of the bony thorax.

Halsted supported his theory with statistics on the survival of his own patients. In a retrospective case series, he reported five-year "cures" in 75% of the 60 patients whose cancer had been confined to the breast, 31% of the 110 patients who had had axillary metastases, and 10% of the 40 patients who had both axillary and supraclavicular lymph node involvement. The operative mortality was just 1.7%, an astonishingly low figure for the time.

The numbers certainly appear impressive. Clearly, Halsted was a skillful operator and a careful reporter. But no case series provides a synchronous control group with which its outcome can be compared. Halsted's results appeared better than those of his contemporaries. But better results could be due to a number of biases inherent in the manner in which the patients were selected or the data interpreted. On what scientific basis did Halsted claim that his patients' outcomes were better than what would have been achieved with other (e. g., less radical) approaches?

In arguing for the superiority of radical surgery, there was an unspoken assumption that meaningful comparisons were made to other practices (published or unpublished case series), past hospital records, or other historical data. This, as it turns out, was not a reasonable assumption. Biostatisticians today routinely expound the many biases inherent in case series or historical comparisons (52).

In fact, even at the time there was a growing awareness of the statistical deficiency of Halsted's argument. Major Greenwood complained that Halsted failed to consider age distribution when he reported statistics on the success of his operation. In a letter, he observed that "surgeons ... are mostly at the intellectual level of plumbers, in fact just well-paid craftsmen. I should like to shame them out of the comic opera performances which they suppose are statistics of operations ... a really decent set of figures from such a panjandrum as Halsted would go a long way" (44).

It would be decades before the criticism of biostatisticians carried any weight with the surgical profession. In the interim, Halsted's radical approach spread from Johns Hopkins Hospital around the world:

"Halsted's intellectual approach to the surgical management of cancer was widely adopted and eventually applied in one form or another to most solid tumors" (47).

The radical operation was primarily an American innovation. "The attention given scientific advances was especially great in a culture that had always placed a high value on tangible results. Physicians, it seemed, were at last exhibiting the 'can do' dexterity that was the essence of American ingenuity," wrote one historian of cancer (58).

This "can do" attitude soon routed the "therapeutic nihilism" that had characterized much European thinking about cancer in the nineteenth century. For example, surgical resection of head-and-neck cancers became more common, especially in the 1940s and 1950s under the leadership of Dr. Hayes Martin of New York and his students. In 1906, Dr. George Crile, Sr. of Cleveland pioneered the radical neck dissection. By the 1950s, this was performed en bloc with the resection of the tumor itself.

Dr. Chevalier Jackson (1865–1958) of Philadelphia refined the techniques of tracheostomy. The first excisions of the abdominal colon took place in the decade between 1894 and 1903. This involved creation of a colostomy, followed by staged tumor excision and bowel closure. In 1908, W. Ernest Miles of London developed abdominoperineal resection for rectal cancer. Until recently, this remained the "treatment of choice" for this disease. "This operation was truly radical," according to two surgeons, "committing all patients to a permanent end colostomy and at least half of the male patients to sexual disability" (47).

Halsted himself and then Dr. Allen O. Whipple (1881–1963) of New York carried out a radical operation for pancreatic cancer called pancreaticoduodenectomy (83). This **"Whipple procedure"** is still in use. But it was Dr. Alexander Brunschweig (1901–1969), also of New York, who took radical surgery to its ultimate extreme with the **hemicorporectomy** (translumbar amputation). This operation, which involved removal of half of the human body, was attempted in a few unfortunate patients. As one textbook comments:

"This practice was a logical, albeit extreme, extension of the doctrine that surgical resection of cancer can result in cure provided a satisfactory margin of normal, uninvolved tissue is taken beyond the limits of tumor spread" (47).

None of these treatments was established because of randomized controlled trials, or anything approaching what we would today consider proof of effectiveness. They were based on a widely held theory that cancer was a local disease and that the more extensive the surgery that was attempted, the better would be the survival results. This became the prevailing dogma of cancer surgery for decades.

But where was the experimental justification by which so many people were cut open, or even cut in half, in the name of radical surgery? There was an almost complete lack of controlled studies. Naturally, we can hardly demand randomized trials from an era in which they were all but unknown. However, after World War Two, and especially after 1962, RCTs became routine in the pharmacological field, yet were still almost unknown in the arena of cancer surgery.

The ultimate in untested, unscientific practice involved the treatment of malignant melanoma. "For much of this century," Moffat and Ketchum of the University of Miami School of Medicine wrote in 1994, "the surgical management of primary cutaneous malignant melanoma was based on a detailed clinicopathological description of a single case by William Sampson Handley in 1907 ... Surprisingly, with no other supporting evidence, Handley's principles became established in surgical teaching and practice and defined the surgical

standard of care for melanoma for many decades" (47, 49).

These firmly held ideas hardened into dogma. Richard Evans, MD, a cancer surgeon, has recalled his own medical education in the 1960s and 1970s:

"Surgeons seemed to work by a rigid set of rules meant to be heeded, but seldom questioned. Cancer surgeons relied upon ideas that had been passed down for almost a century. The number one rule of cancer surgery was to remove every single cancer cell, and every cell that may become cancerous. This was called radical surgery. Radical surgery was considered necessary in order to control the disease and ultimately cure the patient. Though this sounded reasonable, its functional and cosmetic consequences were sometimes devastating" (17).

A brake was finally put on radical surgery by a combination of advances in scientific understanding (derived in part from RCTs) and a widespread rejection on the part of patients and the general public of what were seen as surgeons' excesses. The public's mood was already summarized in 1906 by playwright George Bernard Shaw in the Preface to *Doctor's Dilemma*:

"The test to which all methods of treatment are finally brought is whether they are lucrative to doctors or not. ... Nobody supposes that doctors are less virtuous than judges; but a judge whose salary and reputation depended on whether the verdict was for plaintiff or defendant, prosecutor or prisoner, would be as little trusted as a general in the pay of the enemy. To offer me a doctor as my judge, and then weight his decision with a bribe of a large sum of money and a virtual guarantee that if he makes a mistake it can never be proved against him, is to go wildly beyond the ascertained strain which human nature can bear."

Shaw also noted the **lack of scientific proof** for the radical surgery of his day: "The large range of operations that consist of amputating limbs and extirpating organs admits of no direct verification of their necessity."

The public grew increasingly concerned about the functional and social consequences of cancer operations (47). Some people, faced with radical operations, refused treatment. In fact, despite numerous and vociferous assertions to the contrary, increasing the magnitude of operations had not been scientifically demonstrated to result in a proportionate increase in "cures" or improved survival rates for solid tumors.

The 1970s and 1980s were marked by the ascendance of a more humane philosophy of more **limited or "conservative" surgery**. This type of surgery attempted to preserve body form, function, and parts. Surgeons, commented one textbook, "were initially slow to grasp the need for less radical surgery ... (49)." Eventually, conservative surgery became standard treatment for a number of malignancies, most prominently breast cancer.

Critics of radical surgery resorted to RCTs to prove that alternative and competing methods were equally, if not more, effective than radical operations. As Major Greenwood anticipated, the clinical trial became a weapon in the fight to reign in unwarranted claims of success and to make surgery a more scientifically based discipline. For many kinds of cancer, the conservative approach (sometimes supplemented by radiation and chemotherapy) won out. But the overall effectiveness of surgery still rests more on common sense than it does on randomized clinical trials.

▬ Radiation as a Cancer Therapy

Roentgen rays were discovered at the end of 1895 by Prof. Wilhelm C. Roentgen of the University of Würzburg, Germany. He was rewarded with the first Nobel Prize in Physics for this epochal discovery. By 1896, early investigators (including Thomas Alva Edison in America) found that these mysterious rays could not only visualize the interior of solid objects, such as the human body, but could have a destructive effect on living tissues.

The first attempts to use radiation as a cancer treatment were conducted in January 1896 by a homeopathic medical student in Chicago, Emil H. Grubbé. In Europe, better equipped laboratories were not far behind. On 3 February 1896, J. Voigt of Hamburg treated a case of carcinoma of the nasopharynx and reported for the first time pain relief through radiation therapy (79). In France, V. Despeignes applied roentgen rays to two patients, one of whom had cancer of the mouth, the other of the stomach. In the first case, severe pain ceased almost immediately. In two patients with inoperable breast cancer "daily irradiation soon relieved the excruciating neuralgic pain ... (22)." It is generally accepted that Dr. Leopold Freund of Vienna (21) was "the first to use roentgen rays logically and scientifically within the limits of the age" (53).

Two facts stand out from the early experiments with roentgen rays and later with radium (discovered by the Curies in 1902): they could often relieve pain and palliate other symptoms of cancer; and they could sometimes shrink or even destroy established tumors. Thus, it is not surprising that radiation therapy grew in popularity and that enormous hopes were invested in this new form of treatment. For the first time, an alternative to surgery seemed possible and the mood of pessimism that characterized nineteenth-century thinking about cancer began to dissipate.

The reputation of radiation therapy rested, and continues to rest, on these two obvious facts. However, pain relief and tumor destruction does not tell the whole story of radiation treatment. For radiation, as was soon discovered, was a two-edged sword, with many harmful effects on the body.

It was soon noted that roentgen rays could burn the skin or irreparably damage internal organs or structures. In 1896, Dr. D.W. Gage of McCook, New Brunswick, writing in New York's *Medical Record,* noted cases of hair loss, reddened skin, skin sloughing, and strange growths or lesions. "I wish to suggest," he wrote mildly, "that more be understood regarding the action of the roentgen rays before the general practitioner adopts them in his daily work" (81).

Roentgen rays also turned out to not just "cure" cancer but to *cause* it as well. In fact, hundreds of radiologists and technicians died horribly, many of them of cancer, as a result of underestimating the dark side of their new technique. It was also found that tumors obliterated by radiation often recurred, sometimes in distant organs, and that these recurrences were difficult to treat with any conventional technique. After the explosion of the atomic bombs at Hiroshima and Nagasaki, detailed studies over decades showed that those exposed to radiation suffered many long-term harmful effects. In making an evaluation of the positive or negative effects of radiation, therefore, one simply cannot make a judgment based on its immediate impact on tumors. One needs to study the effects of the exposure over a period of time, preferably for decades.

Such questions can best be answered by evaluations conducted in the course of randomized controlled trials. But RCTs are difficult and expensive to conduct. Since they are not legally required for radiation by the FDA, they are often lacking. The vast majority of evaluations of the effectiveness of radiation therapy are based on reports of case series, not RCTs. When RCTs have been performed, they sometimes show that radiation is ineffective in prolonging overall survival of the participants. Thus, as a general rule, the safety and effectiveness of either adjuvant or therapeutic radiation therapy has not been adequately demonstrated through rigorous trials.

▄ Chemotherapy as a Cancer Therapy

Chemotherapy is more scientifically based than either radiotherapy or cancer surgery. In the five years between 1999 and 2004, over 75 000 peer-reviewed articles have appeared in Medline (PubMed) on the topic of cancer chemotherapy. An additional tens of thousands of abstracts have been presented at the American Society of Clinical Oncology (ASCO) and the American Association for Cancer Research annual meetings. Out of this vast amount of research, over 115 new approvals have been made by the US Food and Drug Administration (FDA) for drugs used in the treatment of cancer patients (see http://www.fda.gov/cder/cancer/druglistframe.htm). All of these are based on clinical trials of some sort. But what is the nature and quality of these trials? Has the current generation of anticancer drugs been proved to improve the overall survival of cancer patients?

In fact, *randomized* controlled trials (RCTs or phase III studies) are inconsistently performed in conventional oncology before or after the approval of a new drug. It is very rare for a trial to compare a drug with placebo (sham treatment) or even best supportive care (BSC). When studies are reported as positive that is usually in comparisons with other agents, or it is a measurement of improvement in surrogate markers rather than of increased overall survival.

Drugs may be reported to increase survival, but upon closer examination this sometimes turns out to be an increase in "relapse-free survival," or "time to recurrence," and not an actual increase in median overall survival. The latter are important figures, to be sure, but the most important and reliable figure is that of overall survival. Otherwise, the patient may experience an increase in the relapse-free period, but no increase in his or her actual life expectancy. Such a patient may only be benefited in a psychological sense. Yet real improvements in overall survival for the solid tumors

of adults are rarely demonstrated in rigorous trials with chemotherapy.

Surveys have shown that the two outcomes that cancer patients seek from chemotherapy are: first, an improvement in quality of life; and second, an increase in their actual survival. Tumor shrinkages in and of themselves are not a high priority (6). The "**Grand Illusion of Chemotherapy**" is the idea that the shrinkage of tumors, improvement in tumor markers, or increased relapse-free survival, necessarily correlates with actual benefit to patients.

But developmental oncologists tend to concentrate on the shrinkage of tumors or perhaps relapse-free survival. "Responses" are often defined in terms of tumor shrinkage, and drugs that shrink tumors are called "active agents." The FDA defines a complete response as a complete disappearance of all clinical and radiographic signs of cancer for one month or more. A partial response refers to a 50 % or greater decrease in measurable tumor size for one month or more. In the past, the FDA also required proof of life prolongation. But this stringent requirement led to very few drug approvals. From the 1940s to the mid-1990s, in fact, only about three dozen anticancer drugs were approved by the FDA, less than one per year. The FDA's reluctance to approve drugs based on shrinkages angered the pharmaceutical industry, as well as some oncologists and patient activists. So, in the mid-1990s the government relaxed these requirements, and since then FDA has approved many new drugs.

Finally, there is a huge economic dimension to the pharmaceutical treatment of cancer. Treating cancer with drugs has become big business. The following news item from the *New York Times* Website (12 October 2000) speaks for itself:

"Genentech, Inc. on Wednesday reported a 27 % gain in third-quarter profits . . . driven by sales of cancer drugs, Herceptin and Rituxan. Third-quarter sales of Herceptin increased 52 %, to $ 72.6 million ... Sales of Rituxan increased 62 %, to $ 117.9 million."

In other words, just this one pharmaceutical company is earning about US$ 750 000 000 per year from the sale of two of its anticancer agents. In the first years of the twenty-first century, it became common to hear talk of billion dollar sellers in the cancer drug field. By 2006, global spending on cancer drugs is predicted to total $ 31.7 billion, up from $ 22.3 billion in 2004, according to the consulting firm of Bain & Co. That makes cancer the fastest growing drug category (89). Bristol Myers should therefore quickly recoup what seemed like a ridiculous research investment of US$2 billion in a very short time, thanks to the FDA's compliant policy of accelerated approval. Oncologists who sell anticancer drugs in their offices—the so-called "chemotherapy concession"—will also benefit from this largesse (64).

The prediction the author made at the German Society of Oncology meeting in 1997 that the cancer chemotherapy market would reach US$13.8 billion by the end of the millennium now seems like a serious underestimation. The actual figures by 2005 were nearly twice that modest projection.

The Conventional Treatment of Non-Small Cell Lung Cancer

I would now like to examine the actual record of these three approaches in the treatment of one particular kind of cancer. Lung cancer is one of the most prevalent causes of cancer death worldwide. In the United States, there were an estimated 186 550 new cases of cancer of the respiratory system in 2004 (4). By another estimate, the world market for cancer therapeutics passed US$42 billion in 2004 and is expected to post rapid annual growth in the next five years, according to a study by Kalorama Information, New York, NY. New biologics and adjunctive therapy products are said to be the main growth drivers (68a).

Annually, cancers of the lung and bronchus accounted for 91 930 US deaths among men and 68 510 among women (2004 figures). It is three times as prevalent a cause of death among men as its nearest contender, prostate cancer (with 29 900 deaths) and has long since overtaken breast cancer as the leading cause of cancer death among women as well (68 510 vs. 40 580). In Germany, in recent years it has accounted for approximately 40 000 deaths annually (28 675 in men and 9296 in women) (84).

There are numerous books and thousands of scientific articles on the treatment of primary non-small cell lung cancer (NSCLC). However, most discussions are descriptive in nature. They accept and describe the therapeutic practices that are generally performed. Few of them examine the question of therapeutics in a critical way, with an eye on the quality of the evidence that is put forward to justify the claims of various treatments.

One exception to this rule is the Physicians' Data Query (PDQ) system of the National Cancer Institute (NCI). This US government database attempts to assess the quality and rigor of studies on which treatment decisions are made. The PDQ statements attempt to introduce a more scientifically based evaluation of the evidence. These statements also represent the official position of the US government on the treatment of cancer in its various stages. It is arguably the most influential body of literature on cancer treatment on the Internet. For these reasons, I will most often cite its statements in discussing the conventional treatments of this disease. (Note: in 1999, the author was appointed an advisor to the PDQ Adult Treatment Editorial Board.)

The PDQ editorial board sometimes uses a **formal ranking system** to help the reader judge the strength of evidence linked to the reported results of a therapeutic strategy. (Unfortunately, the application of this system remains sporadic.) We shall therefore follow its presentation on the effectiveness of the various conventional treatments, with a focus on the results attained through RCTs.

One problem we immediately encounter is the existence of different **staging systems** for this disease. We have followed the PDQ nomenclature of four stages, with stage III divided into two substages (IIIA and IIIB). The PDQ also recognizes and discusses a "stage 0" disease. However, each stage can also be characterized according to the **TNM system** as well (which classifies a tumor by its size, its regional lymph node involvement and distant metastatic spread). In addition, the American Joint Committee on Cancer (AJCC) and the Union Internationale Contre le Cancer (UICC) have proposed changes that will essentially divide stages I–III into two substages apiece. This will be more accurate but will make historical comparisons even more problematical.

The Surgical Treatment of Non-Small Cell Lung Cancer

The surgical treatment of lung cancer has evolved over a period of 100 years. In the late nineteenth century, extensive surgery was virtually impossible, but, then again, lung cancer was rarely encountered. The rising occurrence of lung cancer in most countries (tied to increased tobacco use during and after World War One) coincided with technical landmarks in its treatment. These were the first individual ligation of the hilar vessels (1912), the mass ligature of hilar vessels, the individual dissection and ligation of vessels (1932), and finally in 1933 the first successful radical pneumonectomy, or surgical removal of an entire lung. By the end of the 1930s, **pneumonectomy** was widely performed and for decades was considered the only acceptable treatment for this disease.

"The surgical removal of the entire lung is the only method of treatment that has been employed to date that has been at all efficacious for primary pulmonary carcinoma," wrote William Francis Rienhoff, Jr. in a 1940 cancer textbook. He cited a dozen experts in Europe and America, all of whom agreed that "the ideal procedure for the treatment of carcinoma of the lung is total pneumonectomy (66)." In 1947, another cancer textbook asserted that total pneumonectomy should be "carried out as radically as possible … ." In appropriate patients, "it should be done without hesitation" (2)

Yet the mortality rate of the operation itself ranged from 12–30% at the better centers (2). Deaths were caused by the accidental perforation of large vessels, pulmonary edema, arrhythmia, and heart failure, various types of infection, including pneumonia of the remaining lung, or the opening of the bronchial stump.

Astonishingly, we learn that over a five-year period Dr. Rienhoff had only tried this operation on 20 patients. No survival figures were given in his article and it was thus impossible to form even a crude idea of its effectiveness. As to safety, the figures were almost as primitive: since two deaths (out of 20 patients) occurred immediately after the surgery "the mortality rate must be considered as 10%," said this Johns Hopkins surgeon. Such was the quality of medical statistics on the eve of World War Two.

The procedure was first questioned in the 1950s because of its appalling side effects (8, 35). In a large case series from the Veterans Administration Surgical Oncology Group, the long-term survival was essentially the same following more **limited lobectomy** (the surgical removal of a lobe, in this case of the lung) as total pneumonectomy (74). However, this was not a randomized trial, and selection biases may have clouded the results.

Today, pneumonectomy has largely yielded to more limited surgery such as lobectomy or segmentectomy. But textbooks continue to laud surgery. A 1996 textbook chapter by Memorial Sloan-Kettering Cancer Center (MSKCC) thoracic surgeons repeatedly called surgery the "most effective method" and the "treatment of choice" for early-stage disease (43). Another textbook said that "best results are obtained for stage I to stage IIIA tumors if complete resection is performed …" (29). We are told by some authors that "resections less extensive than lobectomy and no lymph node dissection had adverse effects on recurrence" (43).

What is lacking, in all these arguments, are RCTs to support these positive assertions. One might think that sometime during the last 100 years surgeons might have arranged a clinical trial in which surgery in any form was compared with no further treatment (or best supportive care). To my knowledge, this has never been done. There is an implicit assumption that surgery has to be better than doing nothing of an aggressive nature.

Nor do we really know, based on RCTs, if one surgical approach yields better long-term survival results than another. This too is amenable to scientific experiment. At MSKCC, they routinely dissect the mediastinal lymph nodes as part of their standard surgical operation for lung cancer, believing that this provides the best possible staging of the disease. But two of their surgeons admit: "Whether this technique provides a greater opportunity of cure … has never been demonstrated in a randomized trial." They even assert that "one must believe" that it is superior, "without scientific proof" … a strange way of arguing in a scientific textbook (43).

The value of surgery over no surgery, of lobectomy over pulmonectomy, and so forth, is based overwhelmingly on the retrospective analysis of case series. These yield certain survival figures, which are sometimes naively contrasted to one another. But there is really no way to compare one such case series with another and it is not surprising that we find great variation in the results achieved at different centers and a welter of conflicting opinions on the proper treatment of the disease.

Stage 0 non-small cell lung cancer (NSCLC) is the earliest stage of the disease. The PDQ states that these tumors "should be curable with surgical resection." This statement is true as far as it goes. But, in their own words, "these tumors are by definition noninvasive and incapable of metastasizing." Thus, one would like to know whether they could be treated in some other way, or left untreated at all ("watchful waiting" or "anticipatory management"). No such studies are cited. The scientific value of surgery for stage 0 NSCLC has not been established through RCTs.

Stage I NSCLC

In stage 1 NSCLC, the cancer is only in the lung with normal tissue around it.

Surgery

The PDQ summary states that "surgery is the treatment of choice for patients with stage I non-small cell lung cancer (NSCLC)." Most textbooks agree with this. It is unclear, however, whether the term "treatment of choice" indicates current practice (descriptive) or is a value judgment on the part of the PDQ board (prescriptive). No RCTs are cited to support this recommendation, nor do there appear to be any.

There has been one RCT to compare lobectomy to a more limited excision. According to the PDQ, the results showed a reduction in the local recurrence rate for patients treated with lobectomy compared with those treated with limited excision but no significant difference in overall survival (24).

We have certainly become accustomed in the last fifty years to finding that the results of RCTs sometimes are counterintuitive. If surgery is indeed life saving or life prolonging, one might logically expect a more extensive operation (lobectomy) to convey a life-prolonging effect. Yet, in stage I NSCLC and many other cancers, this is apparently not the case. This has led some surgeons to conclude that radical surgery is never more effective than conservative surgery since the real battle takes place in the bloodstream between remaining tumor cells and the immune system (17).

We can conclude that the surgical treatment of stage I NSCLC is based on logic and inference, rather than scientific experiment. It seems "obvious" and "commonsensical" to all concerned that surgically resecting the tumor in question is necessary. However, we do not know this as a fact. The crucial experiments have never been done and, given the current mindset, probably will never be done.

Radiation Therapy

Certain patients with stage I NSCLC are deemed inoperable or have refused surgery. Some of these patients have then been treated with radiation therapy "with curative intent" (43). It is sometimes asserted that "a definite prolongation of life" may result from radiation therapy. Five-year survival rates of 6–33 % have been reported. A 32 % five-year survival rate was also reported for **brachytherapy** (the use of internal radiation).

There is a single report of patients older than 70 years of age who had resectable lesions that were smaller than 4 cm who were treated with radiation therapy. Survival at five years was comparable to a historical control group of patients of similar age who were surgically resected with curative intent. But historical comparisons are notoriously unreliable and would certainly not be accepted as the basis for claims made about nonconventional treatments (57).

There are a number of retrospective reviews (case series) in which radiation therapy was employed as a primary treatment for early-stage NSCLC. These form an inadequate basis for treatment decisions, since they report on a highly selected group of patients (16, 23). Because there is no scientific basis of comparison with other approaches, such series are not very valuable and certainly not definitive.

As stated, survival in case series may and do differ widely among themselves. For example, while Smart and Hilton reported a 33 % five-year survival rate with radiation therapy, Cooper et al. reported a survival rate of just 6 %. You might suppose that the higher rate was due to better techniques or more modern equipment. However, paradoxically, the higher survival figure dates from the early 1950s (76), while the 6 % figure dates from nearly 30 years later, when far more powerful and focused equipment was in use (10).

It bears repeating that one cannot meaningfully compare retrospectively analyzed case series. Nor can one rely on historical controls. This approach leads to hopeless confusion. Such confusion is quite common when there are no RCTs to formally compare approaches and establish (or contradict) the value of radiation therapy for stage I NSCLC.

Adjuvant Radiation Therapy

Radiation therapy has also been used as an adjuvant treatment after surgery in such patients. One need not review all the studies. However, a 1998 *Lancet* meta-analysis of nine randomized trials evaluating postoperative radiation vs. surgery alone showed a 7% *reduction* in overall survival with adjuvant radiation in patients with stage I or II disease (60).

Thus, adjuvant radiation appears to *decrease* survival after surgery. The PDQ holds out the hope that "these outcomes can potentially be modified with technical improvements, better definitions of target volumes, and limitation of cardiac volume in the radiation portals." Perhaps. But this is the standard response of all dedicated therapists, of any technique, whenever a rigorous study determines that their technique is ineffective or even harmful.

To claim that results using older techniques are necessarily invalid provides a ready-made excuse for the failure of clinical trials to demonstrate the effectiveness of radiation treatment. Since technique is always evolving, radiation can apparently never be proved ineffective. One can always argue that the latest machine, dose, regimen, etc., will do what previous treatments were unable to do. Thus, like a system of religious or philosophical dogmas, apologies for radiation generate statements that are "amenable only to confirmation" and never to rejection (78). By contrast, truly scientific theories, as philosopher Karl Popper (1902–1994) showed, have testable implications which, if false, will falsify the theory itself (59). Indeed, as of 2004, according to the PDQ, there have been no rigorous studies performed that undercut the *Lancet* meta-analysis conclusions.

Adjuvant Chemotherapy
According to three oncologists, writing in the sixth (2001) edition of the DeVita textbook, adjuvant chemotherapy has been "under investigation for several decades." However, "few randomized studies of adjuvant chemotherapy in NSCLC have been published" (13). Trials of adjuvant chemotherapy regimens have also failed to demonstrate a consistent benefit, says the PDQ. In that time, however, there has been no proof that it conveys any survival advantage.

For example, the Lung Cancer Study Group compared four cycles of CAP (cyclophosphamide + doxorubicin + cisplatin) chemotherapy to no further therapy in 269 patients with stage I disease. No benefit was seen for chemotherapy (only 53% of patients were even able to complete the chemotherapy) (13). A study testing a lower-dose CAP regimen in T1 T3 N0 disease seemed to show a benefit in time to recurrence and survival. How-

ever, the test was flawed: a subsequent analysis showed that more patients with advanced disease had been assigned to the observation arm, thereby making the chemotherapy arm appear better (54). In addition, meta-analysis of 52 trials using adjuvant chemotherapy failed to show a decided advantage to this approach (55).

By the 1990s CAP was no longer considered the most "active" combination (where "activity" is defined by tumor shrinkages that may be temporary and partial). Therefore, clinical trials were launched to test the combination of cisplatin + etoposide plus concomitant radiation therapy vs. radiation therapy alone. The results of these trials are not yet known. However, in stage II and III NSCLC, it was found that, after surgery, adding cisplatin + etoposide chemotherapy to radiation therapy did not prolong survival. In fact, treatment-associated mortality was *slightly higher* in the chemotherapy-added group (1.6% vs. 1.2%) and survival was slightly lower (38 months vs. 39 months), according to a study in the *New England Journal of Medicine* (38).

In an accompanying editorial, Desmond N. Carney, M.D., at Mater Hospital in Dublin, Ireland, and Heine H. Hansen of the Finsen Center in Copenhagen, Denmark, conclude that adjuvant chemotherapy in patients with tumors that have been completely removed "should not be considered standard care" (7).

Stage II NSCLC

Stage II NSCLC is defined as cancer that has spread to nearby lymph nodes.

Surgical Treatment
"Surgery is the treatment of choice for patients with stage II non-small cell lung cancer " says the PDQ. Once again, however, it is not clear if the phrase "treatment of choice" is descriptive or prescriptive. In either case, there is no scientific documentation of the beneficial effects of surgery for this stage of NSCLC. In fact, many of the patients who are surgically treated develop second, or recurrent, lung cancers despite the treatment.

Radiation Treatment
The PDQ states that "inoperable patients with stage II disease and with sufficient pulmonary reserve may be considered for radiation therapy

with curative intent." The PDQ notes that "among patients with excellent performance status, up to a 20% three-year survival rate may be expected if a course of radiation therapy with curative intent can be completed" (40).

No RCTs are cited in support of this statement. However, to select a group of patients who already have "excellent performance status" and then to cite survival figures for them, does not seem like a fair test of a procedure. That is because patients with "excellent performance status" are, by definition, likely to have improved survival, regardless of what treatment they are given.

Instead of RCTs, the PDQ cites retrospective reviews showing a five-year overall survival rate of 10%. It claims that a subset of 44 patients with T1 tumors achieved an actuarial disease-free survival rate of 60%. Despite a lack of rigorous scientific support, the PDQ states that "primary radiation therapy should consist of approximately 6000 cGy …" (In this case, the word "should" is definitely prescriptive.)

The PDQ points out that there was one controlled trial of postoperative radiation therapy. However, this failed to demonstrate an overall survival benefit for patients with carefully staged squamous cell carcinoma who received postoperative radiation, although local recurrence rates were reduced (82). It is a common observation in a variety of cancers that radiation therapy may reduce the local recurrence rate without significantly improving the overall survival rate. The PDQ does not comment on this paradoxical situation. One logical hypothesis is that the short-term and long-term side effects of radiation (18) lead to the earlier demise of as many people as those whose lives are extended by the treatment itself.

We have already mentioned the **PORT meta-analysis** of nine randomized trials evaluating postoperative radiation vs. surgery alone that showed a 7% reduction in overall survival in stage I or II patients given adjuvant radiation therapy (60).

Chemotherapy

What is the result of combining postoperative radiation and chemotherapy? This question has indeed been subjected to a rigorous trial. But, here too, results have been negative. In 2000, a multicenter RCT compared postoperative radiation therapy alone to postoperative radiation therapy with concurrent use of the drugs cisplatin and etoposide. It did not demonstrate either a disease-free or overall survival advantage with the combined therapy (38).

An NCI media release of 26 October 2000 concludes: "Adding chemotherapy to radiation therapy does not prolong survival in operable, non-small cell lung cancer, according to a large, randomized study that compared the chemotherapy/radiation combination to radiation alone."

Stage III NSCLC

Stage III NSCLC includes all locally advanced tumors that do not have evidence of distant metastatic disease. It has been subdivided into stage IIIA, which designates tumors that are potentially resectable through surgery, and stage IIIB, which includes tumors that are usually considered unresectable (69). But both of these categories encompass many different types of patients, with possible involvement of the chest wall, pericardium, diaphragm, or proximal airways. No standard of care has yet been established for stage III NSCLC.

About 30000 patients are diagnosed each year in the US with stage III NSCLC. The overall situation with stage III lung cancer is not encouraging: the overall, five-year survival rates range from 0–30% (depending on the series and the extent of disease). Most patients with extensive disease have a 10% or less "chance of cure."

The full armamentarium of conventional treatment, namely, radiation therapy, chemotherapy, and surgery, or combinations of these modalities, are used against this stage of NSCLC. The question is whether any of these have been scientifically established to extend life.

Surgical Treatment

It is often stated that surgical resection leads to long-term survival in carefully selected patients. However, this is based on retrospective series, which offer no dependable basis of comparison with any other treatment (or nontreatment) approach. It is not necessary to discuss these series in detail. They show a wide variation in results. The results are also very confusing, since they employ many different approaches to characterizing these diverse patients. They vary by the size of tumor, tumor extensions, surgical treatments employed, etc.

In all, there have been at least 15 series reporting on five-year survival for patients with stage IIIA

N2 disease (extensive lymph node involvement). These report five-year survival rates ranging from 0% to as high as 50%. Obviously, such series are not comparable to one another. As two lung cancer specialists state:

> "Many reported series present an inappropriately optimistic view of the benefit of surgical resection . . . because they focus on highly selected groups of patients" (69).

The whole concept of using surgery as the primary treatment of stage III disease has now been challenged by the results of two RCTs employing chemotherapy in that capacity. These shall be discussed below.

Radiation Treatment

Radiation can be used as either a primary or an adjuvant treatment for stage III NSCLC. According to the PDQ, there is a "reproducible long-term survival benefit in 5–10% of patients treated with standard fractionation to 6000 cGy," and significant palliation often results. Patients with excellent performance status and those who require a thoracotomy to prove that surgically unresectable tumor is present are most likely to benefit from radiation therapy (40).

The PDQ, which pioneered the use of a formal ranking system to help the reader judge the strength of evidence linked to the reported results of a therapeutic strategy, fails to append a rating score for this pivotal article: it is, however, a retrospective review of 410 patients who were treated in the 1970s. It is clearly not a rigorous RCT. How the PDQ can contradict its own principles and assert that there is a "reproducible long-term survival benefit" based on such a study is puzzling.

The PDQ also claims that "radiation therapy given as three daily fractions improved overall survival compared with radiation therapy given as one daily fraction." The source for this is the so-called **CHART study** (continuous hyperfractionated accelerated radiotherapy). This shows that those who received the hyperfractionated form of radiation had a two-year survival of 29% compared with 20% in the standard radiotherapy group. However, side effects were concomitantly higher. During the first three months, severe dysphagia occurred in 19% of the CHART group vs. the conventional radiotherapy group (3%).

There have been several randomized phase III trials to compare radiation alone and the combined treatment of radiation therapy and chemotherapy. The problem here is that the results of these various trials are difficult to compare since they include patients with different stages of the disease. Nevertheless, they do yield some interesting information.

Sequential Chemotherapy and Radiation Therapy

There have been a number of trials of sequential chemotherapy + radiation therapy vs. radiation therapy alone. Sequential chemotherapy is also called "neoadjuvant" chemotherapy. The idea is that the use of chemotherapy before surgery might lower the systemic tumor burden and prevent the growth of microscopic systemic disease. As one textbook has written, "The concept of neoadjuvant therapy has become very popular and is now often used outside the setting of clinical trials" (69).

In the first trials, chemotherapy did not appear very effective. For example, in the so-called **Mattson study** of 238 patients, the median survival was 10.3 months for the radiation group vs. 11.0 months in the combined chemotherapy–radiation group, an advantage of several weeks (46). In the **Morton trial**, the median survival advantage for chemotherapy was similarly less than one month (50). In that study, *fewer* patients receiving chemotherapy were alive at five years (5% vs. 7%). In the **Le Chevalier study**, the difference in median survival was two months and the difference at five years was 3% (3% vs. 6%) (41).

Y. Sekido, et al., writing in the sixth edition (2001) of the De Vita textbook, cite "the poor design or execution of many of the randomized trials" in this area (71). It consequently ignores most of these studies and focuses on two studies performed by the Cancer and Leukemia Group B (CALGB), a large network of university medical centers and physicians, that sponsors clinical trials (32). In the first **CALGB study**, patients given chemotherapy had a median survival of 13.7 months vs. 9.6 months for radiation alone. Their two-year survival was double (26% vs. 13%) and their five-year survival was 17% vs. 7% (14). Accrual to this study was closed early after identification of a statistically significant difference in survival.

A confirmatory CALGB study was then undertaken (40, 70). The results of this larger study were also positive, but not nearly as positive as the first CALGB study. In this second CALGB study, the median survival was 11.4 months for those receiving standard radiation therapy, 12.2 months for hyperfractionated radiation therapy, and 13.7 months for standard radiation preceded by chemotherapy. In other words, there was a survival advantage of *about 1.5 months in the chemotherapy group,* about a third of the benefit seen in the first CALGB study. Five-year survival was 5% for standard radiation vs. 6% for hyperfractionated radiation vs. 8% for the radiation plus chemotherapy group ... half of the 17% five-year survival seen in the first CALGB trial.

However, on the basis of this series of tests, Sekido et al. have concluded that "induction chemotherapy has been shown in large randomized studies to increase survival rates of patients with unresectable stage III NSCLC" and that "induction chemotherapy is a current standard therapy for these patients" (71). Not everyone agrees. Another textbook concludes: "... the long-term survival advantage of neoadjuvant therapy over more conventional forms of treatment, such as radiation therapy alone, remains incompletely proved" (69).

Sekido claims that "the addition of one month of chemotherapy to radiation resulted in a four-month prolongation of life" (71). This is a selective interpretation of the facts. First, the RCTs themselves have been sifted and certain trials have been declared to have an acceptable level of design and execution for consideration. (In this instance, the selected trials happen to be those that yield results favorable to chemotherapy.) These selected trials are then further sifted and those that yield the most favorable results (in this case, the two CALGB studies) are taken to represent the whole. Then the far more favorable of the two CALGB trials is made the basis of conclusions, even though it was smaller and recruitment was stopped early.

The idea that chemotherapy adds four months' prolongation of life, promoted by the influential DeVita textbook, has been widely repeated, although it is in fact the outcome of a single study. In the larger of the two CALGB studies, as we have seen, the difference in median survival between those receiving hyperfractionated radiation therapy and those also receiving induction chemotherapy was only 1.5 months. Thus, one could more equitably say that in exchange for one month of toxic polychemotherapy patients receive on average 1.5 months of increased overall survival and an increase of 2% in the five-year survival rate. One must leave it to the reader to decide whether such benefits justify the side effects, mental anguish, and financial expenditures involved in this intensive treatment.

One must also note that in none of these trials was there a placebo or no-treatment arm. Thus, we do not know how a comparable group that did not receive chemotherapy would have fared compared with these intensively treated groups. We do not know the absolute value of chemotherapy, only its value relative to radiation therapy.

Concomitant Chemoradiotherapy

The concomitant (simultaneous) use of chemotherapy and radiation has also been tested in several RCTs. This has also become a very common treatment for patients with stage III NSCLC. Most of these studies have compared radiation therapy vs. radiation plus a single chemotherapeutic agent. However, according to Sekido, these have shown no survival benefit: "Concomitant chemoradiotherapy using single agent cisplatin or other drugs has largely failed to improve the survival rates of patients with locoregionally advanced NSCLC" (71).

There have also been some studies of combination chemotherapy using various schedules of radiation therapy. Most of these have been uncontrolled phase I or phase II studies. Results uniformly show increased toxicity, but some of these studies suggest that there might be a therapeutic benefit as well.

Randomized phase III studies have been limited. However, there have been two studies (from the same group) suggesting that carboplatin + etopiside, when added to hyperfractionated radiation therapy, yielded a median survival of 18 months vs. eight months for hyperfractionated radiation therapy alone (33, 34).

According to the PDQ, a 1995 meta-analysis of patient data from 52 clinical trials showed a modest survival increase for cisplatin-based drug combinations plus radiation therapy. Chemotherapy plus surgery gave an absolute benefit of five percentage points at five years compared with surgery alone. (However, this benefit did not reach statistical significance and thus may have been due to chance). Chemotherapy plus radical radiotherapy gave an absolute benefit of 4% at two years (56).

Chemotherapy Before Surgery

In the mid-1990s there was a considerable amount of excitement over the prospect of using chemotherapy before surgery for stage III NSCLC to improve results. This is called **preoperative or neoadjuvant chemotherapy**. Two small RCTs indicated improved survival using a cisplatin-based treatment regimen before surgery. These trials were terminated early, however, because the results in one arm were turning out to be statistically better than in the other arm.

In the M.D. Anderson study, patients treated with preoperative chemotherapy and surgery had an estimated median survival of 64 months compared with 11 months for patients who had surgery alone. The estimated two-year and three-year survival rates were 60% and 56% respectively for the perioperative chemotherapy patients and 25% and 15% respectively for those who had surgery alone (68).

Another small study (from the University of Barcelona) used a different chemotherapy regimen but reached similar conclusions. The median period of survival was 26 months in the patients treated with chemotherapy plus surgery, as compared with eight months in the patients treated with surgery alone; the median period of disease-free survival was 20 months in the former group, as compared with five months in the latter. The rate of recurrence was 56% in the group treated with chemotherapy plus surgery and 74% in the group treated with surgery alone (67).

These tentative results were encouraging. However, the problem in extrapolating from them are obvious. The trials were small and used different chemotherapy regimens. Notice that the median survival in the combined treatment group of the Barcelona trial was less than half of what it was at M.D. Anderson. In all, a total of 120 patients were treated, and only 60 received chemotherapy. A further complication is that in the Barcelona study, all but one of the patients were men. The trials were terminated early (for ethical reasons).

There are other reasons to doubt the effectiveness of preoperative chemotherapy. A small RCT performed in 1998 by the National Cancer Institute of Canada did not confirm the value of preoperative chemotherapy. In this study, 31 patients with stage IIIA (N2) non-small cell lung cancer were randomized to receive radiation therapy alone or chemotherapy with cisplatin + vinblastine followed by surgery. The response rates to both pre-

operative chemotherapy and radiation therapy were both high (50% and 53.3%, respectively). However, the median survival time was 16.2 months for radiation therapy alone and 18.7 months for chemoradiotherapy. This difference was not statistically significant, and there was "no long-term improvement in survival seen with combined modality treatment." Notice that the median survival for the combined treatment group was not the extraordinary 64 months of the M.D. Anderson trial, nor even the very good 26 months of the Barcelona study, but a modest 18.7 months (73).

The authors of the M.D. Anderson study refer to the benefits of preoperative chemotherapy as only "probable." A few years later there was a follow-up on the same patients, which confirmed the positive findings (89). In addition, a phase III intergroup trial has been undertaken to answer a different question: whether the results achieved with induction chemotherapy + radiation followed by surgery are equivalent to those of chemotherapy + radiation *without surgery*. By jumping to this more advanced question, they ignore the obvious need for a larger, more protracted, confirmatory study of the whole concept of presurgical chemotherapy. The treatment thus remains promising but unproved.

Stage IV NSCLC

Stage IV NSCLC is defined as cancer that has spread beyond the lungs. Metastases to the brain is a common characteristic of this stage of the disease.

Surgery

Being essentially inoperable, curative resection is not an option, although surgery may be used as a palliative measure.

Radiation Therapy

Radiation has long been used to treat stage IV NSCLC. A 1947 cancer textbook states that the administration of radiation therapy quite often results in a "diminution of the tumor, a re-establishment of bronchial permeability, disappearance of … pain, improvement of the general condition, and a sensation of well-being." Radiation, we are further told, "has a definite place and contributes definite, sometimes unexpected, results" (3).

This palliative aspect of radiation therapy has been noted innumerable times, beginning with some of the very first treated patients. There is no reason to doubt that radiation therapy can be a highly effective palliative for many of the symptoms of late-stage NSCLC. It can be used to treat tracheal, esophageal, or bronchial compression, bone or brain metastases, pain, vocal cord paralysis, hemoptysis, or superior vena cava syndrome. However, no single mechanism of action has been demonstrated to account for this wide range of effects. While it is not my intention to deny such striking palliative effects, the almost total absence of sham radiation-controlled trials limits our knowledge of the actual physiological contribution of radiation to the control of symptoms in this and other cancers.

Chemotherapy

Chemotherapy is widely used for the treatment of stage IV NSCLC. The PDQ points out that platinum-containing combination chemotherapy regimens produce "objective response rates" (i.e., partial or complete shrinkages of measurable tumors by 50 % or more for one month or more) that are higher than those achieved with single agent chemotherapy regimens. The outcome is similar with most of the cisplatin-containing regimens. In fact, a randomized trial comparing five cisplatin-containing regimens showed no significant difference in response, duration of response, or survival.

However, the question one would like answered is whether or not any chemotherapy, platinum-based or not, actually increases median overall survival compared with placebo or to best supportive care (BSC). There has been a considerable amount of activity around this question. It appears likely (but not certain) that advanced chemotherapeutic regimens do yield a small survival advantage over BSC.

There have been about a dozen such trials. Most of them were underpowered, i.e., did not contain enough patients to yield significant results. They also used different chemotherapeutic regimens, which further complicated the issue. But let us look at some representative trials.

- The largest to date was that of Cullen et al. who used the MIC regimen (mitomycin + ifosfamide + cisplatin). They randomized 351 patients, 176 to receive best supportive care (BSC) and the other 175 to receive MIC. The median survival was 21 weeks in the BSC group and 29 weeks in the chemotherapy group, a net gain of about two months (11).

- The study that is most frequently cited is the one that yielded the best results. This was a comparison of two regimens vs. BSC. It showed a doubling of survival time from 17 weeks to 33 weeks between BSC and the VP regimen (vindesine + platinum). This represents a survival gain of four months.

However, in none of these studies was overall survival more than 37 weeks in any of the groups, treated or untreated. In all of these studies the trend was toward modest increased survival in the chemotherapy groups. Not surprisingly, then, four meta-analyses showed about a six to ten week survival advantage to chemotherapy. The largest of these combined the results of 11 studies, eight of which were cisplatin based. It showed a median survival of six months with best supportive care vs. eight months with chemotherapy, *for an average overall survival gain of two months.* The data were best for the cisplatin-based therapies (56).

More recently, University of Toronto scientists published the results of an RCT comparing docetaxel (Taxol) vs. BSC in patients with stages IIIB and IV lung cancer who had previously been treated with platinum-containing drugs. Again, the results were modestly positive. Out of 103 patients, there were six partial responses. The median survival was 7.0 months for the docetaxel group vs. 7.6 months for the BSC group, a gain of about two and a half months. Paradoxically, survival was somewhat better in patients receiving the lower of two doses of docetaxel. There were serious complications (febrile neutropenia) in 12 of the patients in the docetaxel group, and three of them died of this. The authors conclude that "the benefits of docetaxel therapy outweigh the risks" (73). A study from the UK similarly showed a median survival of 6.8 months in the docetaxel group vs. 4.8 months in the BSC group (62).

Thus, it has frequently been observed that advanced NSCLC patients who receive intensive chemotherapy have an *increased survival of approximately two months* compared with those who receive best supportive care alone, although no specific regimen is presently regarded as standard therapy (20). This gain must be weighed against the considerable toxicity, anxiety, and cost of treatment, including the risk of toxic death.

The recommendation for chemotherapy cannot and should not be made universally. Simes reviewed the Eastern Collaborative Oncology Group

(ECOG) experience in non-small cell lung cancer. He showed that median survival was 4.2 months (in 1985) and that 50% of the survival time was spent on treatment by the protocol. Thirty-nine percent of patients experienced at least one episode of "severe or worse" toxicity from therapy. Simes suggested that subgroups of patients were identified who would likely receive no benefit from treatment (75).

The PDQ cautions: "Outside of a clinical trial setting, chemotherapy should be given only to patients with good performance status and evaluative tumor lesions who desire such treatment after being fully informed of its anticipated risks and limited benefits."

Jimmie Holland of Memorial Sloan-Kettering Cancer Center has stressed "the importance of obtaining a clear understanding of the patient's wishes in this situation in which encroachment on quality of life during expected short survival had to be weighed against the slight benefit" (31).

In fact, a survey of Canadian oncologists, who themselves refer NSCLC patients for chemotherapy, found that the majority of them would reject chemotherapy if they themselves had NSCLC. Eighty-one percent said they would not take part in a drug trial if the regimen contained the highly toxic drug cisplatin (42). In an editorial, Heine H. Hansen of the Finsen Institute commented: "Based on the existing literature, it is difficult not to concur with our colleagues in not taking treatment." He added: "One can question the justification of continuing therapeutic trials along these lines in non-small cell lung cancer (28)." In my opinion, nothing has happened in the intervening years to change the accuracy of this judgment.

Iressa

On 5 May 2003, the US Food and Drug Administration (FDA) approved gefitinib (Iressa) as a treatment for advanced non-small cell lung cancer (NSCLC). Iressa is intended to treat patients whose cancer has progressed despite treatment with other forms of chemotherapy.

Iressa was evaluated in a multicenter US clinical trial in patients who had advanced NSCLC. All patients entered the trial after their disease had already progressed or they had experienced intolerable toxicity with platinum-based drugs.

One hundred and forty-two patients received Iressa at a dose of either 250 or 500 mg/day. Partial tumor "responses" (shrinkages) occurred in 15 of 142 evaluative patients, yielding an overall response rate of 10.6%. Responses occurred in nine of 66 patients receiving 250 mg/day (13.6%) and in six of 76 patients receiving 500 mg/day (7.8%). In other words, the lower dose seemed to work better than the higher dose. The median duration of response was seven months.

Two other large RCTs in the first-line treatment of NSCLC showed "no benefit from adding gefitinib to doublet, platinum-based chemotherapy," according to the PDQ.

In patients who received Iressa alone as a treatment for NSCLC, the most common adverse drug reactions reported were diarrhea, rash, acne, dry skin, nausea, vomiting, and pruritus. These were generally mild to moderate. But more serious instances of interstitial lung disease (ILD) have also been observed in patients receiving Iressa. The overall incidence was about 1%, but in approximately one-third of individuals this proved to be fatal. (The reported incidence of ILD was about 2% in the Japanese postmarketing experience.)

FDA gave its accelerated approval on the basis of a relatively small percentage of partial responses. There was no indication of either complete responses or of increased survival with this drug. Iressa (gefitinib) was subsequently subjected to rigorous clinical trials (INTACT 1 and 2). The results were essentially negative. "Gefitinib in combination with gemcitabine and cisplatin in chemotherapy-naive patients with advanced NSCLC did not have improved efficacy over gemcitabine and cisplatin alone", the authors concluded (91, 92). In April, 2005, the US National Cancer Institute (NCI) decided to discontinue all further clinical trials with Iressa.

Psychosocial Impact of Placebo and "Nocebo" in Advanced NSCLC

One must wonder about the psychologically beneficial effect of being given a powerful and promising new treatment vs. the contrary "nocebo" (negative placebo) effect of being abandoned to one's fate without further attempts at therapy (26). What is the effect on longevity of these two dramatically different pathways? There are comparisons of aggressive treatment to best supportive care (which means no further attempts at cure). To my knowledge, however, there are no single-blinded or double-blinded studies comparing chemotherapy for NSCLC to any sort of sham treatment. This being the case, the RCTs that have been cited leave unanswered the question of what psychological impact, if any, chemotherapy (or its denial) have on patients with advanced NSCLC.

The issue is not trivial. The difference between the results in treated and untreated patients in all of these studies is so small that even a minor impact of mental state could vitiate the seemingly positive effect of aggressive treatment. We do know that a study at the Radium Hospital in Oslo has shown that the greatest predictors of survival among NSCLC patients were general symptoms and psychosocial well-being (36, 37). Lung cancer patients in fact tend to have very high levels of distress (seen in 43.4 % of patients) (86). One needs to gauge the psychological as well as the physical effects of treatment or nontreatment

We know that with a number of other cancers, a patient's state of mind can influence survival.

- Steven Greer has showed that psychological response is related to **breast cancer** outcome at five, 10, and 15 years. Recurrence-free survival is significantly greater in patients who have a "fighting spirit" than in those who react with helplessness and hopelessness. At the final follow-up, 45 % of the patients who responded to their diagnosis with a fighting spirit were alive and well, compared with 17 % who exhibited hopeless responses (25). Questions have more recently been raised about the positive effect of a fighting spirit, but there is little disagreement that helplessness and hopelessness have a detrimental effect on survival (80).
- Similarly, David Spiegel of Stanford University has shown that psychological support, relaxation, and self-hypnosis have a profound effect on the survival of patients with stage IV **breast cancer**. Such women who received psychological support lived twice as long as control patients (77). A larger follow-up study is underway.
- A study by UCLA psychiatrist Fawzy showed that patients with **melanoma** who received psychological support had a significantly lower rate of tumor recurrence than controls (21 % vs. 38 %) and a dramatically lower death rate (9 % vs. 29 %) (19).

- Similarly, Jeanne Richardson showed that patients with **leukemia and lymphoma** who participated in a modest home-based psychological intervention lived significantly longer than those who did not: there was a 39 % reduction in the death rate (65).

It is entirely possible that the very modest positive effect of chemotherapy sometimes seen in advanced NSCLC is due to the opposing, positive or negative psychological impact of chemotherapy or no further treatment (BSC) in these trials. This question has apparently not been studied but is amenable to experimental proof.

Recurrences of Stage IV NSCLC

Much the same can be said about the treatment of recurrences of lung cancer as has been said about stage IV disease. Radiation therapy is well known to provide excellent palliation of symptoms from a localized tumor mass.

Recurrence frequently occurs as brain metastases. In such a case, it may be possible to remove a solitary cerebral metastasis through surgery. The PDQ states that this may lead to "prolonged disease-free survival" although it is unclear if this results in any increased overall survival. The PDQ also cautions that "because of the small potential for long-term survival, radiation therapy should be delivered by conventional methods" and that higher doses "should be avoided because of the high risk of toxic effects observed with such treatments." Selected patients should be considered for a form of radiation known as stereotactic radiosurgery.

What is lacking is an RCT demonstrating increased overall survival from any of these methods, although the palliative benefit can be a worthwhile goal in itself.

The use of chemotherapy in recurrent lung cancer is largely palliative. It has produced objective responses and "small improvement in survival" for patients with metastatic disease. While the survival benefit is small, improvement in subjective symptoms has been reported to occur more frequently than an objective response. Whether this occurs because of a physical reduction of the tumor burden or because of psychological factors has not been explored.

Conclusions

The conventional treatment of early-stage NSCLC consists primarily of surgery, supplemented by radiation therapy and/or chemotherapy in various combinations. In late stages there is more reliance on radiation and chemotherapy as primary treatments.

The use of surgery is time-honored and rests on the commonsensical assumption that resecting a primary tumor en bloc leads either to cure or to significant prolongation of life. This may or may not be true. There is a remarkable lack of RCTs to support this fundamental tenet of modern oncology.

Reliance on common sense as a guide to medical practice has to be tempered by the frequency with which its conclusions are confounded by experimental science. History books are filled with innumerable instances in which the "common sense" of one era becomes the nonsense of another. For example, within living memory it was common sense that radical surgery for breast cancer necessarily yielded better results than more limited options. We now know that is not true. For several decades, it was common sense that pneumonectomy was the only acceptable surgical option for lung cancer. This is no longer believed. No matter how long standing a belief, no matter how obvious it may be to its proponents, it still has to submit to scrutiny through rigorous and controlled phase III trials before it can be established as a fact.

Lung cancer surgery seems almost without any basis in RCTs. The few trials that exist compare radical to conservative treatment and generally reveal no differences. But one seeks in vain for rigorous trials comparing surgery to no surgery. Beliefs about the efficacy of **surgery** are not based on the rigorous testing of carefully drawn hypotheses, but rather on broad assumptions about the biology of cancer that are implicitly shared by doctors and patients alike. In fact, they form part of the fabric of the culture. Such widespread agreement does not make these ideas true. Indeed, critical steps in the argument are often missing. However, this general agreement on, for example, the necessity for prompt treatment of early-stage tumors makes the performance of rigorous clinical trials difficult: if a great majority believe in the effectiveness of a treatment then, naturally, few patients will be willing to forego such treatment for the sake of an experiment. In addition, most such trials would be indignantly rejected as unethical by Institutional Review Boards (IRBs).

Even today, the spoken or unspoken rationale for surgery (and radiation therapy) harks back to an earlier era, in which it was assumed that cancer was a local-regional disease rather than fundamentally a systemic one. Its justification is primarily based on the presentation of a doctor's experiences in the format of retrospectively analyzed case series. There is often a naïve assumption that figures attained through such means can be meaningfully compared with other series or historical data. In some cases, even a single anecdote (as was the case with malignant melanoma) has set the treatment course around the world, for many decades (49).

As to **radiation therapy**, the best evidence is that it has no beneficial effect on survival. Justification for the entire concept suffered a major blow in 1998 when the multicenter European "PORT group" published a meta-analysis in the *Lancet* showing that radiation was not only ineffective in late stages but actually lead to decreased survival in stage I and II patients (60).

Whether this careful study will have a long-term effect on radiotherapeutic practice is not certain. Some radiologists believe that the negative results demonstrated in this summation of clinical trials were the consequence of the outdated methods and equipment used in earlier trials. With modern methods, they say, radiation will be effective. This is another unproved hypothesis. At its worst, this sort of argument makes a dogma out of radiation's efficacy and does not allow for its negation (falsification).

The modern era of chemotherapy arose contemporaneously with the randomized controlled trials, and the centrality of the "gold standard" RCT is part of the ethos of medical oncology. In general, one finds a more sophisticated argument for the value of chemotherapy than for the other two treatments. However, it is deplorable that clinical trials in the last decade often terminate at phase II, and rarely involve placebo-controlled, blinded and/or randomized phase III trials (51).

In the past, however, chemotherapy for NSCLC (especially in conjunction with radiation therapy) was studied through numerous phase II and even phase III clinical trials. Cisplatin-containing chemotherapy does appear to yield a small survival advantage in some stages of the disease. In stage III, for instance, the survival advantage of neoadjuvant chemotherapy, or combined chemoradiotherapy, has at times seemed significant. The overall advantage appears to be about two months of increased survival. (The extent of benefit is colored by which clinical trials one consults.) One must weigh those possible benefits against the considerable toxicity, anxiety, and costs of the treatment itself.

There is a serious need to assess the **placebo and nocebo effects** in standard RCTs that compare chemotherapy (or chemoradiotherapy) with "best supportive care." Providing best supportive care, from the patient's point of view, may be interpreted as a death sentence; conversely, the mere fact of receiving any aggressive treatment may be a profound source of hope. It is known that general well-being and psychological mood correlate with survival in NSCLC. It is also known that psychological interventions can have a profound effect on survival in other kinds of cancer. (NSCLC has not been studied in this regard.) Cancer is more than a physiological phenomenon. The psychological and social dimensions must always been considered in any estimation of treatment efficacy.

In addition, many nonscientific factors also interfere with a dispassionate view of the topic. In most parts of the world, cancer is still "the dreaded disease" (58). Everyone involved in its treatment wants to believe that the time-honored conventional treatments are both effective and reasonably safe. This understandable wish may, however, undermine one's ability to reach sober conclusions regarding the actual effectiveness of these treatments.

One cannot help noticing that researching and treating cancer also provides a livelihood to tens of thousands of medical workers around the globe. In 1999, the average annual income of US oncologists in private practice was US$ 253 000. The *Journal of the National Cancer Institute* (JNCI) commented that "private-practice oncologists typically derive two-thirds of their income from selling chemotherapy," which the *JNCI* characterized as a "chemotherapy concession" (64). The financial interests of the professions involved in the treatment of cancer may militate against any radical reassessments of the effectiveness of established treatments.

Comparisons with CAM

One often hears the argument that complementary and alternative medicine (CAM) are marginalized because its practitioners fail to prove the value of their proposed treatments through RCTs. While clearly there is a great need for high quality RCTs in the CAM field, this assessment is not fair or accurate. A Medline search specifying articles on cancer, that was limited to both "randomized controlled trials" and "complementary medicine," returned a total of 3708 items (accessed 27 May 2005). Even if highly inflated, this shows that RCTs *do* exist in the CAM field; their number and quality are increasing with time.

But the charge is also misleading because it implies that the three conventional methods of surgery, radiotherapy, and chemotherapy are themselves fully proved through positive RCTs. As has been shown, such RCTs are rare or actually provide negative results for many of the treatments that are considered fully "proved."

What one urgently needs in order to make meaningful comparisons of conventional and CAM treatments is a "level playing field," a single standard whereby all potential therapies can be judged. *The need to perform RCTs is urgent for cancer surgery, radiation therapy, and chemotherapy, even when there is no legal requirement to do so.* Regardless of their dominant socioeconomic position, treatments that have not been tested through rigorous trials should be labeled as "unproved" or "experimental." Treatments that have consistently failed to show significant benefit in RCTs should be labeled as "ineffective." They should not be routinely compensated for by government or private insurance companies, unless similarly "unproved" treatments (such as those employed in CAM) are also paid for. Authorities responsible for public information should not anoint such treatments with designations such as "proved," "effective," "orthodox," etc., when clearly they have not been proved effective or reasonably safe by the highest standards of scientific medicine.

The emergence of the **randomized controlled trial (RCT)** was the signal event in the evolution of clinical testing. The RCT is not without practical and ethical difficulties. But although alternative methods of evaluation may eventually emerge, the RCT at the present time provides a level of proof that is unavailable through any other method. When judged by the high standards of the RCT, there is little in the conventional treatment of non-small cell lung cancer that stands up to intense scrutiny.

■ References

1. Aaron HJ, Gelband H (eds): Committee on Routine Patient Care Costs in: Clinical Trials for Medicare Beneficiaries, Extending Medicare Reimbursement in Clinical Trials. Institute of Medicine, National Academy of Sciences. 2000. Available at: www.nap.edu/openbook/0309068886/html/15.html.
2. Ackerman LA, del Regato JA: Cancer: Diagnosis, Treatment and Prognosis. St. Louis: Mosby; 1947.
3. Ackerman LA, del Regato JA: Cancer: Diagnosis, Treatment and Prognosis. St. Louis: Mosby; 1947: p. 461.
4. American Cancer Society, Cancer Facts and Figures. Atlanta, GA: ACS. 2004.
5. Bull JP: The historical development of clinical therapeutic trials. J Chronic Dis. 1959; 10:218–248.
6. Byock I: Completing the continuum of cancer care: integrating life-prolongation and palliation. CA, Cancer J Clin. 2000; 50:123–132.
7. Carney DN, Hansen HH: Non-small-cell lung cancer–stalemate or progress? N Engl J Med. 2000; 343:1261–1262.
8. Churchill ED, Sweet RH, Sautter L, et al.: The surgical management of carcinoma of the lung. J Thorac Surg. 1950; 20:349–365.
9. Cochrane Library Controlled Trials Register. 1999. (Database)
10. Cooper JD, Pearson G, Todd, TR, et al.: Radiotherapy alone for patients with operable carcinoma of the lung. Chest. 1985; 87:289–292.
11. Cullen MH, Billingham LJ, Woodroffe CM, et al.: Mitomycin, ifosfamide, and cisplatin in unresectable non-small-cell lung cancer: effects on survival and quality of life. J Clin Oncol. 1999; 17:3188.
12. Daniel 1:11–14. The Bible–The Contemporary English Version. Nashville: Thomas Nelson; 1999.
13. DeVita VJ, Helman S, Rosenberg SA, et al. (eds): Cancer: Principles and Practice of Oncology. 6th edn Philadelphia: Lippincott; 2001:925–1018.
14. Dillman RO, Herndon J, Seagren SL, et al.: Improved survival of stage III non-small-cell lung cancer: seven-year follow-up of Cancer and Leukemia Group B (CALGB) 8433 trial. J Natl Cancer Inst. 1996; 88: 1210–1215.
15. Doll R: Clinical trials: Retrospect and prospect. Stat Med. 1982; 1:337–344.
16. Dosoretz DE, Katin MJ, Blitzer PH, et al.: Radiation therapy in the management of medically inoperable carcinoma of the lung: results and implications for future treatment strategies. Int J Radiat Oncol Biol Phys. 1992; 24:3–9.
17. Evans RA: The Cancer Breakthrough You've Never Heard Of. Houston: Texas Cancer Center. 2001.
18. Fajardo LF et al.: Radiation Pathology. Oxford: Oxford University Press. 2001.
19. Fawzy F, Canada AL, Fawzy NW, et al.: Malignant melanoma: effects of an early structured psychiatric intervention, coping, and affective state on recurrence and survival 6 years later. Arch Gen Psychiat. 1993; 50:681–689.
20. Fossella FV et al.: Randomized phase III trial of docetaxel versus vinorelbine or ifosfamide in patients with advanced non-small-cell lung cancer previously treated with platinum-containing chemotherapy regimens. The TAX 320 Non-Small Cell Lung Cancer Study Group. J Clin Oncol. 2000; 18: 2354–2362.
21. Freund L: Demonstration eines mit Röntgenstrahlen behandelten Falles von Naevus pigmentosus pilosus. Wien. Klin Wschr. 1897; 10:73–74.
22. Freund L: Elements of General Radio-Therapy for Practitioners. (Translation by Lancashire GH). With an epilog by Clarence Wright, "Notes on Instrumentation." London: Rebman Ltd; 1904.
23. Gauden S, Ramsay J, Tripcony L, et al.: The curative treatment by radiotherapy alone of stage I non-small-cell carcinoma of the lung. Chest. 1995; 108:1278–1282.
24. Ginsberg RJ, Rubinstein LV: Randomized trial of lobectomy versus limited resection for T1 N0 non-small-cell lung cancer. Ann Thorac Surg. 1995; 60:615–623.
25. Greer S, Morris T, Pettingale KW, et al.: Psychological response to breast cancer: effect on outcome. Lancet. 1979; 2(8146):785–787.
26. Hahn RA: The nocebo phenomenon: concept, evidence, and implications for public health. Prev Med. 1997; 26:607 611.
27. Halsted WS: The results of radical operation for the cure of cancer of the breast. Ann Surg. 1907; 46:1.
28. Hansen HH: Advanced non-small-cell lung cancer: to treat or not to treat? J Clin Oncol. 1987; 5:1711–1712.
29. Harvey JC, Beattie EJ (eds): Cancer Surgery. Philadelphia: Saunders; 1996: p. 234.
30. Hill AB: Principles of Medical Statistics. London: The Lancet Limited; 1937.
31. Holland JC: Lung cancer. In: Holland JC, Howland JH, (eds): Handbook of Psychooncology. New York: Oxford University Press; 1990: p. 185.
32. http://www.calgb.org/Public/about/about.html
33. Jeremic B, Shibamoto Y, Acimovic L, et al.: Hyperfractionated radiation therapy with or without concurrent low-dose daily carboplatin/etoposide for stage III non-small-cell lung cancer: a randomized study. J Clin Oncol. 1996; 14:1065.
34. Jeremic B et al.: Randomized trial of hyperfractionated radiation therapy with or without concurrent

chemotherapy for stage III non-small-cell lung cancer. J Clin Oncol. 1995; 13:452–458.

35. Johnson J, Kirkby CK, Blakemore WS, et al.: Should we insist on "radical pneumonectomy" as a routine procedure in the treatment of carcinoma of the lung? J Thorac Surgery. 1958; 36:309–315.

36. Kaasa S et al.: Prognostic factors for patients with inoperable non-small cell lung cancer, limited disease. The importance of patients' subjective experience of disease and psychosocial well-being. Radiother Oncol. 1989; 15:235–242.

37. Kaasa S, Mastekaasa A: Psychosocial well-being of patients with inoperable non-small cell lung cancer. The importance of treatment- and disease-related factors. Acta Oncol. 1988; 27:829–835.

38. Keller SM et al.: A randomized trial of postoperative adjuvant therapy in patients with completely resected stage II or IIIA non-small-cell lung cancer. Eastern Cooperative Oncology Group. N Engl J Med. 2000; 343:1217–1222.

40. Komaki R et al.: Characteristics of long-term survivors after treatment for inoperable carcinoma of the lung. Am J Clin Oncol. 1985; 8:362–370.

41. LeChevalier T et al.: Significant effect of adjuvant chemotherapy on survival in locally advanced non-small-cell lung carcinoma. J Natl Cancer Inst. 1992; 84:58.

42. Mackillop WJ, Palmer MJ, O'Sullivan B, et al.: The use of expert surrogates to evaluate clinical trials in non-small-cell lung cancer. Br J Cancer. 1986; 54:661–667.

43. Martini N, Ginsberg RJ: Treatment of stage I and II disease. In: Aisner J, et al. (eds) Comprehensive Textbook of Thoracic Oncology. Baltimore: Williams and Wilkins; 1996:339–350.

44. Matthews JR: Quantification and the Quest for Medical Certainty. Princeton: Princeton University Press; 1995: p.18.

45. Matthews JR: Quantification and the Quest for Medical Certainty. Princeton: Princeton University Press; 1995: p. 16.

46. Mattson K, Holsti LR, Holsti P, et al.: Inoperable non-small-cell lung cancer: radiation with or without chemotherapy. Eur J Cancer Clin Oncol. 1988; 24:477–482.

47. McKenna RJ, Murphy FP: Cancer Surgery, Philadelphia: Lippincott. 1994.

48. Meinert CL: Clinical Trials: Design, Conduct, and Analysis. Oxford: Oxford University Press. 1986.

49. Moffat FL, Ketcham AS: In: McKenna RJ, Murphy FP (eds): Cancer Surgery, Philadelphia: Lippincott. 1994; p. 20.

50. Morton RF et al.: Thoracic radiation therapy alone compared with combined chemoradiotherapy for locally advanced unresectable non-small-cell lung cancer: a randomized phase III trial. Ann Intern Med. 1991; 115:681–686.

51. Moss RW: The grand illusion of chemotherapy. Dtsch Z Onkol. 2001; 33:15–18.

52. For a discussion of such errors, see: Moss RW: Questioning Chemotherapy. 2nd ed. Brooklyn: Equinox; 2000.

53. Mould RF: A century of X-rays and radioactivity in medicine. Bristol: Institute of Physics, 1993; p. 20.

54. Niiranen A et al.: Adjuvant chemotherapy after radical surgery for non-small-cell lung cancer: a randomized study. J Clin Oncol. 1992; 10:1927–1932.

55. Non-Small-Cell Lung Cancer Collaborative Group. Chemotherapy in non-small-cell lung cancer: a meta-analysis using updated data on individual patients from 52 randomised clinical trials. BMJ. 1995; 311:899–909.

56. Chemotherapy in non-small cell lung cancer: a meta-analysis using updated data on individual patients from 52 randomised clinical trials. Non-small Cell Lung Cancer Collaborative Group. BMJ. 1995; 311: 899–909.

57. Noordijk EM et al.: Radiotherapy as an alternative to surgery in elderly patients with resectable lung cancer. Radiotherapy and Oncology. 1988; 13: 83–89.

58. Patterson JT: The Dread Disease. Cambridge, MA: Harvard University Press; 1987; p. 51.

59. Popper K: The Logic of Scientific Discovery. London: Hutchinson; 1959. (Popper's theory)

60. PORT Meta-analysis Trialists Group: Postoperative radiotherapy in non-small-cell lung cancer: systematic review and meta-analysis of individual patient data from nine randomised controlled trials. Lancet. 1998; 352:257–263.

61. Porter AT: The role of radiotherapy as we approach the next millennium. World Health Organization (WHO). http://www.who.int/ncd/cancer/publications/abstracts/abs9810.

62. Ranson M et al.: Randomized trial of paclitaxel plus supportive care versus supportive care for patients with advanced non-small-cell lung cancer. J Natl Cancer Inst. 2000; 92:1074–1080.

63. Reid DD: Statistics in clinical research. Ann NY Acad Sci. 1950; 52:931–934.

64. Reynolds T: Are physician-scientists a vanishing breed? J Natl Cancer Inst. 2001; 93:490–491.

65. Richardson JL, Shelton DR, Krailo M, et al.: The effect of compliance with treatment on survival among patients with hematologic malignancies. J Clin Oncol. 1990; 14:1128–1135.

66. Rienhoff WF Jr.: Surgical treatment of malignant tumors of the lung. In: Pack GT, Livingston EM (eds). Treatment of Cancer and Allied Diseases. New York: Paul B. Hoeber, Inc; 1940: p. 865.

67. Rosell R et al.: A randomized trial comparing preoperative chemotherapy plus surgery with surgery alone in patients with non-small-cell lung cancer. N Engl J Med. 1994; 330:153–158.

68. Roth JA et al.: A randomized trial comparing perioperative chemotherapy and surgery with surgery alone in resectable stage IIIA non-small-cell lung cancer. J Natl Cancer Inst. 1994; 86:673–80.

68a. RT image. Vol 18, no. 16, 2005. http://www.rt-image.com

69. Rusch VW, Gincherman Y: Surgical management of stage IIIA non-small-cell lung cancer. In: Aisner J, Perry MC, Green MR, et al. (eds): Comprehensive Textbook of Thoracic Oncology. Baltimore: Williams and Wilkins; 1996: p. 351.

70. Sause WT et al.: Radiation Therapy Oncology Group (RTOG) 88–08 and Eastern Cooperative Oncology Group (ECOG) 4588: preliminary results of a phase III trial in regionally advanced, unresectable non-small-cell lung cancer. J Natl Cancer Inst. 1995; 87:198–205.

71. Sekido Y et al.: Cancer of the lung. In: DeVita VJ, Helman S, Rosenberg SA (eds): Cancer: Principles and Practice of Oncology. 6th edn Philadelphia: Lippincott; 2001: pp. 917–1018.

72. Shepherd FA, Dancey J, Ramlau R, et al.: Prospective randomized trial of docetaxel versus best supportive care in patients with non-small-cell lung cancer previously treated with platinum-based chemotherapy. J Clin Oncol. 2000; 18:2095–2103.

73. Shepherd FA, Johnson MR, Payne D, et al.: Randomized study of chemotherapy and surgery versus radiotherapy for stage IIIA non-small-cell lung cancer: a National Cancer Institute of Canada Clinical Trials Group Study. Br J Cancer. 1998; 78:683–685.

74. Shields T, Higgens GA: Minimal pulmonary resection in the treatment of carcinoma of the lung. Arch Surg. 1974; 108:420–422.

75. Simes RJ: Risk–benefit relationship in cancer clinical trials: the ECOG experience in non-small-cell lung cancer. J Clin Oncol. 1985; 3:462–472.

76. Smart J, Hilton G: Radiotherapy of cancer of the lung. Results in a selected group of cases. Lancet. 1956; 270:880–881.

77. Spiegel D et al.: Effect of psychosocial treatment on survival of patients with metastatic breast cancer. Lancet. 1989; 2:888–891.

78. Stanford Encyclopedia of Philosophy. http://plato.stanford.edu/entries/popper/#Pred

79. Voigt J, Ärztlicher Verein Hamburg. Hamburg, Germany; Febr 3, 1896.

80. Watson M, Haviland JS, Greer S, et al.: Influence of psychological response on survival in breast cancer: a population-based cohort study. Lancet. 1999; 354:1331–1336.

81. Weaver JE III: A brief chronology of radiation and protection. 1994–1995. http://www.physics.isu.edu/radinf/chrono.htm#top.

82. Weisenburger TH, Holmes EC, Gail M, et al.: Effects of postoperative mediastinal radiation on completely resected stage II and stage III epidermoid cancer of the lung. N Eng J Med. 1986; 315:1377–1381.

83. Whipple AO et al.: Treatment of carcinoma of the ampulla of Vater. Ann Surg. 1935; 102:763–779.

84. WHO. International Classification of Disease. http://www.depdb.iarc.fr/who/who.htm.

85. Witts LJ: Introduction to Medical Surveys and Clinical Trials, 2nd edn LJ Witts (ed.). London: Oxford University Press; 1964.

86. Zabora J, Brintzenhofe Zoc K, Curbow B, et al.: The prevalence of psychological distress by cancer site. Psychooncology. 2001; 10:19–28.

87. Coghill, Kim. ImClone's Erbitux receives long-awaited FDA approval. BioWorld Online. Retrieved 19 February 2004 from: http://www.bioworld.com/servlct/com.accumedia.web.Dispatcher?next=bioWorldHeadlines_article&forceid=32123

88. Abelson, Reed. Drug sales bring huge profits, and scrutiny to cancer doctors. New York Times. January 26, 2003, p. A1.

89. Gellene, Denise. New cancer drugs are driving up cost of care. Los Angeles Times, May 14, 2005.

90. Roth JA, et al. Long-term follow-up of patients enrolled in a randomized trial comparing perioperative chemotherapy and surgery with surgery alone in resectable stage IIIA non-small-cell lung cancer. Lung Cancer. 1998; 21:1–6.

91. Herbst RS, et al. Gefitinib in combination with paclitaxel and carboplatin in advanced non-small-cell lung cancer: a phase III trial-INTACT 2. J Clin Oncol. 2004; 22:785–794.

92. Giaccone G, et al. Gefitinib in combination with gemcitabine and cisplatin in advanced non-small-cell lung cancer: a phase III trial–INTACT 1. J Clin Oncol. 2004; 22:777–784.

▬ 3 Tumor Immunology

Volker Schirrmacher

▬ Introduction

Tumor immunology deals with the interaction between the immune system and cancer. Its origins can be traced back to Paul Ehrlich at the beginning of the twentieth century. The field developed rather slowly at the beginning, but this changed with the advent of newer technologies. In order to establish tumor cell lineages, methods for culturing cells needed to be established. When transplanting tumors out of mice or rats, they had to descend from inbred lineages to avoid genetic differences that may have had an effect on experimental outcomes. Quantitative studies of antitumor immune reactions in vitro depended on new techniques for tissue culture as well as on the presence of certain growth factors and cytokines.

Further advances were made when monoclonal antibodies became available, which permitted discrimination of cells within the immune system. With the help of flow cytometry and cell sorting these cells could then ultimately be separated.

After the first inbred mouse lineages became available in the 1940s and 1950s, findings for tumor-specific immune reactions against chemically induced transplantation tumors were obtained (14). First, experimental immune therapy studies demonstrated effects against metastases in rat tumor models by vaccination in the autonomous host (23). The existence of so-called **tumor-associated transplantation antigens** (TATA) on chemically induced tumors was shown, but it took sometime before their nature as well as the nature of TATA-detecting receptors on T lymphocytes also became known.

The development of **monoclonal antibodies** using hybridoma technology at first resulted in heightened expectations. It was hoped that the tumor-specific antibodies (or "magic bullets") postulated by Paul Ehrlich could now be discovered. Ever since the 1980s, much effort has been channeled into the identification of tumor-specific antigens using monoclonal antibodies. While some of the antibodies thereby obtained improved the understanding and insight into tumor diagnosis, disappointment was great when it was realized that these isolated tumor-reactive monoclonal antibodies were not really tumor specific. Despite the help of monoclonal antibodies, the nature of TATAs found on chemically induced tumors was not discovered fully.

▬ Identifiable Tumor Antigens

Since it became known that the tumor-transplant rejection process was an immune reaction caused by T cells, T-cell immunology became the focus of subsequent studies. It took many decades of research to fully understand the nature of the antigen-specific **T-cell receptor** (TCR) as well as that of antigens that are recognized by TCRs found, for example, on virus-infected cells or tumor cells. This field of specific anti-tumor T-cell immunology only began when autologous tumor antigens, induced by a combination of cell immunology and genetic methods, were identified.

It was then noticed that TCRs recognize bits of intracellular proteins made up of linear peptides of nine to 15 amino acids on the surface of target cells. The recognition requires the binding of peptide and of so-called major histocompatibility complex (MHC) molecules to the TCR. With the aid of such proteins intracellular peptides are transported to the surface of the cell, where they are then recognized by TCRs.

In the 1990s the first tumor antigens on human tumors were identified (5, 20). These, too, are peptides presented by human MHC molecules (HLA) on the surface of tumor cells for recognition by receptors on tumor-specific cytotoxic T lymphocytes (CTL). Recently an antibody-based method was added that enables identification of new human tumor antigens through serological recombinant expression cloning (SEREX). Using specific CTL as well as the SEREX method, multiple human tumor antigens were discovered on various types of tumors and have been characterized in the last few years.

Studies using animal models showed that the immune system has the ability to ward off tumor cells and that T lymphocytes play a major role in this rejection reaction. With the help of adoptive transfer studies and analysis of those tumor variants that escaped a rejection reaction, the vital role of CTL in vivo was demonstrated. In these immune-escape variants the CTL epitope was lost.

In cancer patients tumor-specific CTL can be activated through in-vitro stimulation of their lymphocytes. The study of melanoma variants, resistant to some but not all of such CTL clones, showed that melanomas were able to express different tumor antigens that can be distinguished by CD8+ T cells. Many such antigens have been characterized and identified at the molecular level (5, 20). The mechanism of expression has also been studied to determine tumor specificity.

There are five main categories of tumor antigens as defined by **CD8+ CTL**:
1. common tumor-associated antigens
2. differentiation antigens
3. antigens caused through mutation
4. overexpressed antigens
5. viral antigens.

The efficiency of a tumor rejection reaction probably depends on the individuality of TATA expression on the tumor cells as well as the absence of mechanisms of tolerance (8). Since CD8+ CTL have been shown to directly lyse tumor cells or destroy even large parts of a tumor in vivo, much effort was directed to the study of immune therapy of cancer using CD8+ CTL. Clinical vaccination trials with tumor antigens defined by CD8+ CTL have given clues as to therapeutic effects, even though the impact of immune response was weak and only temporary.

There are two reasons why interest has shifted to include also tumor antigens recognized through MHC class II-restricted **CD4+ T cells**: primarily, CD4+ T cells are capable of identifying tumor antigens (11) that are distinct from the antigens defined by CD8+ T cells, and additionally, there are known synergistic effects between CD4+ and CD8+ immune cells in tumor regression.

Identification of antigens that stimulate CD4+ T helper cells and attempts to integrate these into an antitumor immune reaction could help to improve immune-therapeutic approaches in the future.

▬ Effector Cells and Mechanisms of Antitumor Immunity

T effector cells play a central role in almost all adaptive immune responses. Activation of mature naïve T cells that have never had antigen contact through professional antigen-presenting cells is the decisive initial step in immune response. A complex series of stimulatory effects results in T-cell activation. Costimulatory molecules play an important role in this process, in which the balance between negative and positive signals determines immune response and tolerance. Antigen-specific triggering, via a **TCR complex** or antibodies against CD3 molecules associated with the TCR, delivers signal 1 of activation (Fig. 3.**1**).

When CD28 molecules are triggered on T cells at the same time, this leads to signal 2 and naïve T cells can be activated. Cytotoxic T cells, (CTL) can effectively be activated by means of combined stimulation with anti-CD3 and anti-CD28 molecules and can expand in culture with the use of cytokines and growth factors. Following direct costimulation of CD8+ T cells through melanoma cells transfected with CD28 ligand (B7), tumor rejection was observed in the animal model (24).

Besides the already mentioned T lymphocytes there are a number of other cells of the immune system that contribute to natural immunity and also display cytotoxic activity against tumor cells. They include the natural killer cells (NK cells) (Fig. 3.**1**), activated macrophages/monocytes, and granulocytes, as well as dendritic cells (DCs). It is generally true that such cells need to be triggered by molecules before they exert cytotoxic effects.

Trigger molecules of cells in the natural immune system include, for example, receptors for the constant region of immunoglobulins, so-called **Fc receptors** (1) (Table 3.**1**), as well as the recently discovered toll-like receptors (TLRs) (13).

Not all of the Fc receptors belong to the activating Fc receptors. Some transmit inhibitory signals.

These receptors are activated physiologically via the constant regions of antibody molecules, which themselves bind to specific cellular targets, thereby generating immune complexes. Normally these are IgG antibodies that serve as a binding link between natural and specifically acquired (adaptive) immunity in antibody-dependent cell-mediated cytotoxicity (ADCC) mechanism. In the ADCC mechanism, effector cells of the natural system (for example NK cells or monocytes or macrophages) are bound through antibody bridges to their specific tumor targets and thereby activated to become cytotoxic.

Antibodies can be found in the serum of patients with cancer; they help identify new tumor antigens using SEREX (21). Some of these antibodies that stem from antigen-stimulated B lymphocytes, or plasma cells, may result in antitumor effects through ADCC mechanisms. Other antibodies, especially of the IgM type, can activate components of the complement system and lead to tumor lysis when directed against tumor cells. Some antibodies can directly activate an **apoptosis** program, which also leads to tumor lysis. It is along these lines that the Fas or Apo receptor molecules, which induce cell apoptosis, were discovered (25).

Even cytotoxic cells can lyse tumor cells via Fas-receptor triggering. This is accomplished via expression of the Fas ligand, not through antibodies.

Perforin, which is stored in cytotoxic granules inside killer cells, is another important transmitter of cytotoxic mechanism in these cells. Upon contact with the tumor cell the killer cell releases perforin, which causes cylindrical holes in the membrane of the tumor cell, similar to those caused by the complement system. The killer cell can release additional toxic mediators, such as granzyme, and thereby damage the target cell (25).

▬ Recognition of Danger Signals by Toll-Like Receptors and DC Activation

During the last few years it has become consistently more evident that the cells of the natural immune system also play an important part in the adaptive immune response. The fundamental need for dendritic cells for the initiation of T-cell immune responses is indisputable (9). Many cells of natural immunity are equipped with receptors on their surfaces for recognition of viral and bacterial

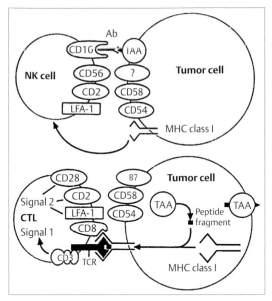

Fig. 3.**1** Schematic depiction of relevant surface structures of human natural killer (NK) cells and cytotoxic T lymphocytes (CTLs) that are involved in tumor-cell binding and possibly in signal transfer. Via their Fc receptor (CD16), NK cells can bind the Fc fragments of antibodies (Ab) that recognize tumor-associated antigens (TAA) and lead to antibody-dependent cell-mediated cytotoxicity. NK cells can also be activated via interactions between the adhesion molecules CD2, LFA-1, and CD56 and their respective ligands on the tumor cell surface. Expression of MHC class I antigens on tumor cells can result in resistance versus NK-cell lysis. CTLs express an antigen-specific T-cell receptor (TCR) that recognizes TAA-peptide fragments in association with MHC class I molecules. CD3 and other accessory molecules play a role in the transduction of activating signals via the TCR (signal 1).

patterns that can be interpreted as danger signals (16, 17). These TLRs, of which nine are known to date, recognize, for example, the CpG sequences of bacterial DNA, whereby a cascade of cytokines is released for fighting off the bacteria (13). Lipopolysaccharides (LPS) in the bacterial cell wall are also

Table 3.1 Activation of effector cells through antibodies against Fc receptors		
Fc receptor	**Activating antibody**	**Type of cell**
FcγRIIIa	Anti-CD16	NK cells, monocytes/macrophages
FcγRI	Anti-CD64	Monocytes/macrophages, granulocytes
FcαRII	Anti-CD89	Dendritic cells, monocytes/macrophages, granulocytes

recognized via TLRs. In the event of a viral infection, double-stranded RNA has become a known danger signal that will lead to interferon-α production via stimulation of the TLR3 receptor on DCs.

In connection with the death of tumor cells, necrosis and tissue destruction are probably essential to the activation of DCs (16). Apoptotic and necrotic cells are ingested and processed by macrophages and DCs. It has not yet been fully established which co-factors play a vital role here and whether or not there is an induction of tolerance or activation of immunity following apoptosis (9, 16, 17). Important signals for distinction between tolerance induction and activation seem to depend on cytokines, but also on stress factors that appear upon the death of a cell and may signify danger (4, 16). Activation of certain heat-shock proteins (HSPs) are evidently interpreted by DCs as a danger signal. A receptor (CD91) has been found on DCs for various HSPs. HSP96 molecules of tumor cells, along with their associated peptides, are thus thought to be especially immunogenic (3). Additionally, activated dendritic cells express CD40 molecules that are recognized in turn by CD40 ligands on the surface of activated T helper cells, leading to reciprocal stimulation between these two cell types. This interaction enables a so-called licensing signal for CD8 precursors of cytotoxic T cells that allows them to express their cytotoxic potential.

These new relationships between recognition of dangerous signals by cells of the natural immune system and the effect on the adaptive immune responses are very important for the development of effective immune therapy strategies (Fig. 3.2). For many years bacterial and viral structures have been added to vaccines as adjuvants (13). It is now within reach, that those patterns that are recognized by toll-like receptors can be tailored along with certain tumor antigens and combined with these to produce highly potent vaccines (Fig. 3.2).

Concomitant Immunity, Generation of Memory Cells, and Tumor Immune Escape

As previously mentioned, dendritic cells play a vital role in T-cell-mediated immune responses. Dendritic cells, being professional antigen-presenting cells of the host's immune system, can take up antigens in proximity to tumors and degrade these over the MHC class II and MHC class I processing pathways. This leads to expression of MHC class I-associated and MHC class II-associated tumor-specific peptides on the surface of DCs. CD4+ as well as CD8+ T lymphocytes found in neighboring draining lymph nodes are specifically sensitized (primed) by such antigen-presenting DCs.

These complex processes were observed in vivo with transplantation tumors in animal models as well as more recently in cancer patients. The growth and extension of a tumor should not be misinterpreted from the outset. The phenomenon of **"concomitant immunity,"** the **concurrence of tumor and antitumor immunity**, has demonstrated that immunity created in tumor-transplanted mice is sufficient to prevent future cancerous growth in another area after transfer of a similar dose of tumor cells, albeit without hindering local tumor growth. In-vitro generation of tumor-specific CTL was possible by restimulation of the spleens of such mice, while this was not effective when utilizing splenic cells from nonimmunized animals.

These various observations can be interpreted as follows: in an immune system not immunized by a tumor, the T cell repertoire entails many TCR specificities. Each single one is only represented in a few instances. Thus, it is a rare incidence that a T cell expressing a receptor for a specific tumor-associated antigen (TAA) will encounter such an antigen when transplantation of TAA-expressing tumor cells occurs. As the pool of TAA-specific T cells must first expand vigorously, it takes several days for a specific immune response to develop. If meanwhile, tumor cells are allowed to grow without hindrance, it is conceivable that a tumor will grow in the area of transplantation, while partial tumor-specific immunity can coexist in other areas.

In such a situation, in which the tumor-carrying organism contains primed antitumor T cells, additional steps are required to activate the previously sensitized T cells into antitumor effector cells. This can occur either ex vivo through stimulation in culture or through early antitumor vaccination attempts (Fig. 3.2). Activated T cells can lyse tumor cells directly as cytotoxic cells, or they can release cytokines that will unfold antitumor activities, or even stimulate other cells to do the same.

Sensitized T cells that are present in immune competent animals with tumor growth are referred to as **memory cells.** They are present even long after the initial antigen contact and can react much faster upon renewed contact with the antigen, providing the basis for a specific secondary response (12). Such memory cells secrete interferon-γ after renewed contact with the antigen, and this can be detected by modern ELISA and ELISPOT tests. With the aid of such tests it has become possible to detect tumor-reactive memory cells in the bone marrow of the majority of women operated on for primary breast cancer (6). Following restimulation in culture for a short amount of time they were capable of producing interferon-γ. After more prolonged stimulation, these cells mature to cytotoxic T cells. The patient's own dendritic cells pulsed with tumor cell lysates are able to reacti-

vate such memory cells derived from bone marrow.

After the transfer of such cells (5×10^6 reactivated T cells + 1×10^6 pulsed dendritic cells) in immunocompetent NOD/SCID (NonObese Diabetes/Severe Combined Immunodeficiency Disease) mice that had previously received a piece of a freshly operated tumor from a breast cancer patient as a transplant, a complete regression of tumor was observed.

Such findings were also observed in a completely autologous system, in which tumor and immune cells were derived from the same patient. The prerequisite for this was that the T cells were taken from the bone marrow. It is possible that in case of a therapeutic effect not only tumor-specific

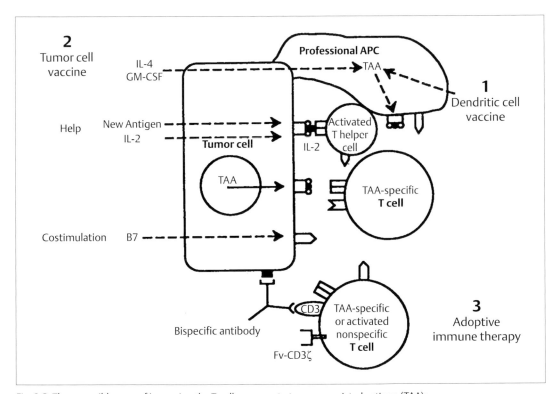

Fig. 3.**2** Three possibly ways of increasing the T-cell response to tumor-associated antigen (TAA):

1. Vaccination with dendritic cells: cultivation of dendritic cells (DCs) in GM-CSF and IL-4, introduction of TAA into professional antigen-presenting cells (APC), processing of TAA, and cross-presentation of MHC–peptides on the surface of this cell.

2. Tumor vaccination: tumor-cell modification through the introduction of new helper cell determinantes, or of cytokine genes (e. g., IL-2), or of costimulatory molecules (e. g., B7).

3. Adoptive immune therapy: Transfer of TAA-specific T cells, or of activated nonspecific T cells, which are bound to the tumor cell via bispecific antibodies or via TAA-binding transfected T-cell receptors (F-CD3) (re-targeting).

T memory cells but also professional antigen-presenting cells play a role in vivo, as cognitive interactions between antigen-specific T cells and antigen-presenting dendritic cells result in multiple reciprocal reactions in which they stimulate one another.

It is becoming more and more evident that the immune system not only reacts to the tumor, but that the tumor also reacts to the immune system. Through the existence of tumor variants and also by the pressure exerted by immune selection, tumor escape variants can develop that are no longer recognized by immune T cells. Often HLA molecules are deregulated or mutant forms develop that are defective during antigen processing (7, 15, 19). The tumor can suppress the immune system by secretion of factors that interfere with the functioning of T cells and DCs. Tumors are able to utilize components of the immune system, such as cytokines, to enhance their growth potential, if they express certain receptors (2). Prehn referred already in 1957 to the possibility of immune stimulation by cancerous growths (18).

▬ Looking Ahead

This short overview demonstrates how tumor immunology has made great strides. Nonetheless, researchers should not put their expectations too high. Even though some basic mechanisms of cellular immune response against tumors have been understood, pressing questions remain unanswered.

In a cancer patient it is difficult to know in advance to what extent the immune system has developed tolerance to tumor antigens, or if it is still sensitive to these antigens, and in how far the immune response can be activated. It is also unclear what characteristics tumor-reactive T cells must possess in order to efficiently ward off a tumor, and how cells gain entry into the cancer and reach this in the first place. Another important question is to find out what is required to sustain a protective immune response over time, and how to maintain an adequate long-term memory.

Generally speaking, it can be said that any immune therapy will achieve the best effect if implemented early on. It is important to activate the immune system of the patient postoperatively in such a way that potentially remaining tumor cells, which are difficult to localize, are hindered in their growth or completely eliminated through specific immune mechanisms. This task is the harder the longer the tumor has existed, the larger it is in size, and the more chance it has had to spread. The biggest adversity to be overcome by any additional form of therapy is that of tumor heterogeneity, i.e., the ability of the tumor cells to change into new variants. One must be prepared for resistance to radiation therapy and chemotherapy as well as mechanisms of immune resistance on the part of the tumor. With the use of gene expression profiling, therapy will become more suited to the individual specificities of the various types of tumors (10). Nevertheless, it is very likely, that given enough time, tumors will always find ways of coming up with new escape variants to evade most types of immune responses. The more aggressive the tumor is, the harder it will be for immune therapeutic measures to effectively hinder its growth.

The following should be noted with reference to immune therapeutic measures:

- they should be broad in range
- they should contain many tumor-specific antigens
- they should possibly offer multiple costimulatory signals
- they should be optimally integrated into the entire concept of a multimodality antitumor therapeutic approach.

Given all of these circumstances, it can be said that, in the future, tumor immunology will provide a vital part in a much improved therapy for cancer.

▬ References

1. Amigorena S.: Fc-receptors and cross-presentation in dendritic cells. J Exp Med. 2002; 195:F1–F3.
2. Balkwill F, Mantovani A: Inflammation and cancer: back to Virchow? Lancet. 2001; 357:539–545.
3. Basu S, Binder RJ, Ramalingam T, Srivastava PK: CD91 is a common receptor for heat shock proteins gp96, hsp90, hsp70 and calreticulin. Immunity. 2001; 14:303–313.
4. Belardelli F, Ferrantini: Cytokines as a link between innate and adaptive antitumor immunity. Trends in Immunology. 2002; 23:201–208.
5. Boon T, Cerottini JC, van den Eynde B, et al.: Tumor antigens recognized by T-lymphocytes. Ann Rev Immunol. 1994; 12:337–366.

6. Feuerer M, Beckhove P, Bai L, et al.: Therapy of human tumors in NOD/SCID mice with patient derived re-activated memory T cells from bone marrow. Nature Medicine. 2001; 7:452–458.

7. Garrido F, Algarra I: MHC antigens and tumor escape from immune surveillance. Adv Cancer Res. 2001; 83:117–158.

8. Gilboa E: The makings of a tumor rejection antigen. Immunity. 1999; 11:263–270.

9. Heath WR, Carbone FR: Cross-presentation, dendritic cells, tolerance and immunity. Ann Rev Immunol. 2001; 19:47–64.

10. Hedenfalk I et al.: Gene-expression profiles in hereditary breast cancer. N Engl J Med. 2001; 344:539–548.

11. Hung K, Hayashi R, Lafond-Walker A, Lowenstein C, Pardoll D, Levitsky H: The central role of CD4+ T cells in the antitumor immune response. J Exp Med. 1998; 188:2357–2368.

12. Kaech SM, Wherry EJ, Ahmed R: Effector and memory T cell differentiation: Implications for vaccine development. Nature Reviews. 2002; 2:251–262.

13. Kaisho T, Akira S: Toll-like receptors as adjuvant receptors. Biochim Biophys Acta. 2002; 1589:1–13.

14. Klein G, Sjoegren HO, Klein E, Hellstroem KE: Demonstration of resistance against methylcholanthrene-induced sarcomas in the primary autochthonous host. Cancer Res. 1960; 20:1561–1572.

15. Marincola FM, Jaffee EM, Hicklin DJ, Ferrone S: Escape of human solid tumors from T-cell recognition: molecular mechanisms and functional significance. Adv Immunol. 2000; 74:81–273.

16. Matzinger P: The danger model: a renewed sense of self. Science. 2002; 296:301–305.

17. Medzhitov R, Janeway CA Jr.: Decoding the patterns of self and nonself by the innate immune system. Science. 2002; 296:298–300.

18. Prehn RT, Main JM: Immunity to methylcholanthrene-induced sarcomas. J Natl Cancer Inst. 1957; 18:769–778.

19. Riker A et al.: Immune selection after antigen-specific immunotherapy of melanoma. Surgery. 1999; 126:112–120.

20. Rosenberg SA: Cancer vaccines based on the identification of genes encoding cancer regression antigens. Immunol. Today. 1994; 18:175–182.

21. Sahin U, Türeci Ö, Pfreundschuh M: Serological identification of human tumor antigens. Current Opinion Immunol. 1997; 9:709–716.

22. Schirrmacher V, Beckhove P, Krüger A, et al.: Effective immune rejection of advanced metastasized cancer. Int J Oncol. 1995; 6:505–521.

23. Takeda T, Kikuchi Y, Yamawaki S, Ueda T, Yoshiki T: Treatment of artificial metastases of methylcholanthrene-induced rat sarcomas by autoimmunization of the autochthonous hosts. Cancer Res. 1968; 28:2149–2154.

24. Townsend SE, Allison JP: Tumor rejection after direct costimulation of CD8 T cells by B7-transfected melanoma cells. Science. 1993; 259:368–370.

25. Tschopp I, Irmler M: Death receptors, apoptosis and cancer. Gann Monograph Cancer Res. 1999; 48: 125–137.

4 Introduction to Medical Biometry
Ulrich Abel

Introduction

Contrary to a commonly held belief, medical biometry does not only pertain to the evaluation of data, but above all, has to do with the methodological aspects of research. These include the planning of trials, their interpretation, and methodological criticism of the study results. In recent years it has increasingly been concerned with meta-analyses of trial outcomes, a necessary component in evidence-based medicine. These tasks have more to do with theoretical reasoning about problems related to medicine than merely with mathematical or statistical procedures.

In this contribution emphasis is placed on questions concerning the methodology of therapeutic research in oncology. A specific focus is given to those aspects that play a role in the evaluation of efficacy of conventional as well as complementary therapies.

The Setting of Therapeutic Research in Oncology

The general epistemological principles that govern medical research also apply to the field of oncology. However, clinical trials in oncology take place in a very special research environment which in turn affects the details of their planning and execution.
- Cancer is a serious, progressive disease that leads to death if left untreated.
- Cancer is a common disease.
- In many instances, the available therapies are of limited efficacy.
- Most of the conventional therapies have many side effects.
- Most of the established therapies are expensive.
- Disease prognosis depends on many factors, especially the initial therapy (operation) and the quality of diagnosis.

Special Features of Research in Cancer Treatment

The circumstances outlined above have a multitude of consequences that characterize the current situation of therapeutic research in oncology:
- **A large number of clinical trials are undertaken.** The total number of trials published to date ranges in the tens of thousands. As can be seen in registries of clinical trials actively recruiting patients is in the order of several thousands. (http://cancertrials.nci.nih.gov, http://controlled-trials.com , www.studien.de).
- **Oncologists often tend to move in a scientific environment and, for the most part, possess a lot of experience with clinical trials.** This is the result of the enormous quantity of studies, many of which are multicenter trials involving numerous oncologists from large clinical centers. Even those oncologists not involved in these studies are required to keep up to date on the latest findings to ensure adequate patient care.
- Oncologists, at least those working in a conventional clinical setting, are mostly well acquainted with the methodological principles of well-designed trials. This simplifies the job for the biostatistical consultant since clinicians with a strong methodological background will more easily accept the–often inconvenient–methodological requirements imposed by a rigorous study design.
- **Drug research is extremely expensive and is dictated by large pharmaceutical companies.** The oncologist W.M. Gallmeier stated in 1994: "In the realm of clinical therapeutic research, industry determines what is done. It is industry that dictates the trends and themes, that chooses who is qualified to cooperate and which clinics are deemed adequate to participate. Questions that are not product-oriented can usually not be financed." (37)
- **Sponsors as well as patients and the public are interested in positive results.** This carries

an increased risk of publication bias or even manipulation of data.

- **One should be skeptical about positive results derived from studies that did not involve careful monitoring and an external center of biometrics.** It has been repeatedly noticed that, among several studies addressing the same question, those involving an external biometrical center produced far less spectacular results than the remaining studies. A rather tragic example in recent years was the treatment of breast cancer with high-dose chemotherapy.

- **The great majority of comprehensive randomized trials yield null results with respect to survival time.** This is simply because there are few true advances in therapy that result in a prolonged survival time. Again, the history of therapy of metastatic breast cancer offers a salient example (1, 25, 26, 36, 50).

- **If there is no firm evidence that a drug extends survival or improves quality of life, approval by regulatory agencies may be given on the basis of antitumor activity (tumor response).** O'Shaughnessy described the politics of the FDA the following way: "The main goal of cancer treatment is the prolongation of life, but the proof that a new drug results in a reduction in tumor growth and an improvement in quality of life in patients can support the approval of a new substance." (62)

- **In oncology there is always the danger of construing dogmas and of reaching epistemological deadlocks.** This danger is present throughout medicine in general, and is not limited to therapy alone, but can be especially pronounced in life-threatening diseases. For a methodological analysis of this phenomenon see reference 6. To put it simply, physicians who are convinced of the efficacy of a certain therapy will not be able or willing to withhold this from their patient, whether their belief is scientifically founded or not. A comparison with nontreated controls can no longer be undertaken, and the belief becomes a dogma.

- **Currently there are numerous widespread interventions in oncology lacking any (sufficient) evaluation.** This holds true for the many untraditional therapeutic approaches in oncology (59, 71, 76, 78), but also, to a lesser extent, for conventional treatment options. Chemotherapy for metastatic ovarian or breast carcinoma was never compared with a no-treatment control. In both cases, it seems impossible to recover the lacking evidence (compare to preceding point).

- **Many patients are prepared to accept considerable side-effects of treatment for even a tiny promise of hope.** Many patients accept serious adverse effects for a little bit of (hypothetical) benefit. Eight percent of patients in a group with operable breast cancer when queried opted for high-dose chemotherapy in the event of metastasis, even assuming that this treatment would extend survival by merely one month (55, 70).

- **In clinical trials, even small effects are of interest.** On the individual level, a small benefit is of interest because of the life-threatening situation. On the population level, small effects may be important because of the large incidence and prevalence of cancer.

- **In many situations, studies are necessarily large but possible (even if expensive).** The necessity follows from the fact that one cannot realistically expect major effects in most instances.

- **Studies can normally only be conducted in large institutions.** Only these are generally able to provide the adequate apparatus and personnel.

- **Conventional nonrandomized studies are of very limited value.** This at least holds true, as we will see, for simplistic historic examples of comparisons in which changes in the prognostic starting position can never be excluded.

- **Blinded studies are almost impossible to conduct.** The attempt to study therapeutic efficacy on quality of life is problematic. Given the characteristic side-effects and routes of administration of most cancer therapies, blinding is often impossible. However, subjective impressions (quality of life ratings) may obviously be biased if the study is not blinded.

- **Clinical trials are rarely designed as equivalence studies.** Of course, studies aimed at showing equivalence (or, at least, non-inferiority) of treatments do exist. This is especially the case when it is clear from the very beginning that the test therapy is not expected to show a distinct advantage with respect to efficacy and that one is even prepared to accept a small disadvantage as long as this is compensated by some other aspects (such as fewer side effects or other benefits for the patient). Nonetheless, it is relatively rare that such questions are addressed in oncology. The main interest is prolonging the patient's life.

- **Interim analyses are almost always necessary:** Since advantages and disadvantages of the therapies are of vital importance to the patients involved in clinical trials, it is generally not ethical to postpone any evaluations of treatment efficacy until all patients have been recruited.
- **In general, one-sided testing for treatment effects is inadequate.** One-sided testing in the usual superiority studies comparing a new therapy to a standard regimen has consequences: If the therapy to be tested appears to be inferior, one is no longer allowed to clarify and publish whether this inferiority is treatment-related or merely a random effect. One-sided testing is generally only acceptable if inferiority of the tested therapy is biologically impossible.

In the context of what will be discussed below, and specifically the last two points just mentioned, the following should always be kept in mind: No matter how plausible the active principle of a cancer therapy may be, how strong the immediately observed antitumor effects are, and how harmless the side effects may appear, one should never exclude a priori the possibility that the therapy may actually shorten the patient's life.

Examples of therapeutic procedures that shorten survival times according to meta-analyses of randomized studies include adjuvant therapy of non-small cell lung cancer using alkylating agents and postoperative radiation therapy of non-small cell lung cancer (61, 66).

Problems of Conducting Studies in Complementary Oncology

If one takes a closer look at the difficulties we have just described, it becomes evident why well-designed trials of complementary cancer treatments are infrequent. Often, proponents of complementary therapies are concerned about the "experimental situation" created by clinical trials and, in particular, by randomized allocation of patients to the treatment groups. Sometimes, they may be reluctant to do the study in the first place, fearing that a (well-founded) null-result might harm their

interests. Sometimes it is the fear of a well-founded negative result. Another point to consider is that research in complementary oncology mostly does not take part within traditional university research centers. Therefore, research culture may be less developed in comparison to conventional medicine, in which high-quality publications play a decisive role in career advancement. Finally, it should also be taken into consideration that certain nonmedical procedures are not under any regulatory pressures.

On the other hand, there are multiple reasons for the dearth of well-designed studies that proponents of complementary procedures cannot be held accountable for. According to the experience of the author, it may be impossible to implement a study, even with the best intentions of all participants involved. Here, four major reasons will be given: For a more detailed discussion see reference 2:

- **Research environment and infrastructure.** Research outside of university settings usually does not have access to established collaborations with methodological centers. Also few, if any, students are available to keep the trial going by working with little or no pay. Many institutions applying complementary medicine are companies that have to count the work and time dedicated by members of the staff to a clinical trial as expenses. Additionally, the available equipment may be insufficient to meet the standards required by a protocol of a multicenter trial.
- **Access to research funding.** Sponsors of respective therapies are often small companies that are unable to come up with the necessary funding for carefully conducted studies. Access to public grant funding is difficult. Regulators of studies often harbor negative feelings toward these procedures, or they have doubts (sometimes well founded) that the trial will be conducted successfully at the applicant's institution.
- **Patient numbers**. Well-designed studies are large, in particular when it comes to complementary therapies where expected treatment effects may be small. Patient numbers required for such trials can greatly surpass the capacities of the mostly humble and small institutions of complementary oncology.
- **Fragmentation of therapeutic approaches.** The therapeutic approaches in complementary oncology are extremely heterogeneous. Since

doctors usually swear by their treatment, even if it is only marginally different from another approach, it will be difficult to unite a group of investigators from different institutions who are prepared to apply identical therapies. This makes multicenter trials difficult. However, heterogeneity of treatment is a problem for monocenter trials, as well, namely for the relevance of the study results: for if a treatment evaluated at one institution is only one of many variants used in other places, then a result will say little about these variants. From the point of view of an external sponsor, the study may not seem to be of much value.

Nonetheless, it does happen that well-designed, randomized trials of complementary cancer therapies are carried out and published. Examples include trials of high-dose vitamin C, laetrile, fever-inducing substances (e. g., OK-432), enzyme preparations, Polyerga, Resistocell, active specific immunotherapy and therapy with mistletoe extracts or preparations.

▬ Primary Outcome Measures in Therapeutic Trials in Oncology

A study is nothing else but structured observation and experience. Clinical studies aim at obtaining data on efficacy and tolerability of therapies under transparent, predetermined, circumstances. We will limit our focus to the aspect of efficacy.

The goal of therapies in oncology is ultimately the prolongation of survival time and the improvement in quality of life of patients. These are the most important primary endpoints in therapeutic studies, gathered through the use of adequate tools. Apart from that, there are other outcome measures that are used in therapeutic studies in oncology, of which the following are the most common:
- tumor response rate and duration of tumor response
- immune response (rate)
- disease-free interval/survival
- progression-free interval/survival
- local recurrence-free interval/survival.

The two categories "disease-free interval" and "disease-free survival" differ in one point: the latter accounts not only for tumor recurrences, but also for deaths, both of which are counted as failures. The same is true for the last two outcome measures listed above.

Which endpoint is most relevant in a therapeutic trial depends on the type of cancer, the stage, and the type of therapy and questions posed by the study. It should always be realized, however, that increase in quality of life and survival time are ultimately of predominant importance to the patient, and all other outcome measures are secondary efficacy parameters.

Some of the methodological problems of the efficacy criteria will now be discussed.

Survival Time and Quality of Life

While *survival time* does not present any specific problems, the outcome measurement *quality of life* does prove problematic, starting with its definition. The difficulties of defining quality of life are similar to those encountered when defining "intelligence": most people have only intuitive and nebulous ideas as to its meaning, and are unable to give a precise definition. As is the case with "intelligence," one is forced to content oneself with operational definitions, in which quality of life is defined by the tools and instruments used to measure it.

In Table 4.**1**, some of these tools are listed. Two types should be differentiated:
- One-dimensional scales, based on clinical observations that may be precise and comprehensible, but only serve to show one aspect of a patient's complex well-being.
- Multidimensional instruments in the form of questionnaires that attempt to capture the diverse aspects (such as symptoms of disease, physical functioning, moods etc.) of a patient's condition.

Table 4.**2** lists the main methodical problems of the measurement of quality of life. Thus, in case of multidimensional instruments it may be difficult to determine which items should be included, and which scales and weights should to be used for the items. It is, for instance, not clear whether it is appropriate to aggregate the components "hope," "pain," and "family well-being" in a single number and, if so, whether they should be given the same weight.

Table 4.1 Instruments of measuring quality of life in clinical studies
Clinical observations
• Karnofsky Index (Performance Index)
• Toxicity (according to WHO criteria)
• TWIST (Time WIthout Symptoms of disease and subjective Toxic effects of treatment)
Self-report by the patient based on questionnaires
• Spitzer Index, composed of five items: "activity, daily living, health, support, outlook"; rating from 0–2 depending on a fixed set of answers
• Functional Living Index: Cancer (linear analogue scales)
• Breast Cancer Chemotherapy Questionnaire
• Cancer Rehabilitation Evaluation System
• Ferrans and Powers Quality of Life Index: Cancer Version
• Southwest Oncology Group Quality of Life Questionnaire
• Personal Functioning Index
• EORTC QLQ-C30 (EORTC = European Organization for Research and Treatment of Cancer) (74)

Table 4.2 Problems of measureing quality of life
• Choice of variables
• Scaling of variables
• Weighing and aggregation of variables
• Validity and reliability of instruments
• Timing of inquiry into health condition
• Influence of physician on patient response behavior
• Bias as a result of dropping out (death) of patients with particularly low quality-of-life measurements
• Bias as a result of nonresponse

More generally speaking, it needs to be clarified whether the instruments used for measuring quality of life are reliable and valid, i. e., whether their measurements are stable (when repeated) and reflect our common notion of "quality of life" and its changes.

A further methodical problem is the timing of measurement that does not necessarily reflect the actual dynamics of quality of life. Of course, patients' responses will be strongly influenced by the most recent impressions. That is why study outcomes depend largely on timing of questionnaires. In a chemotherapeutic study, for example, it will have an impact whether the questioning is done at the start or the end of a cycle (1).

The last three points in Table 4.**2** concern possible biases when measuring quality of life. The most pertinent bias occurs when the patient answers—completely unaware of the fact that he is doing so—according to what he assumes the doctor wants to hear. This has nothing to do with placebo effects, and it should not be confounded with the improvements of quality-of-life ratings due to expectation of long-term cure. (Note that the latter effect also poses a methodological problem, in particular in studies involving a no-treatment control group.) These biases are impossible to evade, unless the study is blinded, but blinded studies, as we have mentioned before, are rarely performed in oncology.

The deaths of patients can bias the true picture of the chronological development of quality of life and it can lead to biased comparisons of the groups of a clinical trial. Usually, cancer patients who die mostly had very low quality of life ratings prior to their death. Their death (and removal from their treatment group) will, therefore, lead to an immediate improvement of the average score of their group, which is surely an unwanted consequence that leads to inaccurate portrayal of the results of a trial.

In a study of 587 patients with advanced lung cancer, the quality of life was shown to improve due to death and, thus, exclusion from the trial (41).

It is not hard to imagine how failure to respond to a question, or the entire questionnaire, will lead to bias in the evaluation, since compliance or ability to respond will likely depend on the state of the patient's health.

These points are meant to be only a brief introduction into the problems of quality-of-life measurement. For a more detailed discussion, including methods developed for eliminating or mitigating the sources of bias, the reader is referred to the following articles: *Oncology* 5, No. 4, 1990; *Controlled Clinical Trials* 18, No. 4, 1997; *Statistics in Medicine* 17, Nos. 5–7, 1998.

The Problem of Secondary Efficacy Parameters

Tumor response will be discussed as an example of a secondary efficacy parameter (surrogate variable). It serves as the main measure of outcome in phase II trials, most of which consist of only one treatment group, that try to evaluate the antitumor activity of a therapy. When discussing the benefits of cancer therapy this particular outcome measure is not very useful; it represents a soft variable. Observed response rates depend on the type and quality of diagnosis, and show considerable oberserver variability. They are also not safe from attempts at embellishment. In comparative studies, the assessment of tumor response should therefore be blinded, i.e., the judgment should be made without knowing the patient's treatment assignment. This is especially important in those cases where response rate forms the basis for deciding whether the therapy should be used as a routine treatment.

The response rate depends on a number of other influencing factors (34). For one and the same type of treatment, the published response rates often show an enormous variability (1, 50). Therefore, nonrandomized comparisons, especially comparisons with rates that have been published, are of little value.

From the methodological point of view, the following question is of central importance: "Is it possible to causally relate the different response rates of cancer therapies to differences in efficacy regarding survival or quality of life?"

In neither instance does this hold true. It is clear that response rate by itself cannot predict quality of life, since potential reduction in pain symptoms due to tumor regression must be weighed against therapeutic side effects.

Ever since the 1980s, oncologists have attempted to correlate differences in response rates to improved survival time. Their line of argument was simple: chemotherapies can induce regression of malignancies, and without exception studies clearly show that responders live longer than nonresponders. These two findings were used as definite proof for the life-prolonging effects of certain therapies. This deduction was certainly also responsible for some types of cancer never being tested in randomized comparative trials with untreated controls.

Doubt concerning this argumentation probably developed due to two disturbing observations: Firstly, there were several studies in which the chemotherapy group was compared with a non-treated control group without any effect on survival time. Secondly, when looking at innumerable randomized comparative trials of aggressive treatment regimens (e. g., comparing two different dose intensities of the same cytostatic drug or comparisons of combination chemotherapy vs. mono-therapy) it became evident that the aggressive regimens almost always correlated with a higher response rate, without any visible effect on survival time (36). This effect was particularly pronounced in randomized evaluations of high-dose chemotherapy.

There are three possible explanations for differences in prognosis between responders and nonresponders, that all do not imply positive effects of therapy on survival (1):

- First of all, responders must live a minimum interval after the onset of therapy to be classified as such, in contrast to nonresponders. Nathan Mantel, a famous biostatistician, provides an amusing and extreme example that demonstrates this "**time-to-response bias.**" (52) Mantel reports on a clinical study conducted on the cancer drug Krebiozen. In this trial patients were defined as responders when they had survived a minimum time period. Early deceased patients were classified as Krebiozen nonresponders. It is therefore not surprising that responders fared better than nonresponders in terms of survival, which proponents of Krebiozen took as evidence of efficacy. According to Mantel, the manuscript was not accepted for publication in the *Journal of the National Cancer Institute.*

- Secondly, it is possible that responders constitute a **favorable prognostic subgroup,** who would have lived longer than nonresponders whether they had received the treatment or not. There is empirical data to support this claim. In a comprehensive analysis of trials of chemotherapy for advanced colorectal carcinoma, it was shown that persons in a worse general condition prior to starting therapy had both a shorter survival time and a lower probability of tumor response (21).

- Thirdly, one can imagine a type of **compensation** in which responders actually do profit from therapy in terms of survival time, but that in the total group this is counterbalanced by overtreatment of nonresponders, who suffer from the toxic effects but (by definition) have no tangible benefit from the treatment (49, 56, 67, 75).

Today it is understood and generally accepted amongst oncologists that the described argumentation (ridiculed by Moertel as the "responder vs. nonresponder maneuver") is a misconception (56). Most clinicians are well aware of the fact that they cannot convince colleagues with this type of reasoning, and that advancing it in support of a therapy would rather give an impression of incompetence (or lack of professionalism) on their part.

The argumentation was further discredited in the mid-1980s when the FDA and renowned medical journals pronounced that they would no longer accept that prolonged survival outcome among responders was proof of efficacy of therapy (13, 46).

By the 1990s, comparisons between responders and nonresponders had become rare. Nonetheless, such comparisons have revivals from time to time, albeit sometimes in linguistically disguised form (14, 58).

Much that has been said about tumor remission also holds true for the other **surrogate variables** mentioned above: These, too, are soft endpoints that are dependent on many influencing factors. Fallacies similar to the "responder vs. nonresponder maneuver" can also be found for these outcome measures:

- Some therapies such as active specific immunotherapy (ASI) of cancer, for example, cause immune responses in a group of patients that can be detected by means of a skin test. In numerous studies it has been shown that patients who respond to ASI with an immune response live longer than those who do not respond, even though there is no visible benefit in survival in patients receiving ASI compared to an untreated control group (8). This can be explained because patients with an immune reaction make up a subgroup with a beneficial prognosis compared with patients whose immune system no longer responds to treatment (53).
- Postoperative radiation therapy of non-small cell lung cancer prolongs remission-free survival, but, as has been mentioned previously, a meta-analysis that appeared in 1998 demonstrated that it actually reduced survival outcome (66). Once again, we can offer a simple explanation: radiation therapy affects health (leading, e. g., to radiation pneumonia) and does not prevent distant metastases, which are more important to survival than local tumor response.

▬ Evaluation of Efficacy

Objectives and Types of Trials

From a methodological point of view it makes sense to divide the question of efficacy of cancer therapy into three parts:

1. Is the therapy able to induce tumor response in the first place?
2. Does the therapy demonstrate any promising antitumor activity?
3. When compared with "standard therapy"—or untreated controls if no standard therapy exists —does it prolong the time until emergence of an unwanted event, specifically survival time, or does it improve the quality of life of the patient?

What trials are needed to clarify these questions? Generally, any statement on the efficacy of a therapy must be based on general experience (11). The methodological requirements for answering these three questions, however, are very different.

With respect to **question 1**, any prior knowledge, based on general experience for example, may suffice. Since spontaneous remissions, especially complete remissions, are rare events in advanced cancer stages, regardless of the patient characteristics, it is certainly possible to attribute a high proportion of regressions under therapy to its antitumor effects (40). This holds true not only for prospective noncomparative studies but may also apply to retrospective studies, based e.g. on clinical registries, or even to a mere collection of case reports.

Of course, case histories must satisfy a number of requirements (3, 39, 76), most of which were laid out by the NCI, in order to be able to furnish evidence of antitumor effects. These conditions are listed in Table 4.**3**. With the exception of the last point, all are usually fulfilled in prospective planned therapeutic trials.

One case series that meets these criteria is that of Coley dating back to 1893: he treated 10 cases of advanced solid tumors, six of which were sarcomas, with live pathogens of Erysipelas. He noticed a complete remission and two distinct tumor regressions. In a further three patients he witnessed a slight decrease in tumor size. The characteristics and results of the treatment were described in great detail for all patients involved, with photographic evidence supporting the results. One

Table 4.3 Credibility of antitumor therapeutic effects in case series

- T (the therapy) is precisely described
- Diagnosis of patients treated with T is well documented and verifiable. (If possible, pathological samples should be available for survey.)
- Patients' medical histories are well documented.
- The modality of T is well described.
- The "success" of T (tumor remission) is well defined, objectively measured, and verifiable (images).
- For cases with a tumor response all therapies administered prior to T or in combination with T are documented. It must be certain that the response cannot be attributed to these therapies.
- It is known how many similar patients the author of the case series actually treated with T (or some other therapy) within the time interval covered by the series.
- Useful information exists on maximal incidence rate of "successes" in untreated patients of the same cancer site and stage.

should note, that tumor regression at that time could not have been attributed to other treatments given prior or simultaneously to the therapy in question (28).

It is natural to ask of what interest it may be to determine the mere existence of antitumor effects. After all, if no data on the size of the effect (e.g., the prolongation of median survival) are available, antitumor activity per se is no basis for expecting a relevant benefit. However, the determination of the presence of antitumor effects of a treatment can be important for at least three reasons:

- It serves to motivate further research into this therapy. Clearly, a therapy that is capable of inducing tumor response is a more promising candidate for further research than a therapy that does not have any apparent antitumor activity. This applies not only to clinical studies but also to research into the underlying biological mechanisms.
- Evidence for antitumor activity of treatment certainly strengthens the credibility of, and acceptance of, potential results of randomized trials that show survival benefit of such treatment.
- This is benefical in the routine use of the treatment, since the knowledge of antitumor activity can induce hope in the patient.

One should always keep in mind that all three aspects may also play a role in established cancer therapies such as chemotherapy and radiation therapy.

Question 2 can be answered in a single-arm prospective study of a relatively homogenous group of patients in which antitumor effects can be roughly estimated. In drug development this is part of the so-called phase II. It follows phase I which focuses on pharmacology and toxicology (rather than on efficacy), aiming at, e.g., establishing acceptable doses.

Estimating a therapy's antitumor effects can be useful when trying to make a well-founded choice from a selection of drugs or treatments before starting costly and long-term efficacy studies. Phase II serves as a sort of screening of promising therapeutic approaches. Observed response rates are then compared with those of previously studied therapies. The estimate of antitumor activity also serves as further preparation for comparative randomized trials in that the foregoing of standard therapy, or even the higher burden of side effects that goes along with the new therapy, is more easily accepted if the treatment being studied has been shown to have been some biological activity of its own.

In order to answer question 3 (therapeutic benefit), well-designed confirmatory studies are needed. Reliable inference regarding therapeutic efficacy cannot be based on personal experience with single cases, but requires comparative trials with study groups that have no systematic differences whatever. In drug development, these studies are part of "phase III," for which regulatory agencies generally request carefully planned, large prospective studies with random allocation of the patients to the study groups ("randomized trials").

The Problem of Comparability

The following will elucidate the fundamental concept of comparability without delving into statistical analysis (11, 12). Simply stated, the groups in a therapeutic trial are comparable if the groups, apart from the treatment, do not show any differences in factors or conditions that might affect the study endpoint. Any such difference may lead to a biased measure of causal treatment effect, and it may contribute to, or be responsible for, the observed effect of a trial, i.e., the differences between the treatment groups with respect to an outcome variable.

In other words: comparability of groups is of essential importance for the persuasive power of a therapeutic comparison.

The reasons for (nonrandom) differences between treatment groups with respect to an outcome measure have been discussed in several publications and illustrated by examples (mostly in reference to discussions revolving around "bias" in nonrandomized studies). Table 4.**4** lists the various categories of the origins of these biases.

The problem of structural inequality, or differences of the composition of groups with respect to "prognostic factors," is especially pertinent to trials in oncology. Imbalance in the treatment groups regarding the distribution of prognostic factors can have several reasons. The most important ones are listed in Table 4.**5**.

Some of the points listed in Table 4.5 relating to definitions and diagnosis need further clarification.

A spectacular example of problems that can arise in nonrandomized trials is the story of **vitamin C in cancer treatment**.

In the year 1976, E. Cameron and the Nobel Prize Winner L. Pauling published a matched-pair study, in which a group of 100 terminally ill cancer patients was compared with 1000 historical controls who did not receive vitamin C treatment (10

terminally ill controls per case, selected from the patient files in the same hospital and matched with the cases for age, gender, tumor site, and histology). The results were as follows: the time between the determination that the patient was "untreatable by standard therapies" and death was highly significantly longer in the vitamin C group than in the control group ($P < 0.0001$) with a median survival time of 210 vs. 50 days. Cameron and Pauling came to the conclusion that the study presented strong evidence of life-prolonging effect of therapy with vitamin C (23).

Some years later, these impressive results were challenged by a Mayo Clinic group, who did two randomized, double-blinded trials with the same inclusion and exclusion criteria used in the study by Cameron and Pauling (30, 57). Both studies yielded practically identical survival curves. In the second study, survival in the placebo group was even slightly longer than that of the vitamin C group.

It is difficult to say today where Cameron and Pauling made a mistake. A crucial problem was the vagueness in the definition "untreatable by standard therapies" that was used both for specifying the groups and the starting point of measuring the survival time. In addition, the question of whether or not this imprecise criterion was satisfied by the patients of the control group had to be decided on the basis of historical records (72).

A shift of the starting point of time measurement may even occur if the study is done prospectively and comprises only newly diagnosed patients. Improvements in diagnosis and early detection of malignant disease, and possibly the growing awareness of the population, lead to a shift towards earlier diagnosis both of the disease itself and of metastases. As a result, survival from the time of diagnosis will appear longer when compared with historical controls, even if no progress in treatment has been made.

Another bias known as **stage migration** is caused by progress in the sensitivity of diagnostics. This is a somewhat paradoxical phenomenon that has been first described in the mid-1980s, but is still widely underestimated or even ignored. In historical comparisons it is a major source of bias.

Let us take a look at the historical development of cancer patient survival: the continuous improvement in diagnostic sensitivity through application of more advanced diagnostic techniques results in a shift in the stages of cancer towards

---

Table 4.4   Sources of bias in a comparative trial

- Structural inequality (differences in prognostic factors of the study groups)
- Differences in quality of treatment and doctors' commitment
- Differences in patients' motivation
- Differences in general patient care and in the experimental environment
- Differences in definition, measurement, or documentation of outcome

---

Table 4.5   Some factors that can cause structural inequality in therapeutic groups

- Definition of disease
- Diagnosis (stage migration, specification of starting point)
- Characteristics of patients admitted to the trial center with the disease under investigation (sociodemographic variables, co-morbidities, selection in referral, etc.)
- Selective allocation to treatment groups through the physician (e. g., exclusion of cases with poor prognosis from one of the groups)
- Self-selection by patients (e.g., due to selective refusal of one of the treatments by certain patient groups)
- Type and quality of previous therapies

more advanced stages. On first appearance, this has the paradoxical result of improving the prognosis both in the subgroups of patients with early-stage and advanced disease, even though overall survival may not change at all. The early stages profit in that fewer of the patients with poor prognosis (metastatic disease) are erroneously attributed to them, and the advanced stages benefit, as cases with a relatively good prognosis are also included (namely those in whom metastatic disease would have gone unnoticed earlier) (35).

Whenever stage migration may play a role in historical comparisons, any *forced* balancing of groups—for example, through matching with respect to stages, or through stage-by-stage comparison—is not only doomed to fail but is even counterproductive, when comparing seemingly identical stages, which in truth are different due to stage migration, these differences are "fixed," and the analysis is inherently biased.

Bias due to the **selection of patients** can be no less extreme. It may occur when the criteria for the application of a treatment, such as those that relate to the patient's general condition, are especially stringent, and when one then compares the patient groups who receive the therapy with those who don't, no matter whether the comparison is between parallel groups or relies on historical controls. Such types of studies were frequent in the early phase of research into high-dose chemotherapy and have led, without doubt, to a completely unfounded optimism regarding the efficacy of this approach (68, 73).

Selection bias also affects the studies of the association between dose intensity and survival time with respect to chemotherapy (44). Such a positive correlation is always to be expected, even when the chemotherapy does not prolong life, since trials with high-dose chemotherapy are restricted to patients in an especially good general condition. The bias will even occur if the therapy groups on which the correlation is based are all from randomized trials. Here, the randomization does not provide balance since the trials are different.

As for possible imbalance due to the primary treatment (which, in oncology, will mostly be tumor resection), it is clear that the quality of this treatment is of utmost importance for the patients' prognosis. This is highlighted by a recent study which found that the survival of lung cancer patients following primary surgery was positively correlated with the annual number of operations of this type carried out in the hospital (15).

From all that has been said, it is clear that the structural differences are of crucial importance for group comparability with respect to mean survival. Historically controlled studies are most affected by bias, and this can not be prevented through matching or through adjustment during the evaluation, specifically if the bias results from the type and quality of diagnosis. Bias may be inevitable, even when the comparative groups are selected to be as similar as possible.

This became apparent in an investigation by the British biostatistician, Stuart Pocock, which was based on the comparison of identical treatment groups in 19 pairs of successive randomized trials in cancer chemotherapy. In each of theses pairs, both studies were done by the same cooperative group and used the same entry criteria. Thus, Pocock compared treatment groups that apparently differed only with respect to the time-interval of patient recruitment. Pocock found that the differences in the annual death rates obtained from the 19 comparisons ranged from −46% to −24%. Four comparisons yielded differences that were significant at the 2% level, and the smallest P-value was 0.0001 (!) (63,64).

Randomization and Feasibility of Randomization

The only procedure that is able to even out any imbalance between prognostic factors—known and unknown or undetermined—is randomization, a process in which patients are randomly allocated to the treatment groups of the trial. This ensures that groups will only show random differences in all initial characteristics. It is not without reason that randomization has become the established gold standard for therapy evaluation. Not only does it offer epistemological advantages, but also pragmatic and "metascientific" benefits, since it simplifies the defense of study results (shifting the burden of proof) (12). Consequentially, most clinicians doing therapeutic research have accepted the maxim that studies should be randomized whenever possible.

However, randomization alone does not render a study convincing! Randomization only serves to balance structural inequalities. It does not affect the other sources of bias listed in Table 4.**4**, which remain problematic unless the trial is blinded (even though the danger may be less acute than in nonrandomized studies). This may explain the finding, made in numerous meta-analyses of randomized trials, that the results of studies investigating of identical treatment comparisons often show considerable and seemingly inexplicable heterogeneity. Randomization also does not safeguard against manipulation and fraud (69, 81, 82).

Conversely, nonrandomized studies are also not inherently flawed, as recent studies have shown (16, 20, 29, 48, 51, 54, 65).

An example of a well-designed nonrandomized parallel-group study was published by Cassileth et al. in 1991. In this matched-pair study, which compared an unconventional approach with conventional treatment, a convincing null result was obtained (24). (It should be noted that for many reasons, null results are generally more convincing than positive results.) (4) The methodology of nonrandomized studies has greatly advanced in recent years. In particular, according to recent suggestions (using e. g., the concept of the so-called synthetic-prospective study [5, 9]), even clinical databases may be suitable for studies of the therapeutic efficacy.

Besides, randomized studies are not always feasible and not always appropriate, especially in unconventional and surgical cancer therapies. The reasons for this shall be mentioned briefly here (7, 18):

- **Physicians' beliefs:** there is consensus that a randomization of patients is only ethically justified if there is sufficient uncertainty regarding relative values of the treatment options to be compared. If a doctor, who is convinced of the superiority of one therapy over another, refuses to conduct a randomization, he or she is acting in an ethically correct manner, regardless of whether this conviction is based on preconceived notions, considerations regarding the plausibility of the treatments, published data, or personal experience with the therapies. The early formation of firm beliefs is fostered by the fact that a new therapy cannot be tested under standardized conditions before all physicians involved in the study are capable of effectively managing it. This is especially important in therapies that require a lot of manual skill such as certain surgical techniques.
- **Patients' preferences:** patients may also decline random allocation if they have a positive opinion based on media releases or discussions with physicians on a particular therapy. If they have put hope into a novel therapeutic approach they will likely not be willing to forego the chance of getting this treatment for the sake of scienfific advancement.
- **Expectations regarding the type of treatment ("label" of an institution):** this argument differs only slightly from the last one. It is particularly relevant in unconventional medicine. Patients who place their fate in the hands of a therapist using unconventional approaches expect and demand this kind of therapy. It would probably be unrealistic to assume that they can be persuaded to participate in a trial in which they have a 50 % chance of receiving quite a different therapy or no therapy at all.
- **Non-availability of one of the study therapies:** this may be due to the fact that the doctors in this institution lack expertise with the treatment, that it has been abandoned in favor of a different standard treatment, or that it requires special equipment that is unavailable in the institution.

Implementation of Therapeutic Trials

> As a general rule, studies are only well planned if they are medically relevant, transparent, potentially conclusive, ethical, and feasible.

The core of a study is the protocol. All imaginable aspects of preparation and conduct of the trial are to be laid down in advance. The methodological and administrative requirements regarding **trial protocols** have enormously increased in the past years. (This is another reason why the burden of planning and conducting a therapeutic trial can only be taken over by large academic research institutions with the financial backing of affluent sponsors.)

A number of recommendations have been published on how to write a study protocol. Of particular importance are the ten detailed guidelines by the **ICH** (International Conference on Harmonization of Technical Requirements for Registration of Pharmaceuticals for Human Use: http://www.emea.eu.int/htms/human/ich/efficacy/ichfin.htm) that has been developed in Europe by the **EMEA**

(European Agency for the Evaluation of Medicinal Products: http://www. emea.eu.int).

The ICH guideline E6 contains the general principles for Good Clinical Practice, E9 deals with statistical principles for clinical trials, for example, and E10 gives recommendations for choosing control groups.

For the special cases of therapeutic studies in oncology, various groups within the German Cancer Foundation (Deutsche Krebsgesellschaft) have developed general Standard Operating Procedures (SOP) for studies, that have been published in a special edition of the journal *Oncology* in June 1998 (47). The magazine contains 13 SOPs, checklists, a model CRF, patient information and informed consent.

Biometrical expertise is not only needed for sample size determination, patient allocation (randomization), analysis and documentation, but for a number of further aspects, such as the formulation of the main hypothesis, the type of the study, the evaluation of treatment success, the definition study endpoints, and criteria for early termination of the trial. We will discuss only three methodological aspects here.

Choice of Outcome Measures

Generally, there is a distinction to be made between primary and secondary endpoints in a study. Confirmatory analysis is only valid for primary endpoints; for secondary endpoint, P-values resulting from statistical testing merely have a descriptive character. Sample size calculations are generally done for one primary endpoint.

Primary outcome measures *must,* **secondary outcome measures** *should* be relevant, objectively determined, measurable in a precise way, and available for a large number of patients. It is advisable to limit oneself to only one primary endpoint, if possible. Otherwise, adjustments must be made in the analysis for the multiplicity of testing (see below).

The Intention-to-Treat Principle

The ITT principle states that no patient is to be excluded from analysis once the treatment decision has been made for this patient. In randomized studies, this basic principle is applied even more rigorously: they should be evaluated as randomized. In other words, patients who did not even begin therapy or who stopped it prematurely must be included in the evaluation. At least this holds true for primary outcome measures, on which the definition of efficacy is based (83). The same applies to patients who did not continue with follow-up procedures for one reason or another. These patients should not be excluded from analysis, because their reasons for dropping out of the study could be related to the effects or side effects of the therapy or to the patients' state of health. Patients should even be included in the analysis if it is later discovered that they violate the criteria for admission to a study, since the study is meant to portray as accurate a picture of reality as possible. The Intention-to-Treat principle guards against manipulations that may arise when retroactive exclusions are permitted. To summarize, post-hoc exclusions, whatever their reason, may counteract the balance produced by randomization and should, therefore, be avoided.

An extreme example of a violation of the ITT principle was apparent in a multicenter trial of adjuvant active specific immunotherapy of lung cancer, in which a statistically significant survival advantage was claimed for the ASI group (43). Initially 264 patients were recruited. In the first analysis of the study results, published in 1987, only a subset of 126 patients was included, providing the basis for the authors' positive judgments of the therapy. Subsequent reports of this study did not even mention the fact that the original sample size of the study was much larger (42). Those study centers in which the patients' reactions in the skin test was too weak (it is unclear how this was defined precisely, and which centers were affected exactly) were excluded entirely from the final analysis. The authors argued that these centers did not adhere to the treatment protocol in a strict way (as evidenced by the weak delayed hypersensitivity reactions). Possibly they were unaware that, by doing so, the results were strongly biased, since patients with a worse prognosis were thereby excluded. In fact, when no patients were excluded from the analysis, a perfect null result was obtained, a fact that was only mentioned briefly in the 1987 publication, and not mentioned at all in later reports.

One should note that the great difference in survival favoring the ASI group in the analysis of the 126 patients was only possible if in the remaining 138 patients the ASI group fared distinctly *worse* than the control group. The respective results were not reported by the authors. For further examples, see reference 8.

Avoidance of Inflation of False-Positive Results

There are at least four—more or less subtle—mechanisms and "maneuvers" that can lead to an increase in the probability of statistically significant results in the data analysis. While, of course, they are not confined to studies of unconventional medicine, they are relatively frequent in this field.

Two common approaches that may result in an inflated type-one error are the simultaneous investigation of multiple endpoints (multiple testing) and subgroup analyses. These multiple analyses are particularly disturbing if a statistically significant result for one of the endpoints or groups is presented, post-hoc, as the finding that was of original interest in the study (60).

An almost bizarre example for this occurred in a randomized, multicenter, double-blinded trial of active-specific immunotherapy of stage 2 malignant melanoma (79, 80). In their publications, particularly the one of 1966 (which expressly focused on subgroup analyses), the authors contended that in the subgroup of male patients aged 44 to 57 years and with 1–5 positive lymph nodes, the ASI treatment conferred a 30% advantage in the four-year survival rate compared to the control group. This was termed "an encouraging survival benefit." One should note that the study gave a null result both for the disease-free interval ($P = 0.99$) and for the overall survival time ($P = 0.88$), and that the proclaimed differences in rates were subject to an extreme random variation, since they were calculated at the end of the survival curve.

Another source for the inflation of significant study results is the early termination of the study after a positive interim analysis. At least this holds true if the level of significance is not adjusted for the multiple testing implied by the interim analysis (45).

The danger is subtle in instances when multivariable models are applied in evolution of clinical study outcomes. Such models are employed in order to adjust the main treatment effect for confounding due to imbalance in prognostic factors. Occasionally, they are even used in randomized trials, where only chance imbalance can occur. Multivariable modeling contains a hidden danger of multiple testing because if the model building process is not precisely specified in the protocol, one has considerable freedom in selecting a model type and the variables to be included, and in the particular way these variables are accounted for in the model. The peril is then that many models are tried and the one yielding the most desirable results for the therapy effect is ultimately presented in the publication.

The proportion of studies with positive result increases dramatically if only *published* studies are considered. This phenomenon is called **publication bias**. This is a selection bias of published material that can be explained by preferential publication of studies with "positive" results (e. g., significant differences between the treatment groups) vs. those with null results. This phenomenon has been extensively studied (e. g., 17, 19, 32). The selection effect is more prominent in observational studies than randomized studies, and it is stronger for small than for large studies. One study that highlights the strength of publication bias was published by Easterbrook et al. in 1991. In this retrospective survey, research projects approved by the Central Oxford Ethics Committee between 1984 and 1987 were studied for evidence of publication bias. Among the 285 studies for which data analysis had been completed, those with a statistically significant result were much more likely to be published than those with a null result, with an estimated relative "risk" of publication of 1.7 (33).

There are several causes for publication bias. On the one hand, investigators and sponsors may withhold the publication of null results. The reason for this may be that they are frustrated and disappointed with the results, which did not meet the expectation, or because they reckon that the publication might negatively affect the application and the commercialization of the therapy. These seem to be the main reasons for publication bias in clinical studies. It is also conceivable that investigators, being convinced of the efficacy of the (new) study therapy, simply cannot accept and believe the null result and, instead of publishing it, first try to refute it in another positive trial. Selective submitting of studies acts invariably in favor of positive results. It can be (partly) prevented in the planning stage of trials by specifying a clear and obligatory publication rule.

There are, however, other causes of publication bias that investigators cannot influence. Publishers and reviewers preferentially select those trials from the submissions that show apparent or even spectacular results. This selection arises not only from the—legitimate—desire to boost the circulation of the journal, but it naturally and almost unavoidably follows from the asymmetry in the importance of positive and negative results in medicine. Obviously, positive results, in the sense of evidence for the efficacy or superiority of a therapy, is important per se, especially in life-threatening disease like cancer, whereas true null results are mostly of less interest to the patient, and their relevance for the community depends on the specific treatment comparison.

According to recently published studies, the extent of publication bias seems be country-specific and subject to cultural norms. A review of 252 controlled trials of acupuncture published between 1966 and 1995 and registered in Medline showed that all fifty trials originating in China, Japan, Hong Kong, and Taiwan were positive, whereas among the 47 trials published in the USA, only 25 (53%) gave the test treatment as superior to control. Similar results were found for other therapies (77).

▬ References

1. Abel U: Die zytostatische Chemotherapie fortgeschrittener Karzinome; 2nd ed. Stuttgart, Germany: Hippokrates Verlag, 1995.
2. Abel U: Spezielle Forschungsprobleme, Teil 1: Warum gibt es in der unkonventionellen Medizin so wenige aussagefähige Studien? In: Bühring M, Kemper FH (eds): Naturheilverfahren und unkonventionelle Medizinische Richtungen. (Loose-leaf edition, March 1995.) Section 1.08, Part 1. Berlin, Germany: Springer Verlag; 1995:1-8.
3. Abel U: Spezielle Forschungsprobleme. Teil 3: Zur Bedeutung von Kasuistiken für die Wirksamkeitsbeurteilung medizinischer Therapien. In: Bühring M, Kemper FH (eds): Naturheilverfahren und unkonventionelle Medizinische Richtungen. (Loose-leaf edition, March 1997.) Section 1.08, Part 3. Berlin, Germany: Springer Verlag; 1997:1-19.
4. Abel U: Die Bedeutung statistisch signifikanter Ergebnisse klinischer Studien. In: Bühring M, Kemper FH (eds): Naturheilverfahren und unkonventionelle Medizinische Richtungen. (Loose-leaf edition, March 1999.) Section 1.08, Part 6. Berlin, Germany: Springer Verlag; 1999:1-12.
5. Abel U: Erkenntnisgewinn mittels nichtrandomisierter Studien. In: Tietze B, Weinschenk S (eds): Naturheilkunde und Umweltmedizin in der Frauenheilkunde. Hippokrates-Verlag, Stuttgart 2000, pp. 3-13.
6. Abel U, Windeler J: Erkenntnistheoretische Aspekte klinischer Studien. 1. Irrtümer in der Bewertung medizinischer Therapien–Ursachen und Konsequenzen. Internist Prax. 1995; 35:613-629.
7. Abel U, Windeler J: Comprehensive Blinded Prognostic Rating–eine Studienform für die nichtrandomisierte Bewertung von Therapien. In: Hornung J (ed.): Forschungsmethoden in der Komplementärmedizin. Schattauer Verlag, Stuttgart 1996, pp. 153-163.
8. Abel U, Windeler J: Erkenntnistheoretische Aspekte klinischer Studien. 3. Fallstudie ASI–Fehlurteile und unfundierte Schlüsse in klinischen Therapieprüfungen. Internist Prax. 1997; 37:619-629.
9. Abel U, Koch A (eds): Nonrandomized comparative clinical studies. Düsseldorf, Germany: Symposion Publishing; 1998.
10. Abel U, Koch A: Spezielle Forschungsprobleme: Teil 5: Nichtrandomisierte vergleichende Therapiestudien In: Bühring M, Kemper FH (eds): Naturheilverfahren und unkonventionelle Medizinische Richtungen. (Loose-leaf edition, April 1998.) Section 1.08, Part 4. Berlin, Germany: Springer Verlag; 1998:1-16.
11. Abel U, Windeler J: Erkenntnistheoretische Aspekte klinischer Studien. 4. Vergleichbarkeit in klinischen Studien. A. "Strukturgleichheit" und die Bedeutung der Randomisation. Internist Prax. 1998; 38:613-624.
12. Abel U, Koch A: The role of randomization in clinical studies: myths and beliefs. J. Clin Epidem. 1999; 52:487-497.
13. Anderson JR, Korzun AH: Chemotherapy versus hormonal therapy in advanced breast cancer. Correspondence. N Engl J Med. 1986; 315:1092-1093.
14. Anonymous: Therapiestrategien nach adjuvanter oder neoadjuvanter Therapie. In: Aktuelle Behandlungsstrategien beim fortgeschrittenen Mamma- und Ovarialkarzinom–Therapie des nichtkleinzelligen Bronchialkarzinoms im fortgeschrittenen Stadium. Der Onkologe. 2000; 6: Supplement for Oncologists, issue 5.
15. Bach PB, Cramer LD, Schrag D: The influence of hospital volume on survival after resection for lung cancer. N Engl J Med. 2001; 345:181-188.
16. Benson K, Hartz AJ: A comparison of observational studies and randomized, controlled trials. N Engl J Med. 2000; 342:1878-1886.
17. Berlin JA, Begg CB, Louis TA: An assessment of publication bias using a sample of published clinical trials. J Am Stat Assoc. 1989; 84:381-392.

18. Black N: Why we need observational studies to evaluate the effectiveness of health care. Br Med J. 1996; 312:1215–1218.

19. Boissel JP, Haugh MC: The iceberg phenomenon and publication bias: The Editor's fault? Clinical Trials and Meta-Analysis. 1993; 28:309–3015.

20. Britton A, McPherson K, McKee M, et al.: Choosing between randomised and non-randomised studies: a systematic review. Health Technology Assessment 1998; 2 (13).

21. Buyse M, Piebois P: On the relationship between response to treatment and survival time. Stat Med. 1996; 15:2797–2812.

22. Byar DP: Why data bases should not replace randomized clinical trials. Biometrics. 1980; 36:337–342.

23. Cameron E, Pauling L: Supplemental ascorbate in the supportive treatment of cancer: Prolongation of survival times in terminal human cancer. Proc Natl Acad Sci. 1976; 73:3685–3689.

24. Cassileth BR, Lusk EJ, Guerry D, et al.: Survival and quality of life among patients receiving unproven as compared with conventional cancer therapy. N Engl J Med. 1991; 324:1180–1185.

25. Chlebowski RT, Lillington LM: A decade of breast cancer clinical investigation: results as reported in the ASCO proceedings. Abstract 92. Proc Am Soc Clin Oncol. 1994; 13:72.

26. Chlebowski RT, Curti M, Lillington LM: Trends in prostate and breast cancer clinical research as reported in the ASCO proceedings. Proc Am Soc Clin Oncol. 1999; 18:A1213.

27. Coates A, Gerski V, Stat M, et al.: Improving the quality of life during chemotherapy for advanced breast cancer. N Engl J Med. 1987; 317:1490–1495.

27. Coley WB: The treatment of malignant tumors by repeated inoculations of erysipelas; with a report of ten original cases. Am J Med Sci. 1893; 105:487–511.

29. Concato J, Chah N, Horwitz RI: Randomized controlled trials, observational studies, and the hierarchy of research designs. N Engl J Med. 2000; 342: 1887–1892.

30. Creagan ET, Moertel CG, O'Fallon JR, et al.: Failure of high-dose vitamin C (ascobic acid) therapy to benefit patients with advanced cancer. N Engl J Med. 1979; 301:687–690.

31. Dannehl K: Naturwissenschaftliche Methode und (alternativ-)medizinische Forschung. In: J. Hornung (ed.): Forschungsmethoden in der Komplementärmedizin. Stuttgart, Germany: Schattauer Verlag; 1996:176–188.

32. Dickersin K, Chan S, Chalmers TC, et al.: Publication bias and clinical trials. Contr Clin Trials. 1987; 8: 843–853.

33. Easterbrook PJ, Berlin JA, Gopalan R, Matthews DR: Publication bias in clinical research. Lancet. 1991; 337:867–872.

34. Edler L, Flechtner H: Remission in Phase-II- und Phase-III-Studien: Kriterien und Voraussetzungen. Onkologie. 1987; 10:330–339.

35. Feinstein AR, Sosin DM, Wells CK: The Will Rogers phenomenon–stage migration and new diagnostic techniques as a source of misleading statistics for survival in cancer. N Engl J Med. 1985; 312:1604–1608.

36. Fossati R, Confalonieri C, Torri V, et al.: Cytotoxic and hormonal treatment for metastatic breast cancer: a systematic review of published randomized trials involving 31 510 women. J Clin Oncol. 1998; 16:3439–3460.

37. Gallmeier WM: Interview in: Der Spiegel 1994; 25:189.

38. Hager ED: Komplementäre Onkologie: adjuvante, additive, supportive Therapiekonzepte für Klinik und Praxis. Stockdorf, Germany: Forum Medizin; 1997.

39. Hawkins MJ, Friedman MA: National Cancer Institute's evaluation of unconventional cancer treatments. J Natl Cancer Inst. 1992; 84:1699–1702.

40. Heim M, Schwarz R (eds): Spontanremissionen in der Onkologie. Stuttgart, Germany: Schattauer Verlag; 1998.

41. Hollen PJ, Gralla RJ, Cox C, et al.: A dilemma in analysis: issues in the serial measurement of quality of life in patients with advanced lung cancer. Lung Cancer. 1997; 18:119–1136.

42. Hollinshead A: Active specific immunotherapy and immunochemotherapy in the treatment of lung and colon cancer. Seminars in Oncology. 1991; 7: 199–210.

43. Hollinshead AC, Stewart THM, Takita H, et al.: Adjuvant specific active lung cancer immunotherapy trials. Cancer. 1987; 60:1249–1262.

44. Hryniuk W, Frei III E, Wright FA: A single scale for comparing dose-intensity of all chemotherapy regimens in breast cancer: summation dose-intensity. J Clin Oncol. 1998; 16:3137–3147.

45. Hughes MD, Pocock SJ: Stopping rules and estimation problems in clinical trials. Stat Med. 1988; 7:1231–1241.

46. Johnson JR, Temple R: Food and Drug Administration requirements for approval of new anticancer drugs. Cancer Treatm Rep. 1985; 69:1155–1157.

47. Kreuser ED, Fiebig HH, Scheulen ME, et al.: Standard operating procedures and organization. Onkologie. 1998; 21(Suppl. 3):1–70.

48. Kunz R, Oxman AD: The unpredictability paradox: review of empirical comparisons of randomised and non-randomised clinical trials. Brit Med J. 1998; 317:1185–1190.

49. Livingston RB: Stage IV non-small-cell lung cancer: the guides are perplexed. Editorial. J Clin Oncol 1989; 7:1591–1593.

50. Macaulay V, Smith IE: Advanced breast cancer. In: Slevin ML, Staquet MJ (eds): Randomized Trials in Cancer. A Critical Review by Sites. New York, NY: Raven Press; 1986:273–357.

51. MacLehose RR, Reeves BC, Harvey IM et al.: A systematic review of comparisons of effect sizes derived from randomized and non-randomized studies. Health Technology Assessment 2000; 4 (34).

52. Mantel N: An uncontrolled clinical trial–treatment response or spontaneous improvement? Contr Clin Trials. 1982; 3:369–370.

53. McCune CS, O'Donnell RW, Marquis DM, Sahasrabudhe DM: Renal cell carcinoma treated by vaccines for active specific immunotherapy: correlation of survival with skin testing by autologous tumor cells. Cancer Immunol Immunother. 1990; 32:62–66.

54. McKee M, Britton A, Black N, et al.: Interpreting the evidence. choosing between randomised and non-randomised studies. Brit Med J. 1999; 319:312–315.

55. McQuellon R, Muss H, Hoffmann S, et al.: The influence of toxicity on treatment preferences of women with breast cancer. Abstract 107, Proc Am Soc Clin Oncol. 1994; 13:6.

56. Moertel CG : Improving the efficiency of clinical trials: a medical perspective. Stat Med. 1984; 3:455–465.

57. Moertel CG, Fleming TR, Creagan ET, et al.: High-dose vitamin C versus placebo in the treatment of patients with advanced cancer who have had no prior chemotherapy. N Engl J Med. 1985; 312:137–141.

58. Müser M: Strategien zur Immuntherapie bei der Behandlung von Krebs. Der Onkologe. 2000; 5:433–437.

59. Nagel GA, Schmähl D, Hossfeld DK (eds): Krebsmedikamente mit fraglicher Wirksamkeit. Munich, Germany: Zuckschwerdt Verlag; 1989.

60. Nelson RB: Cancer trials: pseudoscience or situation science? In: Buyse M et al. (eds): Cancer Clinical Trials. Oxford: Oxford Univ Press; 1984:3–13.

61. Non-Small Cell Lung Cancer Collaboration Group: Chemotherapy in non-small cell lung cancer: a meta-analysis using updated data on individual patients from 52 randomized clinical trials. Brit Med J. 1995; 311:899–909.

62. O'Shaughnessy JA, Wittes RE, Burke G, et al.: Commentary concerning demonstration of efficacy of investigational anticancer agents in clinical trials. J Clin Oncol. 1991; 9:2225–2232.

63. Peto R: Clinical trial methodology. Biomedicine, Special Issue. 1978; 28:24–36.

64. Pocock SJ : Randomized clinical trials. Letter to the Editor. Br Med J. 1977; 1(6077): 1661.

65. Pocock SJ, Elbourne DR: Randomized trials or observational tribulations? Editorial. N Engl J Med. 2000; 342:1907–1909.

66. PORT Meta-analysis Trialists Group: Postoperative radiotherapy in non-small-cell lung cancer: systematic review and meta-analysis of individual patient data from nine randomised controlled trials. The Lancet. 1998; 352:257–263.

67. Powles TJ, Coombes RC, Smith IE, et al.: Failure of chemotherapy to prolong survival in a group of patients with metastatic breast cancer. Lancet. 1980; 1(8168): 580–582.

68. Rahmann ZU, Frye DK, Buzdar AU, et al.: Impact of selection process on response rate and long-term survival of potential high-dose chemotherapy candidates treated with standard-dose doxorubicin-containing chemotherapy in patients with metastatic breast cancer. J Clin Oncol. 1997; 15:3171–3177.

69. Ranstam J, Buyse M, George SL, et al.: Fraud in medical research: an international survey of biostatisticians. Contr Clin Trials. 2000; 21:415–427.

70. Ravdin PM, Siminoff IA, Harvey JA: Survey of breast cancer patients concerning their knowledge and expectations of adjuvant therapy. J Clin Oncol. 1998; 16:515–521.

71. Richardson MA: Research of complementary/alternative medicine therapies in oncology: promising but challenging. J Clin Oncol. 1999; 17 (November Supplement):38–43.

72. Rosenbaum PR: Observational studies. Berlin, Germany; New York, NY: Springer Verlag; 1995.

73. Schmoor C, Schumacher M: Methodological arguments for the necessity of randomized trials in high-dose chemotherapy for breast cancer. Breast Cancer Res Treatm. 1999; 54:31–38.

74. Senn HJ, Drings P, Glaus A, et al. (eds): Checkliste Onkologie. Stuttgart, Germany: Thieme Verlag: 1998.

75. Smith I: Measuring response in incurable cancer. In: Stoll BA (ed.): Cancer Treatment: End Point Evaluation. New York, NY: Wiley; 1983:23–42.

76. The Office of Technology Assessment, US Congress: Unconventional cancer treatments. OTA-H-405, US. Government Print Office, Washington, DC 1990.

77. Vickers A, Goyal N, Harland R, Rees R: Do certain countries produce only positive results? A systematic review of controlled trials. Contr Clin Trials. 1998; 19:159–166.

78. Vogler-Hinze S: Unkonventionelle Methoden in der Krebstherapie. Stuttgart, Germany: Hippokrates Verlag; 1995.

79. Wallack MK, Sivanandham M, Balch CM, et al.: A phase III randomized, double-blind, multiinstitutional trial of vaccinia melanoma oncolysate-active

specific immunotherapy for patients with stage II melanoma. Cancer. 1995; 75:34–42.

80. Wallack MK, Sivanandham M, Whooley B, et al.: Favorable clinical responses in subsets of patients from a randomized, multi-institutional melanoma vaccine trial. Ann Surg Oncol. 1996; 3:110–117.

81. Weiss RB, Rifkin RM, Stewart FM, et al.: High-dose chemotherapy for high-risk primary breast cancer: an onsite review of the Bezwoda study. Lancet. 2000; 355:999–1003.

82. Weiss RB, Gill GG, Hudis CA: An on-site audit of the South African Trial of High-Dose Chemotherapy for metastatic breast cancer and associated publications. J Clin Oncology. 2001; 19:2771–2777.

83. Windeler J: Das Intention-to-treat-Prinzip in klinischen Arzneimittelprüfungen. Arzneimitteltherapie. 1993; 11:103–111.

5 Expert Systems in Complementary Oncology

Dieter Praetzel-Wolters, Hagen Knaf, and Patrick Lang

Introduction

The human organism is a highly complex system with an intricate network of various interrelated causes and effects. Diagnosis, prognosis, and therapeutic planning require a high level of medical expertise and experience. Due to the complex effects a disease exerts on the human organism, it is generally necessary to sift through of a lot of data in order to provide a good diagnosis and prognosis in any individual. Accordingly, the physician uses an extensive set of rules herein.

The evaluation of such medical data is increasingly supported through adaptive diagnostic systems based on mathematical models. In order to apply mathematics in a sensible way, a **mathematical model** of a section of the reality one wishes to work on is required. A mathematician might emulate the growth of bacteria in culture after an infection in otherwise healthy individuals. This model would in this case be a function or graphic depiction illustrating the time dependent amount of a type of bacteria observed in the blood after an infection present in a certain person. Such a function might look as shown in Fig. 5.**1** (the units in the graphic are chosen arbitrarily). The progression of this function, e. g., time until the start of the immune response, was calculated by the mathematician by taking mean values of lots of data points. The model of bacterial growth obtained in such a way would, of course, be very simplistic, since it would be independent of other parameters like the person's age or the individual characteristics of the immune system.

Mathematical modeling is often a complex, longwinded interactive process between experts from within the context of application and the mathematicians producing the model. Once a model is found it is evaluated and analyzed using mathematical methods. Nowadays the computer plays a large part in this. Without it, many of the models would be far too complex and therefore useless. In the evaluation, visualization is often the initial step for translation back into the specific context of application. This entire process is referred to as **simulation**—its computational part as **scientific computing.**

Mathematical Contribution to Diagnosis and Therapy

The diagnosis and therapy of diseases can be conceived as regulatory processes. In individual diagnosis, information on the actual disease state is achieved initially by assessing the medical history of and by questioning the patient, and also through a set of targeted procedures such as radiography and computed tomography or ultrasound. This information serves as the foundation upon which the physician, using his knowledge and experience will come up with a diagnosis and initiate therapeutic measures.

Expert systems can now be of manifold value in the diagnostic and therapeutic setting. A well-functioning expert system can guide doctors to the correct diagnosis by delivery of concrete suggestions for diagnosis, as well as supporting accumulation of the physician's own experience. In other instances, a different group of doctors can play a part in the development of an expert system— knowledge can thereby be integrated and made objective.

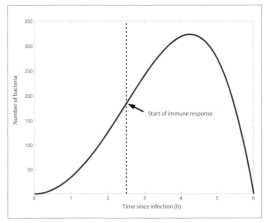

Fig. 5.**1** Model for bacterial growth following an infection.

A large amount of medical data arise from clinics and private practices. Once used for diagnosis and treatment, these data are often not studied further. Here lies a tremendous potential for the extension, improvement, and safeguarding of existing medical knowledge. Through the application of systematic **data mining**, existing medical hypotheses can be verified and statistically validated. Software systems for automatic recognition of patterns in data can provide the impulse and motivation for research in a new direction.

Expert systems and data mining are pillars that provide the basis for computer-supported medical diagnosis and therapy, which has been gaining considerable importance in recent years. This novel medical field requires the intensive and interdisciplinary collaboration of physicians, mathematicians, computer specialists, physicists, and engineers. In addition to utilizing previously existing medical information more effectively, and learning from it through combination with medical expertise, expert systems could serve as integral components of a system that is yet to be constructed, consisting of interlaced medical data banks that would be provided online for physicians for diagnosis and therapy.

▬ What is an Expert System?

> An expert system is a computer program that simulates an expert within a clearly defined area of expertise and terms of functions.

One example is the "Mycin" system developed in 1972, which helps the physician choose the type and dose of antibiotics. This system is made up of three main components:

- **Consultation component** After insertion of patient data and data pertaining to, say, the bacterial types detected in the blood sample, the system proposes an antibiotic for therapy, including suggestions for dosage. It is crucial to understand that data fed into the system may be vague: in this case, a morphological description of the organisms found in the sample can be given. The system tries to identify these through combination with other information.
- **Explanatory component** Following suggestion for therapy, it can be revealed which data and information was used.

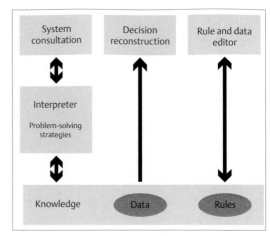

Fig. 5.**2** Structure of an expert system.

- **Acquisition component** This component enables new expert knowledge to be integrated into the existing system, or current information to be edited. Entering new information does not require any knowledge of programing, and can be done entirely by the expert.

The structure of the "Mycin" system is prototypical for an expert system. Generally the structure is as shown in the depiction shown in Fig. 5.**2**, the components of which are to be described shortly. The arrows in the diagram symbolize the flow of data and the direction of flow.

The knowledge of a (medical) expert consists of data and rules, in which the handling of information is defined dependent on specific situations. Data are, for example, the characteristics of bacteria or the effects of certain medications. Accordingly, the fact that certain bacteria can be treated with certain medicines can be defined as a simple rule.

This perspective of expert knowledge is referred to as **rule-based approach** and is used throughout the entire chapter. An alternative is the so-called **object orientation**, in which data and rules are conceptualized as more abstract objects combined.

When considering integration of expert knowledge into a computer program two problem areas should be addressed:

- Data structures must be developed that are well suited for storing and retrieving human expertise—this occurs under the keyword

knowledge representation. The problems surrounding knowledge representation and their possible solutions cannot all be mentioned here, but will be described briefly below, see p. 58, under fuzzy logic, as a possibility of implementing knowledge.

- In association with the implementation of knowledge is its **formalization:** expert depictions of existing knowledge are generally too complex to be directly implemented into respective software. This is due to the complex nature inherent to language itself, but often also due to lack of formal structure. Therefore, before input into the expert system, relevant knowledge must be represented by means of a simple formal language. Ideally, the expert himself performs this translation process. This is especially important, since expert systems should be designed in order to be customized by the user: completeness of knowledge in a certain area can not be expected. This implies that the knowledge can be modified, updated and expanded using a software module, a so-called data and rule editor. Input via this editor ensues in the mentioned formal, but easily written and readable, language. Above all, system users are not expected to have any programming knowledge.

The **expandability of an expert system** is the precursor to learning aptitude: there are various techniques that permit automatic generation of new knowledge from entered data. Such procedures look for structures within the data and interpret them according to the rules of the pertaining expert system. These procedures rely mathematically on multivariate statistics, approximation theory, or cluster analysis. Neuronal networks also play a role.

The actual simulation of experts—the query of a specific situation within the area of expertise of the system—occurs through the **consultation module**. Following entry of data describing the situation, the interpreter analyses these, and compiles the rules needed, then applies these and finally displays the result in a user friendly manner.

Typically, the entered data are not precise. The interpreter must be capable of dealing with poorly delineated situations. Contrary to knowledge, strategies for entry-dependent collocation of the rules are permanently integrated within the sys-

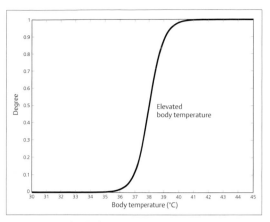

Fig. 5.**3** Example of a fuzzy set.

tem, or more precisely, in the interpreter, and cannot be altered by the user.

For various ends, it is necessary to fully understand the route from given input data to output data within the expert system: controllability of the system should be mentioned, as should applications in expert training or the test of newly to be integrated knowledge. A structured depiction of the routes from entry to output offers a module for reconstruction of decisions.

▬ Uses in Medicine

The use of expert systems in medicine does not differ much from that in other specialist areas. The following formulated areas of application can easily be transferred to other fields.

- **Relief for the doctor of performing routine tasks** The expert system can take over the classification of patient data for diagnostic purposes, including concrete diagnostic suggestions for the physician. A further field of application is the choice of a specific therapy, oriented according to the individual circumstances of a particular patient.
- **Improved availability of medical expert knowledge** An expert system can be used, among other things, as a specialist book or databank. The internet allows the functionality of expert systems to become available to the wider general public who in turn can use it to improve their health-related behavior and the surveillance of their own health.

- **Support of medical education** A complete expert system provides the user with the option of retrieving explanations for specific conclusions, arrived at by the system in a particular situation. The user can compare his conclusions with that of the system and, if necessary, correct them. Medical models are becoming increasingly realistic through interconnection with expert systems.
- **Objectifying knowledge using formalized depictions** The construction of an expert system requires clear and formal depiction of existing subjective knowledge on a particular circumstance. This enables knowledge to be comprehensible and traceable enabling full utilization of functionality of the expert system. The collaboration of multiple experts on a system makes this approach very effective.
- **Facilitation of validation of knowledge** or rather verification of hypotheses.

Since the demands that medicine places in terms of complexity and operational reliability are considerably higher than in the technical–scientific area, a warning should be given: none of the above mentioned points should be misinterpreted to the extent that competency of a medical expert can be replaced by a computer program.

▃ Fuzzy Logic

The formal representation of knowledge in a computer program is problematic due to a variety of reasons: even when limited to a tightly confined area the knowledge to be integrated is too vast and networked too complexly for real-life applications.

Medical knowledge, in particular, is often vague. Transitions between "healthy" and "pathological" behavior can be blurred. The described entities often demonstrate considerable breadth in variety.

When utilizing rule-based representation of knowledge the networking of existing information is presented through logical rules. In the simplest case this occurs through logical implications, such as rules in the form of "A implies B." To assist in the problem of vaguely defined entities, an expansion of the basic prepositional logic is necessary—the so-called fuzzy logic.

Fuzzy Set

Fuzzy set is a concept that helps to determine the blurry entities in a specialist mathematical field. The term "elevated body temperature" is a typical vaguely defined term often found in medicine. It could be defined mathematically, specified as "body temperature above 37 °C." For application, e. g., within an expert system, a continuous transition between normal condition leading up to the condition of increased temperature would be desirable.

An alternative model would be to give a so-called fuzzy set for the characteristic "elevated body temperature" (Fig. 5.**3**):

This diagram gives you the specific amount at each relevant body temperature at which the body temperature should be considered "elevated." This degree of elevation assumes values between 0 and 1. Values close to 0 are to be interpreted as "(almost) not elevated," while values closer to 1 are to be looked at as "definitely elevated." In analogy to this example, any vaguely defined entity can basically be mathematically expressed.

Linguistic Variables

Expert knowledge partially consists of the formulation of characteristics of specific objects in the respective technical terminology. The re-creation of such formulations in fuzzy logic occurs through the use of linguistic variables: the observed object characteristic receives a name under which it will appear within the expert system. In addition, it must be clarified which properties or values this characteristic may assume. Crucial to this specification is that these values can be numeric, as well as technical, in nature.

For example, the linguistic variable "body temperature" can appear in an expert system. The possible values of this variable were temperatures from within the interval 30–45 °C.

Depending on the mode of application the following more complex construction could make sense: as possible values for "body temperature" the terms "normal," "elevated," or "fever" can be used. Each of these so-called **linguistic values** clearly must be defined more precisely. Since these are obviously blurry entities, specification ensues through indication of the respective fuzzy set, as described above in the example "elevated body temperature."

The advantage of this approach is in the increased viability and it allows the formalization of knowledge that as close to technical terminology as possible.

Fuzzy Rules

Fuzzy rules are expert regulations that are grasped based on fuzzy logic. All fuzzy rules can be traced back to a simple basic structure, namely the logical implication:

"If x equals A, then y equals B."

Both x and y are linguistic variables. The letters A and B stand for linguistic values that these variables can assume. Let us take, for example, the aforementioned linguistic variable "body temperature" for x, and "treatment with aspirin" for y with the linguistic values of "none," "moderate," and "high." A fuzzy rule would then be:

(1) "If body temperature is elevated, treatment with aspirin is moderate."

Now both "elevated" and "high" are blurry linguistic values specified through fuzzy sets. With "moderate" each dose of aspirin is related to a respective degree (how "moderate" is the dosing?). With each given body temperature rule (1) should provide the user with a suggested dosing. How this is to be determined, is the next question that needs to be addressed.

Fuzzy Implication

In Fig. 5.**4**, the fuzzy set for the linguistic value "elevated" can be seen. The prevailing body temperature is 37.8 °C as marked through a vertical line. The height of the gray area relates to the degree to which the respective temperature is considered "elevated."

Above and to the right is the depiction of the fuzzy set of the linguistic value "moderate." It is cut off at the height of the "elevated" degree belonging to the temperature of 37.8 °C. The remaining fuzzy set is depicted as blue.

The sense for this operation lies in treating all aspirin doses with a "high" degree (namely higher than the degree of elevated body temperature) in the same way. The particular degrees do not play a major role given the concrete body temperature.

When choosing a recommended dose, the smallest dose is taken at which the remaining fuzzy set shows a maximum as marked by a thick vertical line. With these simple procedures one combines low doses with high efficacy.

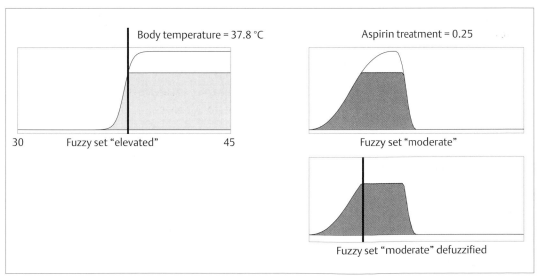

Fig. 5.**4** Fuzzy implication and defuzzification.

The method shown is referred to as "fuzzy implication." The change of the initial fuzzy set, through cut-off and designation of a recommended dose, only offers one possibility from a slew of options from which, oriented according to the respective application, the designer of an expert system can choose. The designation of the recommended doses is generally referred to as "**defuzzification**" because a sharply defined numeric value is determined from a fuzzy set.

Fuzzy-Logical Operations

When generating more complex fuzzy rules the use of logical operators such as "and" and "or" is unavoidable. In the case of basic prepositional logic the meaning of such operations are clear, but not in the event of fuzzy logic: an expression such as "x equals A" is, in this case, always fulfilled to a certain degree that is determined by the respective fuzzy set.

If one constructs expressions of the type "(x equals A) and (y equals B)," one must calculate in each event the degree of fulfillment of "(x equals A) and (y equals B)" from the degree of fulfillment of "x equals A" and "y equals B." This occurs through declaration of a general calculation provision for the fuzzy set of an expression determined through conjunction of "and"—and "or"— interconnections based on the fuzzy sets of its components. All the mathematical details cannot be presented here.

Combination

The complexity of expert knowledge, and thereby also of expert systems, is caused for the most part due to a combination of rules with the same linguistic variables, but opposing influences on the values of these variables.

Taking a look, for example, at the following two fuzzy rules:

1. If body temperature equals fever, then high aspirin dose
2. If trouble with stomach lining, then moderate aspirin dose

In this case, the recommended dose for aspirin must be ascertained from two opposing rules. Basically, this can occur if one determines the degree of the variables for "aspirin treatment" separately

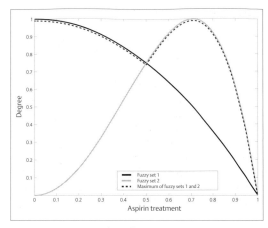

Fig. 5.**5** Aggregation of two fuzzy set. The blue (or gray) line indicates the linguistic value "moderate" or "high" of the co-variable "aspirin treatment." The dotted line indicates their maximum.

for both rules according to the depicted procedure (see above Fuzzy implication). A weighted average of the two values can then be taken. The weights can be adjusted according to the importance of the rules.

However, fuzzy logic uses a more complex approach: as in the case of logic operations, the new fuzzy quantity is first established by superposing the modified fuzzy quantities for the linguistic values "high" and "moderate." One refers to this step as aggregation, and, as with defuzzification, a lot of possibilities exist for the aggregation procedure that can be chosen depending on the specific application. Fig. 5.**5** shows the formation of a maximum of two fuzzy sets in such an aggregation procedure.

▬ Example: Interpretation of Regulation Thermograms

Regulation thermography offers a typical example for the application of a rule-based expert system. This diagnostic procedure of complementary medicine is based on recognition and evaluation of pathological patterns in body temperature. In the field of complementary medicine within oncology, much expert knowledge exists for the detection of breast cancer and gastrointestinal cancers using the methods of thermography. It plays a part, not only when determining patterns to be recognized, but also in their interpretation for diagnosis.

Regulation Thermography

The functions of the human body depend largely on its temperature. In order to maintain an optimal distribution of temperature throughout the body, it possesses a complex control and regulating system, the center of which is located in the hypothalamic region of the brain. For example, in reaction to incoming impulses in this region from cold or warm receptors, the production of heat in the organism can be regulated by increasing or decreasing metabolic activity. Regulatory impulses run from the brain to the skin as well, where they can influence the amount of heat that is perspired through contraction of blood vessels. The nerves through which these impulses pass can interact with nerves running within the spinal column from the internal organs to the brain. In this way a pathological disturbance within an organ can lead to a change in thermal regulation of the skin—this is referred to as a **reflex arc**.

Regulation thermography attempts to measure and interpret these changes in the regulatory behavior. The goal is to associate certain changes in regulatory behavior with specific diseases. According to expert opinion, this is possible: an extensive pool of pathological temperature patterns and their diagnostic interpretation is available.

Regulatory behavior is determined by the twofold measurement of the test person's body temperature on defined parts of the body (**areas**). The first measurement ensues after the test person has undressed in an examination room with standardized temperature and humidity. The room temperature should be below normal body temperature, which induces a cold stimulus that, in turn, stimulates the regulatory system of the body. After a defined period of time the measurement is repeated. The body will then have reacted to the cold stimulus. The comparison between the first and second measurements allows a conclusion to be drawn as to the regulatory activity of the skin.

The entirety of the measured temperatures is referred to as a **regulation thermogram**. Fig. 5.6 depicts an ideal thermogram in form of a histogram: shown as the temperature values of 60 areas. Abbreviated designations for areas can be seen on the horizontal axis above on the diagram, the first temperature measurements are the black rectangles and the second are blue. All rectangles refer to the horizontal black line, the forehead temperature (measured first). The individual tem-

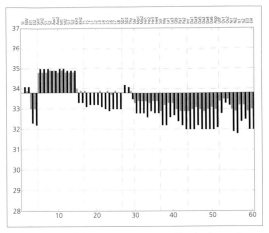

Fig. 5.**6** An ideal thermogram presented in the form of a histogram.

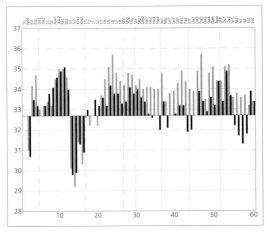

Fig. 5.**7** For comparison, the thermogram of a woman with mammary carcinoma.

perature values can be read on the left vertical axis. Figure 5.**7** depicts a pathological thermogram of a woman with breast cancer.

Fuzzy Modeling of Expert Knowledge

The regulation thermogram encompasses temperature measurements at 110 areas. Expert knowledge of pathological activity in three areas within the thoracic regions—the sternum, as well as the two asymmetrically aligned pectoral muscle areas—serves as an example in the following thermogram.

These areas are used during evaluation of thermograms in reference to breast cancer in women. All further numeric values mentioned are more or less accurate (according to current scientific standards), but are to be taken merely as examples.

The following validation criteria are applied to all three areas:

- **Absolute temperature** For each area, the difference between the first value at the area and the first value on the forehead is tested. Differences in temperature smaller than –0.8 °K and bigger than +0.2 °K are considered pathological. The first event is termed a **cold area**, while the latter case is considered a **hot area**. Overstepping or falling short of the indicated boundaries is considered to be all the more pathological, the more pronounced the deviation.
- **Regulation** In this case, the difference between the first and second measurement is observed for each area. If the difference falls below –1.1 °K, this indicates a so-called **hyperregulation**. Exceeding beyond the value –0.25 °K, a phenomenon known as **paradoxical regulation**, is also considered pathological. When comparing hyperregulation with paradoxical regulation, the first is regarded to be less pathological.

The pathologies of absolute temperature and regulation should be added for a combined overall rating. This occurs according to the following guidelines:

- Regulation pathologies carry more weight than absolute temperature.
- When both pectoral muscle areas exhibit different activities, the more pathological of the two is included in the final assessment.
- Activity of the sternum area and the more pathological pectoral muscle areas are of equal importance.

The valuation rules suggest fuzzy modeling using two linguistic variables: "Abs Temp" as one variable to designate the absolute temperature of one area, with the linguistic values "normal," "cold," and "warm"; "Reg" as another variable with the values "normal," "hyper," and "paradox" to record the observed regulation.

Now these linguistic values need to be specified through indication of fuzzy sets. Figure 5.8 shows the fuzzy amounts of the values of the variable "Reg." These were determined using temperature values denoted in the valuation rules, otherwise modeling was kept fairly simple, since no further information was specified.

An observed regulation of –0.1 °K as measured at the sternum area was classified, for example, as paradoxical with a degree of pathology approximately 0.8, as normal with a degree of approximately 0.2, and as hyperregulation with a degree of 0.

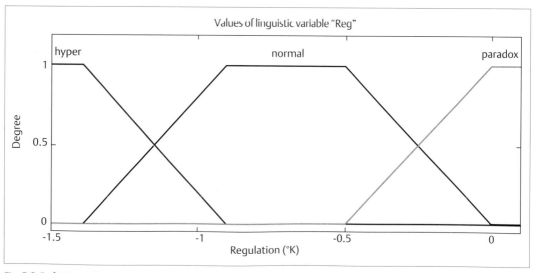

Fig. 5.**8** Definition of linguistic values.

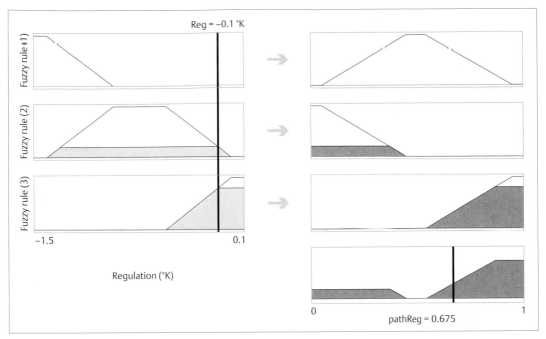

Fig. 5.**9** Evaluation of a block of three fuzzy rules.

The assessment of an area as pathologically active is determined based on linguistic variables, separately for absolute temperature and regulation, respectively. For regulation, "PathReg" is the variable used, for example. Attributed linguistic values would be "negative" (no pathological activity), "positive" (pathological activity is present) and "suspicion" (suspicion of pathological activity). As already described, a fuzzy set is determined for these linguistic values based on pre-existing knowledge.

The expert rulings for assessment of regulation of each of the three respective areas can now be expressed by way of fuzzy rules as follows:
1. If (Reg = hyper), then (PathReg = suspicion)
2. If (Reg = normal), then (PathReg = negative)
3. If (Reg = paradoxical), then (PathReg = positive)

The application of this block of rules should offer the user a "degree of pathology" for regulation observed in the respective area. Figure 5.**9** demonstrates the process for determining the degree of pathology for an entered value of –0.1 °K for the regulation: it is at approximately 0.68, clearly indicating a pathological activity in the observed area (0.0 = nonapplication of a fuzzy assertion; 1.0 = accuracy of a fuzzy assertion).

In Figure 5.**9** the first three lines of the graphic stand for the three fuzzy rules in the sequence of appearance (1–3): on the left side you see the fuzzy sets for each of the linguistic values of the variable "Reg" of the respective rule. The vertical line represents the observed regulatory value of –0.1 °K; the height of the gray areas denote the degree of truth of the denotations "Reg = hyper," "Reg = normal" or "Reg = paradox."

On the right side you see the fuzzy sets for the linguistic values of the variables "PathReg." The heights of the blue surfaces show the true values for "PathReg = suspected" or "PathReg = negative," or "PathReg = positive."

The last line of the graphic entails the result of aggregation and defuzzification: the end result— the degree of pathology of regulation at an area—is depicted by a vertical bar.

Figure 5.**10** gives an overall oversight of the dependency of the degree of pathology on regulation in areas observed.

In a similar way, expert behavior on activity of absolute temperatures can be gathered with the help of linguistic variables for absolute temperatures and likewise linguistic variables for the degree of pathology of absolute temperature.

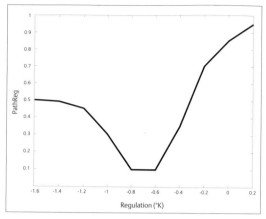

Fig. 5.**10** Correlation between regulation and degree of pathology.

Finally, the determined degree of pathology for absolute temperatures and regulations of all three areas must be combined to yield a single value.

This occurs in two steps: first, a weighted mean value is determined from the degrees of pathology and regulation for each area. The fact that regulation carries more weight is accounted for. In the second step the third line of expert rules are followed by combining the mean with the maximum of the just calculated degree of pathology in the three areas.

The minimum degrees of pathology can be seen to lie between –0.8 °K and –0.6 °K. The visible increment in degree of pathology in the left branch of the function graphic shows the increasing hyperregulation. The right branch shows paradox regulation. According to expert opinion, much higher degrees of pathology are reached here in comparison to the left branch. One can discern the minimum degrees of pathology to fall between the values –0.8 °K and –0.6 °K. The notable increase in degree of pathology of the left branch of the function of the graph indicates the increasing hyperregulation. Paradox regulation is represented by the right branch in the graph. Here considerably higher degrees of pathology are reached than in the left branch.

Design of an Expert System for Regulation Thermography

Regulation Thermography lends itself not only to the presentation of knowledge via fuzzy logic, but also other points important for the programming of a medical expert system can be elucidated with this example.

Creating a Body of Rules

The construction of fuzzy rules on the basis of existing knowledge is basically also possible for the layman. Nonetheless, some steps are necessary during this process, which may require the collaboration between a medical expert and mathematician: the choice of methods to be used for logical implication as well as aggregation and defuzzification. These methods are, for the most part, determined at the beginning of the development process of a system and are left unaltered in the once functioning expert system. Nevertheless, they are dependent on mode of application and must be chosen via engagement with a medical expert.

Specification of linguistic values of fuzzy sets is a different story: in this case expert knowledge is incorporated, and the special structure of fuzzy sets must be determined. In the example of "elevated body temperature" this is given by the curve depicted in blue (see Fig. 5.**3**, p. 57).

The medical expert normally does not have a preconceived notion of such a structure. This frequently evolves either indirectly from existing knowledge or it must be determined through the iterative process of trial and error: a backbone network appropriate for the respective linguistic value is primarily set up, and then changes are made to the details until they show the desired activity within the expert system. The latter can naturally only be appraised in dialogue with a medical expert.

Automatic Generation of Rules/ Hypotheses

The adaptive process for the definiton of fuzzy sets described above can partially be automated, given the appropriate data: a physician must specify the desired output for a sufficiently large amount of input data into the expert system, based on his or her expertise. Following entry of this training data set into the expert system, the actual output is compared with the desired output. On the basis of comparison, the system is modified. This process is repeated until a satisfactory accord between desired and actual output is achieved. The modification does not necessarily need to be performed manually, but can be done using a computer software program.

The process of automation of system modification can be taken even a step further: given a training data set that is extensive enough, fuzzy rules can directly be extracted from the latter using various mathematical procedures, and integrated into the system's rule databank. The physician is then able to read these rules and verify their meaning, possibly even testing them as hypotheses.

Neuronal Networks

Instead of using training data sets to develop fuzzy rules, the desired system output can also be reproduced directly by creating a mathematical mapping. When input and output data are numerical values, they lend themselves well to neuronal networks. They can be easily and swiftly modified to account for additional new training data sets, thereby enabling a constant stream of learning.

The disadvantage vs. the automatically generated fuzzy rules is that the developed depictions using neuronal networks are generally not useful for medical interpretation. Combination of fuzzy rules with neuronal networks is widely used and usually leads to improvement in quality of output.

In the realm of complementary oncology, regulation thermography is used, among others, for

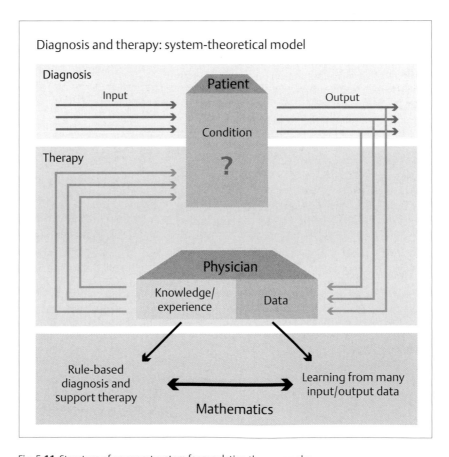

Fig. 5.**11** Structure of an expert system for regulation thermography.

early detection of cancer. Depending on the pathological temperature patterns in the thermogram a six-point scale (0–5) is devised to indicate tumor-cell activity (TCA): A TCA of 0 designates "no trace of tumor-cell activity detectable within the body." The more pronounced the observed pathological patterns are, the higher the value will be for TCA.

From the 220 temperature values comprising the thermogram, the TCA is determined to represent the classification profile. This is a situation in which neuronal networks can be applied directly: a neuronal network trained on the basis of a data set commensurate in size can deliver an approximated TCA classification of new thermograms not entailed within the training data set.

Within the context of expert systems for regulation thermography there is yet another area of application for neuronal networks: expertise for determination of TCA classification can be divided into "global" and "local" rules. The thermogram can be subdivided into 10 groups of areas that do not overlap. For each of these groups of areas there is a set of expert rules that are only used by this group and indicate a "degree of pathology" when taken together. The degrees of pathology of the individual groups are ultimately merged through "global" rules for TCA. These rules are far more difficult to determine than their "local" counterpart. It therefore makes sense to (additionally) utilize well-suited neuronal networks at this point: as input the degrees of pathology of the groups of areas are taken, and as output the TCA of a thermogram is measured.

In total, the result for the case of regulation thermography is the following extension (Fig. 5.**11**) of the expert system structure shown in Fig. 5.**2**: a neuronal network has been added for approximate estimation of TCA directly from the thermogram. A so-called neuro-fuzzy system allows for extraction of rules from a set of data as well as providing a neuronal network for determination of TCA from the 10 degrees of pathology of the area groups. Both components can be delivered and trained with data via a training module as specified by a medical expert.

▬ Further Reading

Bothe H-H: Fuzzy Logic. Berlin–Heidelberg: Springer; 1995.

Kruse R, Gebhardt J, Klawonn F: Fuzzy-Systeme. Stuttgart: Teubner; 1993.

Nauk D, Klawonn F, Kruse R. Neuronale Netze und Fuzzy-Systeme. Braunschweig: Vieweg; 1996.

Pedrycz W. Fuzzy Control and Fuzzy Systems. Winnipeg: John Wiley & Sons Inc.; 1989.

Rost A. Lehrbuch der Regulationstherapie. Stuttgart: Hippokrates; 1994.

6 Observational Studies on Drugs Efficacy

Berthold Schneider

Introduction

As early as 1864, C.A.Wunderlich, a clinician from Leipzig differentiated between "rational medicine" and "empirical medicine." (16) This distinction is still made today, even though proponents of the former still deem themselves superior to the latter as followers of conventional medicine, while followers of empirical medicine point to past successes and to wide acceptance by the population.

In reality, these categories are more complicated. Primarily, medicine, even conventional medicine, is a science based on experience. Insights are conscious beliefs or models that we make, based on perceptions of ourselves and our environment, to help us understand our world better. The way in which we process insights, based on sensory perceptions of our experience, is primarily determined genetically. The actual specifications depend on many historically developed or newly acquired influences and circumstances. Thus, there are various ways of gaining insight, and there are different insights based on the same experiences.

This is also the reason that we have so many different schools and directions within medicine. The designation "complementary medicine" is more accurate than the term "empirical medicine," for example. This serves to clarify that even conventional medicine is based on experience, and that complementary medicine is also based on rational reasoning. The term also means that the methods and the considerations and models behind these methods in complementary medicine do not stand in contrast to, but are an extension to the accepted and established methods and considerations in the traditional school of thought in medicine.

Therapeutic Efficacy and Proof of Efficacy

According to the verdict by the German Federal Administrative Court (Bundesverwaltungsgericht) in October 1993, therapeutic efficacy is "insufficiently established if it does not follow from the documents provided that the application of a certain medicine will lead to a larger number of therapeutic successes than its nonapplication, according to current scientific insights and knowledge." (4) According to this, efficacy is the trait of a drug that can incur more cures in patients, or at least alleviation of symptoms, than would be possible to achieve without it.

The proof of efficacy resides on three pillars:
- **Causality:** changes that are expected in a patient through application are compared with changes without application.
- **Universality:** efficacy must not only be applicable to individually selected patients, but also for all prospective users of the agent.
- **Objectivity:** the procedure with which the assertions are made must be clearly delineated so that they can be repeated and verified.

In order to make a declaration on the future efficacy of a drug, the experiences and observations of previous applications and nonapplications must be taken into consideration. Statements pertaining to efficacy require an inductive reasoning from known observations to unknown, future events, which can be done through the use of probability and statistical analyses.

The probability for a certain result of an event (e. g., curing a patient by use of a particular medicine) is thus a measure of reliability with which a result can be repeatedly obtained and expected in the future. Using this measure of probability, the efficacy of a drug can be described as follows:

> A drug is effective if the probability of therapeutic success given application is higher than without application of the drug.

The proof of efficacy demands a comparison of probabilities for therapeutic success that is defined by determination of a **primary outcome measure**. This can be cure, or at least a visible improvement at the end of treatment. With treatment of symptoms, one can take the symptom being treated as the outcome measure, e. g., reduction of blood pressure when treating for hypertension.

For efficacy, the difference in the distribution of probability of the outcome measure, between treated and untreated patients, is decisive. This difference is termed the **effect size.** This can be, for example, when using the outcome measure "cure," the difference between the probability of a cure in the test group vs. the control group, or the ratio of respective probabilities (meaning the relationship between the "cure rate" and the rate for "no cure"). When dealing with quantitative outcome measures, such as reduction in blood pressure, one often resorts to outcome measures such as the difference in expected values, whereas when dealing with the duration until reaching a cure or improvement in the patient one would choose the difference of median periods until improvement, based on the total of all possible results.

Controlled Clinical Trials

Once outcome measures and effect sizes are determined, the effect sizes and **confidence interval** (CI) are estimated. Given an appropriate testing procedure, it is then decided whether efficacy can be claimed. For this, data from both a **control group** and a **test group** are needed.

Given these, one can only receive a valid (unbiased) estimate, if the patients in both groups are comparable (structurally similar) in relevant starting and treatment terms. This is warranted in controlled clinical trials, in which patient allocation to the test group or to the control group occurs in a **randomized** fashion.

Usually a similar number of patients are distributed to both the control and the test group, but differences in distribution rates are sometimes possible. The patients in the test group are treated with the drug to be tested, those in the control group with a comparable agent (either placebo or a standard drug). Otherwise the treatment terms and evaluation of results should be the same for both groups as is determined and documented in the protocol.

Through the random allocation, and given the equality in all other treatment terms, structural consistency is guaranteed. In order to eliminate the influence of awareness of the assigned treatment, distribution of drug can be performed **double-blinded**, in other words, neither the treating doctor nor the patient receiving the treatment is aware of what kind of medicine he or she is receiving, or what group he or she belongs to (given that this is ethical and feasible).

> The controlled clinical trial is the only type of study currently approved for medicines for which the efficacy and safety is still completely unknown.

Cohort Studies

Particularly within the field of complementary oncology, there are numerous procedures that have been applied for years, whose efficacy and safety has never been tested in controlled clinical trials. Patient records contain information as to results (such as changes in status of disease) achieved by these methods. It lends itself to utilize this information for proof of efficacy and safety. The type of study that would come into question is the epidemiological cohort study.

Study Design

Cohort studies are epidemiological population studies. Using them should help in examining the relations between various procedures and factors that influence health (e.g., treatment measures, habits, environmental factors), and the health condition—or changes thereof—in the population.

These measures or factors are not determined in the study, but emerge out of the actual situation.

Herein lies the essential difference to controlled clinical trials, in which procedures applied to patients are determined at random. Controlled studies are "experiments" on patients in which an answer is wrenched from nature through determination of the general conditions and systematic specification of test and control group treatment. In comparison, cohort studies are "observational studies" in which no artificial situation is produced and nature is not coerced, but simply systematically observed.

Should cohort studies serve as proof of efficacy for a certain drug (test treatment) for a specific type of disease, patients must be chosen that are representative for this disease from the general population.

In addition to the test treatment, other treatments for the disease should be used in this population, and these may then serve as control treatments. Since the treatments are not predetermined, it is not necessary to include only new treatment patients into the study whose findings are prospectively collected and documented. One may also resort to files of aleady documented and completed cases and collect the data retrospectively (8). Given the increasing use of good information systems for physicians and clinics with well-structured databanks, conducting such studies in the future should become much easier.

When planning and conducting **retrospective cohort studies**, the same general guidelines apply as have been established by the German Federal Institute for Drugs and Medical Devices (BfArM) (3):

- The study design must specify the responsibilities (director of the study, coordinator, monitoring, biometrics, sponsor).
- The purpose and precise question of the study need to be formulated.
- The selection of patients (or patient files) has to be determined. For this purpose, a representative selection is to be made of eligible treatment facilities (practices, clinics, outpatient follow-up clinics), in which patients with the disease to be studied can receive the test treatment as well as the control treatment.
- The procedures needed to achieve representation must be described.
- Specific inclusion and exclusion criteria for all patients whose data have been collected must be given.
- Inclusion criteria require determination of period of treatment and reasons for treatment (diagnosis, indications, initial state).
- The findings that are collected through patient files must be clearly named (demographic data, medical history, diagnostic findings, performed procedures, initial findings, progressive findings of treatment course, special events, treatment results). The relevance of these findings for query of the study should be explained. It should be specified which findings are primary, and which are secondary, outcome measures (or are important for determining these outcome measures) and which are concomitant or disruptive measures.
- Test treatments, control treatments, and additional treatments must be named and justified.
- The extent and type of specifications to be documented must be determined (e. g., designation of compounds, pharmaceutical form, dosage, duration, and type of treatment (continuous therapy, intermittent, or as needed).
- Plans for concepts for evaluation as well as regulations (see below) for construction of report.
- The number of patients intended should be justified.
- Data from all patients that are included by the criteria, and do not show any exclusion criteria, are to be collected and documented. In the event that the data are saved on a databank that has been verified for completeness, accuracy, and plausibility, these data can merely be transferred to a data set to be evaluated. If the medical histories are present only in paper form, they must be transferred to case report forms (CRF). The accuracy of the transferal should be controlled through independent monitors. The data of the case report forms must then be entered into the databank system and verified for completeness, accuracy, and plausibility.
- Besides patient data, specifications of treatment centers that are relevant for the query of the study (e. g., specialization of the treating doctors, specification of the treatment center) are to be collected and saved. The type of retrieval and documentation (e. g., the databank system used) is declared in the study protocol.

Concept for Evaluation

In cohort studies, allocation of treatment to patients occurs primarily according to decisions made by physicians or patients. It can be seen as a random incident, whose distribution depends on various parameters of the treatment facility and patients ("co-variables"). These variables will generally also influence the treatment outcome, and a direct comparison between test and control group is no longer possible. Test and control group can no longer be seen as identical in structure. This is the reason, why the effect size (see above) cannot be directly assessed from the data.

One of the main problems in evaluation is to even out the influence of these co-variables on treatment outcome and thereby allow an unbiased comparison of treatment success between the two therapeutic groups.

There are two approaches to accomplish this:

- During **stratification**, subgroups (strata) with similar values in their co-variables are devised. The comparison between control group and test group (estimation of effect size) occurs within the subgroups. The comparative results are summarized in adequate form based on subgroups (9). The **matched-pairs technique** constitutes a special type of stratification in which the subgroup consists of both a patient pair and similar values for co-variables, in which one patient receives the test treatment while the other receives the control treatment.

- In **analysis of co-variance**, the dependency of therapeutic success on co-variables is conceived via an adequate function (usually a linear function of the scaled and transformed respective co-variables). With this function, the observed therapeutic results are converted to a common reference value of the co-variables and these (cleansed) results are then compared between the treatment groups.

Naturally, this adjustment can only be performed for those co-variables that were collected in the study. For a good adjustment, it is therefore necessary to gather as many reliable co-variables as possible. Practical problems arise, however, in both equalization methods. Stratification according to 10 or more co-variables is practically not feasible. If each co-variable has just two characteristics (such as "present" and "not present"), then 1024 combinations already exist, according to which stratification should be performed. Functions for adjustments with many co-variables can lead to problems, especially if interdependent influence of co-variables (so-called reciprocate influences) is also taken into consideration.

These problems are surmounted by use of a **balancing score**. This is a function of all co-variables that could possibly influence treatment allocation, so that at a given value of this function the distribution is independent of the co-variables. To achieve adjustment, stratification according to all possible combinations is no longer necessary: one only needs to stratify according to the values of the function, or clear therapeutic efficacy with the one function of balancing score.

A balancing score that lends itself for observational studies is the probability of the allocation of test treatment as a function of the co-variable ("allocation score" or "propensity score") (12, 13). If the function entails all the co-variables that influence treatment allocation, stratification—or better co-variance analysis—according to propensity score offers an optimal adjustment. In this case,

following adjustment using the allocation score the therapeutic comparison is as unbiased, and valid, as with random distribution.

Beyond that, the propensity score offers other valuable information on the conditions and variables that induce doctors in practice to apply a certain test treatment. Generally, the advantage of cohort studies vs. randomized studies is that they offer a pristine picture of practical application of the medicine, and can also point out risks that cannot be determined in controlled trials (5).

The practicality and effectiveness of a balancing score was demonstrated in several observational studies (2, 6, 11, 14, 15). In an extensive comparison of controlled clinical trials and observational studies it was shown that therapeutic effects estimated by applied observations did not differ in quality, nor were they consistently larger than the results achieved by randomized, controlled studies (1).

Meanwhile, the use of epidemiological cohort studies has gained acceptance as a valid means of verification of efficacy and safety of drugs, at least under certain conditions according to European law. In the aforementioned recommendations of the BfArM (3), it is stated that "the proof of efficacy by observational studies alone is not possible, with the exception of special justified cases"; however, this limitation is put into perspective by a footnote: "as long as substantial, understandably documented, plausible empirical knowledge is available for known drugs, a carefully designed observational study may facilitate the acceptance of efficacy statements for a given indication. Concerning the possible use of observational study results in those special cases in which it is not possible to perform clinical trials, each case must be decided individually."

Guidelines 1999/83/EG of the EG Commission play an even more pivotal role in the proof of efficacy for observational studies, according to which a "bibliographical reference to other sources of information (e. g., postmarketing studies, epidemiological studies, trials conducted with similar compounds) accounts for a valid verification for safety and efficacy of a product—not just trials and studies for proof—given that the applicant has sufficiently explained and given reasons for citing these references." (7) This ruling is now in effect.

Observational studies are not only important for proving efficacy in the accreditation of drugs.

They also play a big part in pharmacoepidemiology.

▬ Example of a Cohort Study in Oncology

With a retrospective cohort study the efficacy and tolerability of a complementary oral enzyme therapy in postoperative treatment of breast cancer patients is studied (2). All records were retrieved between 1991 and 1997 from patients who had received postoperative follow-up for primary, non-metastatic breast cancer in 128 treatment centers (practices, hospitals, outpatient follow-up clinics, oncology practices). Additionally to antineoplastic therapy (radiation, adjuvant chemotherapy, systematic hormone therapy), an oral enzyme therapy was given to some of these patients in these institutions as follow-up treatment. The ages of the patients at the time of follow-up was between 18 and 80 years old.

Patients that fulfilled these entry criteria (non-metastatic breast cancer, follow-up between 1991 and 1997) based on the charts, had their data on medical history, recordings on given treatments, and treatment results transcribed to a standardized report sheet and entered into a databank. The plausibility and accuracy of the data were verified. Patients that additionally received proteolytic enzyme therapy in follow-up in addition to standard

Table 6.1 Effect of proteolytic enzymtherapy during the follow-up after breast cancer surgery. Frequency distribution of various patient and treatment characteristics in test and control groups		
	Test group	**Control group**
Age at start of follow-up (years)	Mean value: 59 (± 10)*	Mean value: 60 (± 12)
Duration of follow-up (days)	Mean value: 609 (± 476)	Mean value: 441 (± 462)
Postoperative condition		
Complete remission	224 (94.9%)	352 (94.9%)
Partial remission	11 (4.7%)	16 (4.3%)
Minimal recovery	1 (0.4%)	3 (0.8%)
UICC Stage**		
0 or I	81 (35.4%)	148 (37.9%)
IIa	92 (40.2%)	129 (33.0%)
IIb	43 (18.8%)	77 (19.7%)
IIIa or higher	13 (5.7%)	37 (9.4%)
Radiation		
No	84 (35.1%)	113 (27.6%)
Yes	155 (64.9%)	297 (72.4%)
Chemotherapy		
No	188 (78.7%)	284 (69.3%)
Yes	51 (21.3%)	126 (30.7%)
Hormone Therapy		
No	145 (60.7%)	180 (43.8%)
Yes	94 (39.3%)	230 (56.1%)
Physical therapy		
No	211 (88.3%)	325 (79.3%)
Yes	28 (11.7%)	85 (20.7%)
Treating physician		
General practitioner	155 (64.9%)	87 (21.2%)
Internist	11 (4.6%)	40 (9.8%)
Gynecologist	20 (8.4%)	47 (11.5%)
Oncologist	1 (0.4%)	151 (36.8%)
Radiologist	49 (20.5%)	85 (20.7%)
Age of treating physician		
Up to 45 years	65 (36.3%)	245 (62.7%)
Above 45 years	114 (63.7%)	146 (37.3%)

* Standard deviation; ** International Union Against Cancer

therapy, made up the test group, patients who did not receive standard therapy comprised the control group. Data from 649 patients were collected for evaluation, of which 239 (37 %) belonged to the test group and 410 (63 %) to the control group.

Since distribution to test group and control group did not occur in a randomized fashion, differences in patient characteristics and characteristics of the treatment facility were to be expected between the two groups. Table 6.1 shows the frequency distribution for some relevant characteristics for the two groups.

The womens' ages were similarly distributed at the start of follow-up. The median duration of follow-up was quite different between the two groups (609 days in the test group and 441 days in the control group). The condition after surgery (response) and postoperative UICC (International Union against Cancer) staging was similarly distributed in both groups.

In terms of applied follow-up treatment there were larger differences to be seen, however. Hormone therapy in the test group was given to 39.3 % while in the control group 56.1 % received this treatment. Particularly pronounced are the differences in treatment centers, especially in the age and specialty of the treating physician. Of the women in the test group 64.9 % were treated by a general practitioner, while this was only the case in 21.2 % of the patients in the control group. The percentage of patients seen by an oncologist was 0.4 % in the test group (one patient) and 36.8 % in the control group. Of the patients in the test group, 63.7 % were treated by a physician over 45 years old, while this was the case in only 37.3 % of patients in the control group.

Due to this lack of homogeneity between the two treatment groups, a direct comparison of the results is not possible, since they were influenced by different starting and ending conditions, and any comparison is therefore likely to be skewed. In order to achieve an unbiased comparison for therapy, the treatment results must be cleared from the influence of any possible disturbance variables. This can occur with the help of the **propensity score**, with the probability for distribution of a patient to the test group as a function of all relevant patient and treatment characteristics.

The propensity score can be estimated using logistic regression analysis based on data in the study. In this regression it is assumed that the logarithm of the ratio for the test group (the ratio of the probability P for the assignment to the group to the probability $1 - P$ for the assignment to the control group) is a linear function of the relevant characteristics. In terms of a formula, this logistic function would look like this:

$$\text{Log } P/1 - P = \beta_0 + \beta_1 x_1 \dots \beta_k x_k$$

Where $x_1, \dots x_k$ symbolize the values of patient and treatment characteristics (influencing variables) and $\beta_0 \dots \beta_1, \beta_k$ represent the respective coefficients of the linear function. For the co-variable x_i, the coefficient β_i designates how far the logarithm of the ratio has changed when the value of the variable is increased by one unit.

Quantitative co-variables, such as the age or the duration of follow-up, can be employed directly.

Categorical co-variables, such as, for example, a physician's specialty or the implementation of radiation, must be re-coded into quantitative variables. This is easy for binary categorical variables, such as implementation of radiation therapy, where a category is either present or not present. If a category is present, the variable is coded with a 1, otherwise with 0.

For categorical variables with more than two categories a category is chosen as a reference (e. g., for specialty the category "family practitioner"). For the remaining categories dummy variables are introduced that are given the value 1 when a category is present, otherwise the value 0. The reference category is present when all dummy variables have the value 0. It is not individually designated by its own variable.

For logistic regression of the co-variables shown in Table 6.1 the following quantitative variable was used:

x_1 – age in years
x_2 – duration of follow-up in days.

For status postoperatively "complete remission" was chosen as the reference category. The remaining categories were coded with dummy variables:

x_3 – 1 at partial remission
x_4 – 1 at minimal increase.

With the UICC stages, stage 0 or 1 was taken as a reference category. The remaining categories were coded:

x_5 – 1 at stage IIa
x_6 – 1 at stage IIb
x_7 – 1 at stage IIIa or higher.

The remaining categories were coded with 1, when the respective therapy was given, otherwise with 0:

x_8 – radiation therapy
x_9 – chemotherapy
x_{10} – hormone therapy
x_{11} – physical therapy.

With the specialty of the treating physician "family practitioner" was used as a reference category. The other categories were coded as follows:

x_{12} – 1 for the internist
x_{13} – 1 for the gynecologist
x_{14} – 1 for the oncologist
x_{15} – 1 for the radiologist
x_{16} – the age of the treating physician, was coded by 0 for an age up to 45 years, and with a 1 for an age above 45 years.

From the study data coefficients β_i are estimated according to maximum likelihood method. The **likelihood** is the probability for the observed random spot check result as a function for the unknown parameters. As a random sample result, it is of interest whether the patient was allocated to the test group or the control group.

The probability that a patient with the influencing variables $x_1, \dots x_k$ is allocated to the test group is:

$$P(x_1, \dots x_k; \beta_0, \beta_1 \dots \beta_k)$$

and the probability that they are allocated to the control group is:

$$1 - P(x_1, \dots x_k; \beta_0, \beta_1 \dots \beta_k).$$

The exact type of these functions is determined by logistic equations. The probability depends on the unknown parameters $\beta_0, \beta_1 \dots \beta_k$.

Since the distribution to the groups is random for the various patients, the likelihood is the product of this probability across all patients in the study, in which P is taken to represent one patient in the test group, and $1 - P$ to represent another patient in the control group.

Table 6.2 Coefficients b_i and odds ratios $\exp(b_i)$ (with 95 % confidence interval and statistical significance P) of the co-variables of the propensity score

Influencing Variable	b_i	$\exp(b_i)$	95% Confidence interval	Significance P
x_1 – age (years)	–0.030	0.971	0.950–0.992	0.008
x_2 – duration of follow-up (days)	0.000	1.000	0.999–1.000	0.991
Postoperative condition				
x_3 – partial remission	–0.250	0.779	0.175–1.455	0.205
x_4 – minimal recovery	0.536	1.709	0.097–30.140	0.714
UICC Stage*				
x_5 – IIa	0.124	1.132	0.654–1.960	0.657
x_6 – IIb	0.217	1.242	0.606–2.548	0.554
x_7 – IIIa or higher	–0.026	0.974	0.368–2.581	0.958
x_8 – radiation	0.064	1.066	0.633–1.796	0.810
x_9 – chemotherapy	–0.810	0.445	0.239–0.827	0.010
x_{10} – hormone therapy	–1.370	0.254	0.148–0.435	<0.001
x_{11} – physical therapy	–0.852	0.427	0.221–0.823	0.011
Treating physician				
x_{12} – internist	–1.292	0.275	0.113–0.668	0.004
x_{13} – gynecologist	–1.282	0.278	0.138–0.557	<0.001
x_{14} – oncologist	–5.244	0.005	0.001–0.041	<0.001
x_{15} – radiologist	–0.293	0.746	0.376–1.483	0.403
x_{16} – physician's age > 45 years	0.570	1.768	1.040–3.003	0.035
Constant b_0	2.651	14.163		

* International Union against Cancer

Estimated values b_0, b_1, ... b of coefficients are those values, in which the likelihood takes on a maximum. Maximization can be performed in an appropriately small statistical packet, such as SPSS or SAS.

The estimated b_i coefficients for the co-variables shown in Table 6.**1** are listed in Table 6.**2**.

For interpretation, the expression $exp(b_i)$ lends itself for binary variables coded with 0 or 1 rather than the coefficient b_i. The term $exp(b_i)$ stands for the odds ratio for distribution to the test group; it indicates by how much the distribution ratio changes, when a certain variable is present (in comparison to the ratio when the variable is missing). With a relative ratio of > 1, the ratio (and thereby also the probability) for assignment to the test group is larger than for the assignment to the control group; with a relative ratio of < 1 it is smaller. In Table 6.**2** $exp(b_i)$ and the 95 % confidence interval are listed in addition to b_i.

If the confidence interval covers the value 1, the influence of the respective variables is insignificant. Additionally, the probability of significance is given by the *P* value. This is the probability that the estimated value $exp(b_i)$ or one larger than that (when estimated values are < 1) is to be expected when the total odds ratio is exactly 1. When the confidence interval does not include the value 1, $P < 0.05$.

The term b_0 is the estimated value of the coefficients ($_0$, that indicates the value of log $(P/[1 - P])$ for the event that all variables x_i are 0. This term is needed for calculation of the ratios $P/(1 - P)$ for the given x_i values.

Table 6.**2** shows that group distribution was particularly dependent on the specialty and the age of the treating physician, on the treatments received (especially hormone treatment), and (to a lesser extent) on the patient's age. The postoperative condition (remission, UICC stage) and the duration of follow-up did not have any bearing on group distribution.

This is consistent with the data in Table 6.**1**, in which the distribution of age and specialty of the physician and the treatment received were particularly different amongst the two groups. General practitioners and older doctors in follow-up treatment particularly prescribed oral enzyme therapy, whereas internists and gynecologists and particularly oncologists decided to forego this. Additional enzyme therapy was rarely given together with application of chemotherapy, radiation, and especially hormone therapy, in contrast to when these treatment forms were not given.

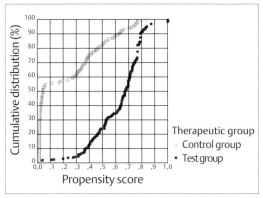

Fig. 6.1 Cumulative frequency distribution of the propensity score in both groups.

Table 6.3 Frequency of some characteristics in test and control groups within strata			
Category	Propensity score	Test group	Control group
General practitioner	0.3–0.6	39 %	45 %
	0.6–1.0	80 %	62 %
Physician's age ≤ 45 years	0.3–0.6	30 %	41 %
	0.6–1.0	39 %	26 %
Radiation	0.3–0.6	71 %	61 %
	0.6–1.0	37 %	42 %
Chemotherapy	0.3–0.6	69 %	77 %
	0.6–1.0	85 %	67 %
Hormone therapy	0.3–0.6	75 %	75 %
	0.6–1.0	21 %	5 %
Physical therapy	0.3–0.6	19 %	17 %
	0.6–1.0	7 %	11 %

Variables incorporated into calculation of the propensity score can help predict the distribution group with 78% accuracy, when the patient has a predicted propensity score of 0.5 or more for distribution to the test group, and less than 0.5 for the control group. This indicates, that the probability for assignment to the test group was very accurately gathered using the variables. This can also be observed in the cumulative distribution of frequency (empirical distribution frequency) of the propensity scores in both groups as seen in Fig. 6.**1**. Of the patients in the control group, 60% had a propensity score of 0.3, while only 5% of patients in the test group had such a low propensity score.

In order to be able to verify the balance between the therapeutic groups within the classes of propensity scores, classes from 0.3 to 0.6 and from 0.6 to 1.0 were made, and the frequencies of selected categories of co-variables for both groups compared within these classes.

The class of 0 to 0.3 was not suitable for observation, since only eight patients had such a low propensity score and the frequencies showed much variability. The results are shown in Table 6.**3**.

The class of 0.3 to 0.6 contained 182 patients, of which 75 belonged to the test group and 107 to the control group.

The class of 0.6 to 1 contained 200 patients, of which 155 belonged to the test group and 45 to the control group.

The frequencies of the selected categories were notably more homogenous within the propensity score classes between the two groups, than in the total count. The bigger differences between the groups in the class of 0.6 to 1 can be traced back to the fact that, in this class, only 45 patients belonged to the control group and therefore there were high rates of variability.

The primary goal of the study was to examine whether disease-related or treatment-related complaints can be reduced by supplementary oral enzyme therapy, compared with no such therapy. Such disturbances included:

– gastrointestinal complaints
– general complaints
– dyspnea
– headaches
– tumor-related pain
– cachexia
– skin reactions
– infections.

Based on patient files it was determined whether a patient suffered such complaints during her fol-

Complaints	Group	Patients n	Success n (%)	Raw odds ratio	Adjusted odds ratio	95% Confidence interval	Significance P
Gastrointestinal	Test	140	59 (42%)				
	Control	203	74 (36%)	1.270	1.843	1.022–3.321	0.042
General	Test	201	49 (24%)				
	Control	322	79 (24%)	0.992	1.113	0.636–1.948	0.707
Dyspnea	Test	52	16 (31%)				
	Control	60	10 (17%)	2.222	3.105	0.972–9.918	0.056
Headache	Test	50	25 (50%)				
	Control	85	25 (29%)	2.400	1.568	0.652–3.773	0.315
Tumor-related pain	Test	51	33 (65%)				
	Control	47	28 (60%)	1.244	0.705	0.266–1.871	0.483
Cachexia	Test	23	15 (65%)				
	Control	14	1 (7%)	24.375	133.95	3.695–4.855	0.008
Skin reactions	Test	85	32 (38%)				
	Control	227	137 (60%)	0.397	3.028	1.371–6.685	0.006
Infections	Test	52	25 (48%)				
	Control	70	17 (24%)	2.887	1.318	0.473–3.672	0.597

Table 6.4 Treatment success for complaints: raw and propensity score-adjusted odds ratio for various complaints

low-up period, and whether the complaints disappeared at the end of follow-up. Each complaint was examined separately. In the evaluation, only patients suffering from that particular affliction were included. If the complaint was no longer present at the end of follow-up, this was taken as a measure of success.

In Table 6.**4**, the number of patients (n) that suffered complaints in the test group and in the control group are indicated in the third column. In the fourth column, the absolute numbers and percentages of successes (i.e., no complaints at the end of follow-up) are indicated.

The odds ratio for each complaint was calculated as a comparative measure based on these. It is the relationship of the ratio of success between the test group and control group (the number of successes to the number of failures).

The raw odds ratio is calculated as follows:

$$(a^*d)/(b^*c)$$

a – number of successes in the test group
b – number of failures in the test group
c – number of successes in the control group
d – number of failures in the control group.

In the fifth column in Table 6.**4** these odds ratio are listed. Values greater than 1 show superiority of the test group, values smaller than 1 superiority in the control group. However, the odds ratios may be skewed through lack of homogeneity in the two groups. In order to counterbalance this, the adjusted odds ratio was calculated by means of logistic regression. It was assumed that the logarithm of the success ratio $P_e/(1 - P_e)$ in the totality is a linear function of the group affiliation x_1 (that is coded by a 1 for the test group and by a 0 for the control group) and the propensity score x_2:

$$\log(P_e/[1 - P_e]) = \beta_0 + \beta_1 x_1 + \beta_2 x_2$$

The value $\exp(\beta_1)$ indicates the adjusted relative success ratio of groups cleared of heterogeneities, in other words the relative success ratio of test group to control group for the same values of propensity scores for both groups. This can be appreciated through a simple mathematical formula: Since the variable x_1 for the test group takes on the value 1 and the value 0 for the control group, the logarithm for the odds ratio is:

$$\log\left\{\frac{P_e(\text{test})}{1 - P_e(\text{test})} \bigg/ \frac{P_e(\text{Control})}{1 - P_e(\text{Control})}\right\} =$$

$$\log\frac{P_e(\text{test})}{1 - P_e(\text{test})} - \log\frac{P(\text{Control})}{1 - P_e(\text{Control})} = \beta_1 + \beta_2(\text{test}) - x_2(\text{Control})$$

When the value of the propensity score x_2 (test) in the test group is the same as the value x_2 (control) in the control group, the difference between both is 0 and the logarithm of the odds ratio is equal to β_1. The value $\exp(\beta_1)$ indicates the relative success ratio that has been adjusted to the same conditions (i.e., the propensity score) for both the test and control group and cleared of any inconsistencies. It is an unbiased parameter for therapeutic efficacy in the treatment of the test group.

The estimated values b_0, b_1, and b_2 of the coefficients are retrieved according to the maximum likelihood method based on data from the cohort study. In Table 6.**4** the estimated values for adjusted odds ratio are given in column 6 as $\exp(b_1)$, in column 7 the 95 % confidence interval is listed, and in column 8 the P value for statistical significance (i.e., the probability that the estimated value is expected to be larger or smaller than the adjusted odds ratio given an adjusted overall odds ratio of 1).

For gastrointestinal complaints, general discomfort, dyspnea, cachexia, and skin reactions the adjusted odds ratio is larger, for headache, tumor-related pain, and infections, it is smaller than the relative ratio.

A significant superiority in the test group vs. the control group was seen for gastrointestinal complaints, cachexia, and skin reactions. It is remarkable that for skin reactions the raw odds ratio was significantly smaller than 1, the adjusted ratio larger than 1, however. The raw odds ratio is here especially influenced by inconsistencies between the two groups.

As has been shown under Concept of Evaluation (p. 69), heterogeneities can be balanced through stratification. Strata are made, and the odds ratio is calculated within each class. These relative ratios are ultimately combined to form an overall ratio following the method of Mantel and Haenszel (10). The prerequisite is, that the strata are homogenous, i.e., the same overall value can be assumed for each stratum for the odds ratio. This procedure is less appropriate for this study, since the distribution of the propensity scores for the two groups is very different and very large classes must be constructed in order to have a sufficient amount of cases from each class. We will still present

Table 6.5 Frequency of successes for gastrointestinal complaints within strata of the propensity score

Propensity score	Group	Patients n	Success n (%)	Odds ratio	95 % Confidence interval
0–0.3	Test	7	3 (43 %)		
	Control	114	50 (44 %)	0.960	0.958–3.056
0.3 – 0.6	Test	45	16 (36 %)		
	Control	65	19 (29 %)	1.336	0.593–3.007
0.6–1	Test	88	40 (45 %)		
	Control	24	5 (21 %)	3.167	1.085–9.239
Adjusted odds ratio (Mantel and Haenszel)				1.711	0.958–3.056

the example of gastrointestinal complaints to demonstrate. The values of the propensity score are separated into three classes: class 1 : 0–0.3; class 2: 0.3–0.6; class 3: 0.6–1. The numbers of patients and successes regarding gastrointestinal complaints within these two groups are shown in Table 6.**5**.

Table 6.**5** shows the calculated odds ratio, which varies from 0.960 to 3.167. Overall, the same odds ratio may be taken for all three classes.

The test for homogeneity (calculated with the program StatXact 4.01) shows no significant deviation from the homogeneity hypotenuse ($P = 0.332$). As an estimated value for the overall adjusted odds ratio according to the method of Mantel and Haenszel, the value 1.711 with a 95 % confidence interval from 0.958 to 3.056 is calculated.

The probability of gaining statistical significance P is 0.069.

When doing stratification using relatively large classes, the cleared odds ratio yields a similar estimated value (with similar confidence interval) as when using logistic regression (cleared odds ratio, 1.843; CI, 1.022 to 3.321). This demonstrates the equivalency of the two methods of compensation.

Summary

In summary of this example it should be noted that through cleansing of the therapeutic results of cohort studies with the help of propensity score, valid statements were made on therapeutic efficacy of a drug.

The quality of the clearing of distribution inhomogeneities depends on the extent to which the propensity score includes all relevant co-variables. The frequency with which the actual distribution

class can be predicted correctly can be taken as a criterion. In the example, the frequency was almost 80 % for the control group given a propensity score of less than 0.5, and for the test group given a propensity score greater than 0.5.

One can therefore assume that the propensity score entails all necessary influencing factors and purges them from their influence on the end result. Through the inclusion of further possible influential variables, an improvement in the score was achieved. Analysis of the completeness of the propensity score is an important step in the evaluation of cohort studies.

Addendum: Basic Terminology of Probability and Statistics

The total of the results or characteristic values that one obtaines in limitless repetitions of a certain procedure or event (e. g., therapeutic success in all possible variations of application of a drug for a given disease) is called the population (R. von Mises has also used the term "collective").

The relative frequency with which a certain singular result (in other words a specific characteristic) or certain amount of results (characteristics) in the population occurs is the probability for the outcome, or the amount of results. It should be noted that the probability is sometimes also interpreted as the "expectation" of a person to an unknown event without any bearing overall. Since such an interpretation of a "personal" or "subjective" probability is not commonly found in the literature, it will not be explained further.

The allocation of probabilities to the possible values of results and characteristics is the **probability distribution** (in short also referred to as "distribution"). It fully characterizes the totality and is therefore the goal of all inductions; that means a conclusion should be drawn from the probability distribution underlying the observations (data) and the certain parameters of distribution. This occurs when **estimated values** or statistics are calculated from the observed values (data) that represent the probability distribution or parameters of interest. In this way, for example, the relative frequency with which a certain event has occurred (e. g., a cure) in a certain number of observations is an estimated value for the probability of this result. These observed results are referred to as a random sample and one assumes that they are random and independently taken out of the overall population.

The number of observations in a **random sample** is called the **random sample size,** which is usually designated as n. The estimated values calculated with data from a random sample represent the distribution, although they are inaccurate, since they only make up a tiny proportion of the overall population. In order to ascertain the accuracy of the representation through the estimated values one assumes that the taking of a random sample is repeated any number of times and that an estimated value is calculated from every random sample. These estimated values will vary randomly. They will make up a new population in which the estimated values are allocated a probability distribution, also called the "**estimated distribution**." With this distribution, the credibility of the estimate is characterized.

The **mean value** (also referred to as "**expected value**" in populations) characterizes the "accuracy" of the estimate. An estimate, in which the expected value of the estimated distribution is in accordance with the actual value of the parameter (that is unknown) is termed unbiased.

The **standard deviation** of the estimated distribution is known as the "**standard error**" of the estimate. It characterizes the precision (more exact the imprecision) of the estimate: the smaller the standard error, the more precise the estimated value is to the real value of the parameter (in unbiased estimates).

A further characterization of precision is offered by the confidence interval for a given probability of confidence designated by γ, usually fixed at 95 %. This is an interval that contains the actual value of the parameter given the probability γ. This means that if one constructs the confidence interval according to the same rules for ever imagined repetition of random sampling, the proportion of the overall intervals (e. g., 95 %) will contain the actual parameter value and the proportion $1 - \gamma$ (e. g., 5 %) will not include it.

The narrower the confidence interval calculated from the exact data of a given sample size, the more precise the estimate.

If the breadth of the confidence interval is specified, the random sample size n can be determined so that these specifications are adhered by. With the confidence interval the hypothesis that the parameter will have a certain value, such as 0, for example, can also be tested. This hypothesis is called the "null hypothesis." If the confidence interval calculated from the data of a given sample includes this value (e. g., 0), then the null hypothesis is accepted; otherwise it is rejected.

The probability of error (type I) of the test is $1 - \gamma$. Were one to repeat this test for any limitless number of times with the actual parameter coinciding with the fixed value of the confidence interval, then the proportion of false rejections would be $1 - \gamma$ (e. g., 5 %).

A test procedure equivalent to this entails calculating a test statistic of the random samples that characterizes the difference between the random samples and the determined value of the parameters of the null hypothesis. With repeated random sampling the value of the test statistics will vary randomly with variation of the distribution dependent on the values of the random samples (and thereby of the actual parameter values) and on the random sample size n. The null hypothesis is rejected when the probability for the calculated statistical value of the test value (based on the observed random samples) or for even greater values (with the null hypothesis being valid) is less than or equal to a small value α, that is usually set at 5 %. This value α equates to the specification $1 - \gamma$ in the test with the confidence interval, which means that α is the **probability of error** (type I) in rejecting the null hypothesis, even though it is correct.

If the probability for the calculated statistical value of the test (or a larger value) with the null hypothesis being valid is larger than α, then the null hypothesis is accepted (**probability of significance**).

If the actual value of the parameters does not coincide with the value determined in the null hypothesis and one decides to accept the null hypothesis, then one commits a type II error. The probability of committing such an error depends on the actual deviation of the parameter value from the fixed value of the null hypothesis and the random sample size n. The larger the random sample size the less the probability to accept the null hypothesis for a given alternative reference value for the parameter. This opens up the opportunity to predetermine the random sample size n in such a way, that, for a given alternative reference value for the parameter, the predicted acceptance of the null hypothesis is at the most a reduced probability β, or the rejection of the null hypothesis at least a probability of $1 - \beta$. This probability mentioned last is called the power of a test procedure. It is often set at 80%.

▬ References

1. Benson K, Hartz AJ: A comparison of observational studies and randomized controlled trials. N Engl J Med. 2000; 342:1878–1886.
2. Beuth J, Ost B, Pakdaman A, et al.: Impact of complementary oral enzyme application on the postoperative treatment results of breast cancer patients–results of an epidemiological multicenter retrospective cohort study. Cancer Chemother Pharmacol. 2001; 47: S45–S54.
3. Bundesinstitut für Arzneimittel und Medizinprodukte (BfArM): Empfehlungen zur Planung und Durchführung von Anwendungsbeobachtungen. Bundesanzeiger 1998; vol. 50, Nr. 229, p. 16884.
4. Bundesverwaltungsgericht, 3rd Senat, File Nr 3C 21/91, Decision of Oct 14, 1993.
5. Cepeda MS: Editorial: The use of propensity scores in pharmacoepidemiologic research. Pharmacoepidemiol Drug Safe. 2000; 9:103–104.
6. D'Agostino Jr. RB: Tutorial in Biostatistics: Propensity score methods for bias reduction in the comparison of a treatment to a non-randomized control group. Stat Med. 1998; 17:2265–2281.
7. EU Commission, Guideline 199/83/EU of Sept 8, 1999. Official Gazette of the European Union of Sept. 15, 1999, L243/9.
8. Feinstein AR: Clinical Epidemiology. Philadelphia: Saunders; 1985.
9. Kant I: Kritik der reinen Vernunft. Philosophische Bibliothek. Hamburg, Germany: Felix Meiner Verlag; 1976: Vol 37a.
10. Mantel N, Haenszel W: Statistical aspects of the analysis of data from retrospective studies of disease. J Natl Cancer Inst. 1959; 22:719–748.
11. Perkins SM, Tu W, Underhill MG, Zhou XH, Murray MD: The use of propensity scores in pharmacoepidemiologic research. Pharmacoepidemiol Drug Saf. 2000; 9: 93–101.
12. Rosenbaum PR, Rubin DB: The central role of the propensity score in observational studies for causal effects. Biometrika. 1983; 70:41–55.
13. Rosenbaum PR, Rubin DB: Reducing bias in observational studies using subclassification on the propensity score. J Am Stat Assoc. 1984; 79:516–524.
14. Rubin DB: Estimating causal effects from large data sets unsing propensity scores. Ann Internal Med. 1997; 127:757–763.
15. Wittenborg A, Bock PR, Hanisch J, Saller R, Schneider B: Vergleichende epidemiologische Studie bei Erkrankungen des rheumatischen Formenkreises am Beispiel der Therapie mit nichtsteroidalen Antiphlogistika versus einem oralen Enzymkombinationspräparat. Arzneimittel-Forschung. 2000; 50:728–738.
16. Wunderlich CA: Die rationelle Therapie. Arch. für Physiologische Heilkunde. 1864; 5:1–16.

7 Electronically Supported Outcome Measurement

Jörg Sigle

Introduction

In the context of the current chapter, the technical term "outcome measurement" refers to studying the outcome of any kind of medical measures. Sensible outcome measurement is not limited to studying the efficacy of medical measures alone, but focuses very specifically on the benefit achieved. As patients search medical advice in order to enjoy either longer or better lives, any medical measure is beneficial only as far as it helps them achieve these goals. With steadily expanding possibilities, options, and costs in medicine, asking for what is actually beneficial for patients becomes more important than ever.

In this respect, the assessment of patients' subjectively perceived quality of life (QoL) has shown to be a valuable tool. This approach may be of interest for small studies and large multicenter efforts alike. In the setting of routine care-based research, however, regular measurement of quality of life is practised merely at a minority of places. This might be due to traditional attitudes of the scientific community, which still prefers "objective" physiological parameters to "subjective" questionnaire results. Although comprehensive scientific sources and validated, practical instruments exist, substantial knowledge of methodology, the significance of results and financial resources may still be deficient. Practical obstacles, in any case, may be overcome by modern tools, and any insight retrieved by their application is indispensable for medical decision making, individual evaluation, and optimization of therapy and quality assurance.

Necessary investments are relatively small compared to other fields of medical science: there are limited monetary expenses for technical equipment and acquisition of know-how, and time must be provided for training, data collection, and analysis and discussion of results. Some non-technical local conditions may merely demand creativity. Just like in any other research or quality assurance project, involved staff have to identify and to exploit available sources of know-how, and to understand and avoid possible sources of bias. This can be facilitated by applying methods from the discipline of evidence-based medicine.

Basic Methodological Considerations

Evidence-Based Medicine

A study design must fulfill certain requirements in order to avoid results which may be biased or misleading.

For several years, the movement of evidence-based medicine has propagated the application of the best available knowledge in the care for each individual patient, at the same time providing methods enabling every medical professional to locate up-to-date knowledge and to identify possible sources of bias in scientific publications.

Whoever uses these methods regularly can also learn to avoid bias in their own studies, and may probably practise reliable documentation and explorative analysis of routine data before calling for another randomized, double blind trial for each upcoming question (10, 11).

Efficacy and Benefit

Occasionally, patients may ask their physician whether a certain measure may actually help. Medical professionals, economists, and politicians do routinely ask whether a certain measure is efficacious (and maybe efficient)—with demonstrated efficacy (or efficiency) they take the resulting benefit for granted. As a consequence, *efficacy* (and maybe *efficiency*) has been studied and demonstrated for a variety of measures, but actual achievable *benefit* has not.

A patient with hay fever, for example, may feel immediate relief of symptoms when using a certain drug. However, the same drug may make the patient so tired that its actual benefit is questionable.

The amount of benefit that a measure can achieve may also depend upon how reliably it is targeted to adequately selected patients: Thus a drug that may lower blood pressure in any given patient by 10–20 mmHg is effective in each of them. One death due to a stroke or heart attack may be avoided by giving this treatment to three patients with a diastolic blood pressure of 115–129 mmHg for 1.5 years. If the same approach, however, is applied to patients with a diastolic blood pressure of 90-109 mmHg, the same result requires treatment of 128 patients over 5.5 years (10).

Prolonged Survival, Historical Controls, Screening

The duration of survival achieved under a recently introduced treatment may be compared to the duration of survival once achieved in historical controls. For example, a study of a new therapy for women with stage II breast cancer (free lymph nodes) might show a five-year survival rate of 78 %, whereas a study of conventional therapy, initiated 12 years ago, resulted in a five-year survival rate of only 65 %.

The second study started seven years after the first one and, in this time, ultrasound and computed tomography (CT) scanning resolution may have improved. Specifically, more advanced devices may have shown some suspicious lymph node, which might have been overlooked using the older ones. Thus, some patients may have been included in the stage II group 12 years ago, while patients with exactly the same level of disease, but examined with better diagnostic technology, would have been included in the stage III group five years ago.

In this scenario, baseline risks of both resulting stage II groups are not comparable at all, and advances in the diagnostic, not therapeutic, field of medicine might cause the observed survival gain. To avoid this **stage migration bias**, experimental and control groups should be studied at the same time, and historical controls should be avoided.

In another example, a study among women diagnosed with breast cancer might find one group who attended regular screening examinations with an average survival time of eight years, and another group without screening and an average survival time of five years. Apparently, screening prolonged survival by three years. This conclusion, however, is invalid: It is generally expected that screening might contribute to the discovery of lethal diseases in an earlier stage, and thereby improve the odds for curative therapy. However, screening might just as well discover the same lethal disease earlier, while it may still be impossible to change the course of the disease in any way. As efficacious screening delivers the diagnosis earlier than clinical symptoms would have done, no matter whether the course of the discovered disease can be changed or not, any introduction of screening will result in longer times between diagnosis and death. Time is absolutely certainly added to the observed interval at its beginning (**lead time bias**), but not necessarily at its end, where we would hope for additional survival. This is especially important as the diagnosis of a malignant disease may itself affect a patient's quality of life.

To avoid this kind of bias, survival time should not be measured from the point in time of primary diagnosis, when studied measures affect this point by themselves. Instead, subjects must be randomized into experimental and control groups before any of the studied events take place. As a consequence, large patient populations must be observed for long periods to obtain unbiased knowledge on the effects of screening.

To assess the benefits of breast cancer screening, such trials have actually been conducted. When their results are discussed, the toolchest of evidence-based medicine should be used: In the age group 50–69 years, let us assume a single woman's risk of dying due to breast cancer is 0.345 % or 0.00345 (**control group event rate**). Let us assume annual screening is able to reduce this risk to 0.252 % or 0.00252 (**experimental group event rate**). Politicians or business representatives might praise such a result as a "reduction by 27 %," or "almost one third" (**Relative Risk Reduction, RRR**), and rather not quote the less impressive absolute difference of 0.093 percent points or 0.00093 (**Absolute Risk Reduction, ARR**). The reciprocal value of that, 1/0.00093, equals 1075, and this is the number of women who would need to be screened (**Number Needed to Treat, NNT**) over 10 years to avoid one death (4). Similar simple math can be used when considering how many women can be screened in the same period before one of them receives a false-positive result, is erroneously treated, and consequently harmed (**Number Needed to Harm, NNH**).

The last example illustrates that the true meaning of an impressive relative risk reduction depends upon the baseline risk (which, in the example of breast cancer, depends upon age), the quality of medical measures and their side-effects. Consequently, recent controverse discussion of breast-cancer screening found a demand for additional data (5, 7).

All of the above examples show that studies on survival time need careful design, and may often turn out to be much more demanding than initially expected.

Spontaneous Course of Disease and Motivation

Some considerations support the assumption that our knowledge about the spontaneous course of many diseases must be limited: A patient experiencing an especially favorable course of a certain disease may possibly not want to see a physician at all. A patient with an especially unfavorable course may possibly not manage to see one in time—and the truly fatal disease may later be overlooked or misdiagnosed. For those patients already selected who actually see a physician, pressure resulting from patients' presentation, expectations, their environment, or from the physician, may cause diagnostic and therapeutic measures by far exceeding anything warranted by scientific literature or professional experience. Also, the fact that activity rather than watchful waiting generates monetary and academic rewards may unfortunately influence treatment decisions and research designs alike.

Applicability of Study Results

Medical studies often enrol highly selected groups of patients, and they are conducted in specialized and well-equipped environments. As a consequence, the studied population and the studied intervention may both be different from everyday settings. Thus, even if a study fulfills every methodologic requirement, it remains difficult to estimate how well its results may apply to an individual case in routine patient care.

Routine Care-Based Research

The mechanisms and consequences outlined above lead to a severe lack of knowledge. This deficit may probably only be alleviated if data from routine care are routinely collected and analyzed. On the one hand, such measures may actively support the evolution of available services through continuous, feedback-controlled, quality improvement, and thus promote the best possible use of limited resources from the patients' perspective. On the other hand, such measures must not place any additional burden on medical staff, who want to excel as medical professionals, not bookkeepers. The practicability of any attempt in this direction will consequently depend upon the use of modern information technology, which, however, needs to be guided by medical competence. Of course, both components must be adequately and reliably financed, according to their fundamental importance.

▬ Quality of Life Measurement

Health-Related Quality of Life

Particularly in incurable diseases, prolongation of survival cannot be the only therapeutic objective. In some cases, patients and physicians may have to choose between the prospects of longer survival or better quality of life during the remaining time.

The importance of quality of life may become especially prominent in palliative care of patients with malignant diseases, or with painful diseases of the musculoskeletal system, where mitigation of symptoms may be sought; also in patients with cardiologic diseases, where treatment shall enhance physical fitness. Apart from being the primary goal of palliative measures, improved quality of life is also a byproduct of successful curative treatment.

Consequently, the term **quality of life** (**QoL**) has been used very often in recent years. Many treatments have been advertised as being "proven to enhance quality of life," while closer examination might reveal that, e.g. only the **Karnofsky Index** has been used to assess the single dimension of physical fitness by proxy rating, or that freedom of movement has been measured for a single extremity in angular degrees.

The term **health-related quality of life** (**HR-QoL**) is usually derived from the WHO definition of health: "A state of complete physical, mental, and social well-being and not merely the absence of disease or infirmity" (28).

Many instruments for QoL measurement assess these areas in separate dimensions, and some assess a variety of symptoms or limitations which are specific for various diseases. The WHO definition itself has been enhanced to include the area of spirituality.

Advanced concepts discern multiple periods of time spent with different levels of quality of life, and blend quality and time into **Quality-Adjusted Life Years (QUALY)**. Economists use data from reference populations to link certain medical conditions with respective levels of "utility" for patients, and try to optimize this measure. Whereas such blending of multiple dimensions of quality of life into simplified measures may be useful for specific tasks, this approach causes a loss of differentiated information for clinical users. To solve this dilemma, some questionnaires report results for individual dimensions as well as aggregated measures or **global quality of life**.

A study conducted among physicians from Finland, Austria, and Germany found that 30–40% were accustomed to the concept of quality of life, that 40–90% accepted certain components of this concept, and that more than 90% considered a common measure to rate the effect in clinical or economic studies as useful. The concept of "health-related quality of life" grown in medicine was more naturally accepted than the concept of economically coined "utility" (6).

Self-Assessment vs. Proxy Rating

Various studies have compared results of self-assessments with results of assessment by relatives, nurses, and physicians (proxy rating). They show that the estimation of external observers can differ substantially and systematically from the patient's view (9).

Only patients know their own internal standards, to which they compare their current situation. An elderly lady, asked to rate her physical health, may answer: "Very good, doctor, I could climb two stairs without having to rest." A 16-year-old boy, however, may answer: "Absolutely poor, doctor, 100 meters took me 12.4 seconds!"

Occasionally, subjective data are considered "soft data," "less valid" or "less meaningful" than objective measures like blood pressure, tumor diameter, and so on. However, when filling in a validated questionnaire, patients transform their subjective experience into objectively measured data. The results actually belong to the hardest and most meaningful parameters available. On the one hand, a formal analysis must appreciate the fact that reduced quality of life is among the key motivations that make a patient seek medical treatment. Consequently, no parameter chosen as a mere replacement can reflect therapeutic success more accurately. On the other hand, some studies have shown that a baseline assessment of quality of life belongs to the most important prognostic parameters (9, 14).

Questionnaire Development

New QoL questionnaires (instruments) should be developed according to established, effective algorithms (16). First, patients and experts are asked to identify relevant areas and questions. Afterwards, prototypes of all questions are generated and their practicability, translatability, and intercultural usability are verified. A prototype of the questionnaire is presented to larger patient collectives, and all collected answers are analyzed in order to identify actually contained separate dimensions. The number of questions is adjusted as a compromise between coverage of all separable relevant issues, sufficient resolution, and a preferable low number of questions. The result undergoes validation in field studies. As this process requires a lot of time and resources, each new development of an instrument should be preceded by a thorough assessment of already available alternatives. An overview of available instruments can be found at http://www.qlmed.org. Unfortunately, when the MAPI Institute took over maintenance of the site, contact details of the authors of listed instruments were removed and access announced to be granted only after a substantial payment. An overview of instruments usable in oncology as well as general advice on how to select a specific instrument for a given project are included in the book *Effect of Cancer on Quality of Life* (8).

Costs of Quality of Life Measurement

Quality of life can be measured without expensive devices or laboratory analysis, just by asking patients simple questions. As early as 1993, costs for an assessment using an electronic questionnaire, including equipment and staff, were calculated to be below $ 2 per assessment. This is about 10 times cheaper than a UCG, 20 times less costly than a single immunologic laboratory test, and 100 times cheaper than a CT (14).

Preconditions of Quality of Life Measurement

- Quality of life should only be measured to answer a clearly defined question. Results can be seen like laboratory results: if they are only collected because "everybody is doing it," they will not provide any benefit at all.
- Quality of life should only be measured if necessary resources are available. Otherwise, collected data will probably be of low quality (incomplete, unreliable, collected with inadequate methodology). The budget should cover technical equipment, staff training, material, and labor required for collection and post-processing of data, analysis, and discussion of results.

Adequate Setting

- Whoever administers QoL questionnaires should be familiar with the instrument used and with any applicable standard operating procedures. Patients should be invited to the measurement in a standardized way. Neither staff nor relatives or other patients should influence patients during the selection of answers.
- Within a given project, the measurement should take place at a well-defined place and at a well-defined point in time (e.g. in the waiting room before a consultation). Measurements may be collected before and after an intervention, or during a series of scheduled visits during a follow-up or research program. An assessment performed in a defined setting in the clinic or practice should be preferred over an assessment taking place in the undefined setting of the patient's own home.

▬ Paper-Based vs. Electronic Outcome Measurement

Whenever there is a transit from paper-based to electronic data processing within a given workflow, a completely paperless implementation may offer an advantage. This is particularly the case when large amounts of data must be handled or when small amounts of data must be processed often, fast, and reliably.

Paper-based administration of questionnaires requires the following steps:
1. Preparation
   - Design of a questionnaire
   - Printout of a sufficient number of copies
2. Data collection
   - Handout of the questionnaire
   - Completion of the questionnaire
   - Return of the questionnaire by the study subject
   - Checking for completeness of answers and, if required, collection of missing answers
3. Post-processing
   - Optional: transfer into a data-processing system
   - Optional: repeated transfer into a data-processing system to reduce the probability of typing errors
   - Scoring of results (optionally: performed by data-processing system)
   - Computation and presentation of results (optionally: performed by data-processing system)

Post-processing can be simplified if for example a data-processing (IT) system using a scanner has been prepared. Perfect data quality (including valid and legible patient identification, completeness of answers, plausibility of collected content, interactively presented questionnaires) cannot, however, be guaranteed in paper-based questionnaire administration, as the data collection phase has usually ended when post-processing begins. Implementations involving manual data entry, scanners, or fax-receivers will consequently be used mainly when small numbers of patients are to be studied, or when financial or organizational restrictions make the visit of patients at an adequately equipped site or the provision of electronic questionnaires at a sufficient number of sites impossible. In such a setting, however, limitations with regard to quality and availability of data are accepted, as is additional labor.

A paperless questionnaire administration, in contrast, includes only two discernable steps:
1. Preparation
   - Design of an electronic questionnaire

2. Data collection
   - Completion of the questionnaire by the study subject

All other steps occur invisibly, fast, and reliably, producing high-quality data contained in an electronic system, or additionally printed on paper, available immediately after the administration of the questionnaire.

Patients accept electronic questionnaires with an adequate user interface very well. Resulting data are more complete than those from paper questionnaires, and more problems can be identified than in interviews. Only with electronic questionnaires can additional labor for handling questionaire results be avoided and, at the same time, interactive and multimedia questionnaires be made feasible. They can record the location, point in time, duration, language and questionnaire revision automatically, and make collected data available immediately for any additionally intended processing. This is essential if results of a questionnaire administration are required in an adjacent consultation. The system can also tell at any time whether a certain patient has been invited to fill in the questionnaire. Only in this way can an outpatient clinic ensure that QoL data is collected from each patient at every visit within a follow-up program—and that this is done reliably before the patient has left the clinic.

Technical Possibilities

Basically, individual electronic questionnaires for specific projects can be realized relatively easily using quite arbitrary development tools, or even common office software packages. Simple text-based systems, interactive forms, or solutions based upon organizers or dedicated hardware may be helpful. However, this approach will most probably generate solutions containing controls easily operated by a programmer, who is accustomed to Window-based user interfaces and little organizers, but not by an elderly lady, for example. Check-boxes, radio-buttons and scroll-bars, the mouse, or multiple small buttons of some special device, all with different functions, need to be identified, understood, and operated reliably— and many actions on these user interfaces require immediate checking of the result on a display which is maybe much too small with much too little contrast. These issues limit the group of patients who

may be studied using such solutions and/or establish the requirement of a time-consuming introduction of the patient to the specific instrument.

Systems that support (even automatic) questionnaire administration via phone are also relatively easy to produce from a technical point of view. Further possible approaches are listed in 14.

Requirements for an Ideal Tool

If a system is created and configured specifically for a project, related know-how must be conserved for the duration of its use and for the possible future data analysis. Availability of continuous support or, alternatively, of complete documentation, is crucial for its usability and sustained possibility to analyze data collected with this system.

- An ideal electronic tool should most importantly offer a patient interface that all patients can use intuitively, without any instructions, even if they are elderly and have restricted cognitive or motor abilities.
- The system should work with arbitrary questionnaires; a library of electronic questionnaires should exist. Persons with basic IT knowledge should be able to transfer new questionnaires onto the system.
- A new electronic system must not be a dead end for data, like the paper questionnaire it is going to replace. Consequently, it should be able to export collected data from various questionnaires in similar format via open, well-documented interfaces, and to communicate with other systems.
- Practical functionality for data analysis and immediately computed results should promote acceptance by professionals and patients alike.
- It should be possible to use the system in a simple, autonomous configuration as well as integrated into existing IT settings. It should be possible to configure it without specialist know-how, and defined configurations should be easy to distribute among multiple users.
- Specific requirements with regard to hardware or software should be low, and existing equipment should be usable.
- The system should be completely documented.
- Upon request, professional support should be available; it should have gathered experience in multiple settings.

- Up to a working application including data analysis, costs should remain limited and predictable, including investment in equipment, operating costs, and labor.

The QL-Recorder

As an abstract concept, this tool makes QoL measurement as simple as recording music with a tape recorder. It meets the requirements for an electronic outcome measurement tool as set out above.

The software AnyQuest for Windows provides a graphical user interface that comes very close to paper and pencil. One question is usually shown at a time, and below it some answer fields to check, some scales, or even images to select from. The patient interface is designed in a very simple layout using relatively large letters. It is a result of numerous practical experiences, e.g.:

- controls that are not required by the patient are not displayed
- questions are answered just by clicking a pen, the mouse, or a finger tip at an answer field or at any point on a visual analog scale
- configurable display of colors, fonts, and images, also as questionnaire background
- support of talking or musical questionnaires
- automatic or manual process after each given answer; possibility to move back or forth within loaded questionnaires
- answers can easily be corrected
- special fields for "cannot answer/do not wish to answer" can be shown
- reasons for difficulties in answering a question can be recorded
- special treatment of multiple inputs within short periods to compensate for lower-quality touch screens without confusing the patient
- for use with touch screens or pen computers: possibility to hide the mouse pointer to avoid a tendency toward the last-used answer position
- possibility to arbitrarily interrupt and resume questionnaire administration, including documentation of such events
- comprehensive included functionality for mathematical and logic computations
- integrated functionality for basic data analysis
- security features to protect configurations at various levels

- low minimum hardware requirements, compatibility with a variety of older and current operating systems or emulators
- support of various input devices without any need to change software or configurations: mouse, trackball, touch-screen, pen-computer
- recording of patient identification manually, semi-automatically, or automatically from external sources (e.g. via a GDT interface), or from barcode scanners or card readers
- support of international language versions and multiple revisions of questionnaires
- co-existence of multiple configurations for different studies on the same computer or network
- wide possibilities of integration in existing IT environments, with regard to data exchange and communication with external programs, e.g. to use automatically encrypted data transfer over the Internet, xDT and SQL, HL7 or XML interfaces.

AnyQuest can compute questionnaire results immediately and provide automatic printouts, including graphical presentation of a patient's course over time in all measured dimensions. Thus, it can support the consultation and the immediate assessment of treatment results in the individual case. It can also aggregate data collected by different researchers with different questionnaires very easily and export them in tabular formats for advanced statistical analysis (e.g. using SAS, SPSS, Excel, and other software). This enables researchers to perform cross-validation, meta-analysis, and other analyses spanning multiple studies using original data collected years ago by various authors.

Depending upon their complexity, QoL questionnaires which are already available e.g. as *.pdf or *.doc files, can typically be transferred onto the system within minutes or a few hours. Generation of questionnaire definition files in multiple languages is simplified by built-in translation support functions.

Pre-Configured Software Packages with Electronic Questionnaires

Completely functional QL-Recorder software and additional material are available online (12). Several packages provide a variety of freely usable questionnaires and do not require any additional configuration. More questionnaire definition files are available as separate files, references to additional packages or contact details in the QL-Recorder questionnaire library (13). Among the most commonly used or most interesting questionnaires available for the QL-Recorder are:

- **EORTC QLQ (QoL Questionnaire)**: It implements a modular concept with a generic core questionnaire of 30 questions and additional modules for specific indications. There are comprehensive manuals and a collection of reference data. Academic studies supported by the pharmaceutical industry may use the questionnaire free of charge; however, any use shall be registered with the EORTC QoL Group. The currently available electronic version eQLQ includes the core questionnaire EORTC QLQ-C30 and the disease-specific modules LC-13 (lung cancer), BR-23 (breast cancer), HN-35 (head and neck cancer), BR-20 (brain tumors), and PAN-26 (pancreatic tumors). Contact details and links to the EORTC website are included in the questionnaire library of the QL-Recorder.
- **SF-36 (Short Form, 36 Questions)**: This is one of the most commonly used QoL questionnaires. The QL-Recorder offers both a regular and a talking version.
- **IBSQOL (Irritable Bowel Syndrome QoL Questionnaire)**: The electronic version eIBSQOL has been supported by Glaxo-Wellcome. In addition to the QoL questionnaire, it contains questions based upon the Rome-II criteria. Apart from the algorithmically generated diagnosis, however, it prints a patient's individual answers, allowing for the specialist's own judgement of the patient's condition.
- **HADS (Hospital Anxiety and Depression Scale):** This instrument can be used to search for clinically relevant states of anxiety or depression.
- **SAQLI (Calgary Sleep Apnea Quality of Life Index)**: This illustrates well how the QL-Recorder can substantially simplify a demanding interview with a quite complicated algorithm for result computation.
- **QWB-7-SA (Quality of Well-Being Questionnaire, Self-Administered Version)**: This is another example of how an assessment originally designed as an interview, then redesigned as a self-administered questionnaire, can be administered in an easily usable electronic version.

Non-Technical Requirements

Research Questions

In addition to being motivated to study the benefit of medical measurements for patients, sensible outcome measurement requires a clearly defined research question, e.g.:

- "How do parameters like physical function or pain change in individual patients while they receive individual therapy?" Here, QoL measurement is used as a monitoring tool in an individual patient exactly like a sphygmomanometer would be.
- "Out of all our patients, can we identify subgroups which benefit especially from a given therapy with regard to parameters like physical function, pain, or emotional condition?" Here, QoL measurement is used to study a group of patients in order to optimize therapeutic approaches in general.

Staff Training

Before outcome measurement is introduced, participating staff must be trained. The importance of collected data for delivering high-quality care in general, and to each individual patient, must be communicated. Additionally, it must be clarified that a QoL measurement is an actual medical test or examination just like any other.

- Staff must become acquainted with the technology used and must be able to help the patient in every way in a competent manner. Before questionnaires are administered to patients, staff should practise this among each other. Just like blood-taking, a questionnaire administration must be carried out reliably and with high technical quality, whenever it is medically justified.
- Just as for the measurement of blood pressure, convenient tools for the measurement of QoL have become available—and very much as with blood pressure, physicians must now learn to use the test results in the individual case as well as for strategic decisions on therapeutic approaches. This requires a process of gathering clinical experience, and the reflection on results of clinical studies.
- As a first step within this learning process, the difference between surrogate parameters (e.g.

blood pressure) and true outcome parameters (survival time, quality of life) should be communicated.

- A competent support team should be available to answer technical or content-related questions.
- A small number of all photocopies should be available so that in exceptional cases data can at least be collected independently of any specific location, time, or availability of technical equipment.

Process Management and Tight Feedback

During the introduction of routine QoL measurement, high-quality data collection must be supported by management measures, including:

- exact definition of the population to be examined and of indications for the examination
- exact description of available examination methodology
- generation and communication of a plan listing all intermediate goals to be achieved
- early involvement of all participating colleagues
- training of all participating colleagues
- informing patients on the objective and the course of the examination
- tight checks to ensure whether target populations are examined completely and, if applicable, feedback to involved staff on the examined proportion, patient reactions, quality and content of results. If patients are "lost," reasons must be investigated and discussed with staff.

Data Protection

Legislation or applicable rules regarding data protection do vary among countries, states, or even institutions. Generally, they do not only apply to efforts using information technology; however, when paper-based methods are used, they are ignored more easily (e.g. like the cart filled with patient files that is left unattended during typical ward rounds). Applicable legislation must be reviewed to learn about specific requirements. In Germany, patient-related data that must be protected are data that may be attributed to a given individual without any additional means. Whenever files are established to collect patient-related

data, it may be necessary to report to a locally responsible person or institution.

Data protection means both protection from unauthorized access and ensuring the permanent possibility of authorized use. Consequently, planning of electronic outcome measurement includes a backup strategy.

▬ Application Examples

The following examples show how outcome measurement using electronic QoL questionnaires has been successfully implemented. Related material may be downloaded from the web-site of the QL-Recorder:

- As early as 1994, the EORTC QLQ-C30 was used at the outpatient clinic for internal medicine at the University of Ulm, Germany; within 4 weeks, 1120 patients (94.8% of the target group, patients of any age except for children) filled in the questionnaire. Collected data were 99.98% complete; the missing answers resulted only from the fact that, very rarely, patients felt they could not answer a certain question. Results were clinically meaningful and valid, and the feasibility of routine QoL measurement with the QL-Recorder was proven (14).
- Patients with malignant diseases visiting an outpatient clinic were regularly queried with the EORTC QLQ-C30 since 1994. The long-term routine collection of QoL data turned out to be feasible, and collected data showed that a satisfactory quality of life of patients cared for with a holistic therapeutic approach could be sustained toward the end of their lives.
- Since 1995, patients of a clinic specializing in pulmonary diseases have been assessed routinely with the EORTC QLQ-C30. Collected data are imported directly into the locally developed tumor documentation system TREG. This system supports the management of long-term follow up, provides facilities for statistical analysis, and can be operated by physicians (17).
- Since 1995, in-patients of a clinic offering conventional and complementary medicine alike were asked to fill in the EORTC QLQ-C30 at admission, at several intervals, and when discharged. Routine assessment was shown to be feasible, and a correlation was demonstrated between baseline QoL and duration of survival

as well as an improvement of QoL in various dimensions during the hospital stay (2a).

- In 1996, QoL was measured repeatedly using the EORTC QLQ-C30+3 in 352 in-patients with hemato-oncologic diseases. Integration of the measurement into clinical routine work was shown to be an essential prerequisite for high data quality. The participation rate was independent of patients' gender, diagnosis, and therapeutic goal (curative or palliative). However, it fell from 80–90% at 65 years to 40% at 90 years. It remains unclear whether higher age itself or the correlating higher reduction of QoL in various dimensions was the reason for this observation. This relation should be kept in mind when QoL-related comparisons are made between groups in which the proportion of patients older than 65 years differs (3).
- Since 1998, electronic QoL questionnaires have been used in the pediatric clinic of the University of Ulm. Children as well as parents have been asked to fill in questionnaires on a mini pen-computer. For this purpose, two separate configurations were prepared so that the questionnaire for children or for parents could be launched by selecting the respective icon on the computer desktop. The solution has been accepted well by children and parents alike, and even children at age eight were fully able to use the electronic questionnaire. In the meantime, the workgroup has received the Lilly QoL award for work using the QL-Recorder (21).
- Since 2000, a practice in Vienna offering complementary medicine has asked all patients treated with whole body hyperthermia to fill in the EORTC QLQ-C30 routinely (22).
- In 2001, the QL-Recorder was used in a study on substance abuse at the department of Clinical Pharmacology at the University of Göttingen.
- In 2001, the author used the QL-Recorder for routine QoL assessments in a rural general practice. Results were automatically imported into the laboratory results page of the practice management software and appeared on the physician's desktop to be used during consultations, both to identify primary problems of patients and to assess effects of therapy.
- In 2005, the German Ministry of Education and Research (BMBF) granted funding for a project designed at the department of General Practice at the University of Göttingen that will introduce similar systems into 25 practices (20).

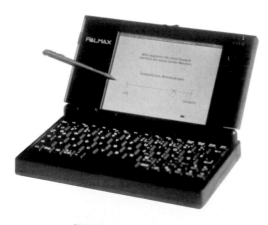

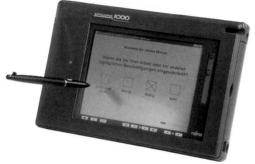

Fig. 7.1 Implementation of the QoL-Recorder on a Palmax PD-1000 Mini-Pen Computer and a Fujitsu Stylistic 1200 Pen Computer.

▬ References

1. Dudeck J et al.: Basisdokumentation für Tumorkranke–Prinzipien und Verschlüsselungsanweisungen für Klinik und Praxis. Munich, Germany: Zuckschwerdt Verlag; 1999.
2. Höhmann D: Klinische Signifikanz von EORTC QLQ-C30 Daten für die Prognose von Patienten mit Mamma-, Pankreas-, Ovarial- und kolorektalem Karzinom. Dissertation, University of Witten-Herdecke, Germany, 2001. (http://www.ql-recorder. com/document)
2a. Höhmann D, Hager ED, Sigle J: Prognostic significance of EORTC QLQ-C30 data for patients with pancreatic cancer; scientific meeting of the Ulm Cancer Center during the Spring meeting of the EORTC-GITCCG: "Prognostic Factors in Colorectal Cancer: Impact of Tumor Biology and Treatment Quality" (Poster) Ulm 2001

3. Holch S: Routinemäßige Messung der Lebensqualität bei stationären Patienten. Dissertation, University of Ulm, Germany, 2000. (http://www.ql-recorder.com/document)

4. Lancet 1993; 341:973–978; cited according to Sackett 1997; p. 137.

5. Olsen O, Gotzsche P: Cochrane review on screening for breast cancer with mammography. Lancet 2001; 358:1340–1342. (Many other articles on this topic have been published in Lancet 349 to 359; available at www.thelancet.com by searching for "mammography screening.")

6. Leidl R et al.: Do physicians accept quality of life and utility measurement? HEPAC 2001; 2:170–175.

7. Cancer institute gives US breast-cancer policy the all-clear. Nature 2002; 415:950.

8. Osoba D et al.: A practical guide for selecting quality-of-life measures in clinical trials and practice. In: Osoba D (ed.): Effect of Cancer on Quality of Life. Boca Raton, Fl: CRC Press; 1991:89–104.

9. Porzolt F: Messung von Lebensqualität–Wie und wozu sie das Wohlbefinden Ihrer Patienten quantifizieren sollten. Der Allgemeinarzt. 1996; 18: 610–625. (Includes extensive references to further information on this topic.)

10. Sackett DL et al.: Evidence-based Medicine–How to Teach and Practice Evidence-based Medicine. New York: Churchill Livingstone: 2001.

11. http://www.jsigle.com/ebintro

12. http://www.ql-recorder.com

13. http://www.ql-recorder.com/libqstns

14. Sigle J: Praktische Aspekte der Lebensqualitäts-Messung–Routinemäßige Messung der Lebensqualität mit einem elektronischen Lebensqualitäts-Recorder. Dissertation, University of Ulm, Germany; 1997. (Includes extensive references to further information on this topic.) (http://www.ql-recorder.com/document)

15. Sigle J, Wilhelm HJ: Medizinisches Qualitätsmanagement. In: Lehmann T, Meyer zu Bexten E (eds): Handbuch der medizinischen Informatik. Munich, Germany: Hanser Verlag; 2002.

16. Sprangers M et al.: The European Organisation for Research and Treatment of Cancer approach to quality of life assessment–Guidelines for developing questionnaire modules. Quality of Life Research 1993; 2:287–295.

17. von Bültzingslöwen F: TREG–a clinical tumor data base with instruments for medical reporting, measurement of quality of life and statistical analysis. Cancer Research and Management, Proc EMBEC, 1999, II, 1560–1561.

18. World Health Organization (ed.): The constitution of the World Health Organization. WHO Chronical. 1947; 1:29. http://www.who.int/rarebooks/official_records/constitution.pdf)

19. Goldbeck L, Braun R: LQ-KID: ein computergestütztes Verfahren zur Erfassung der Lebensqualität chronisch kranker Kinder und Jugendlicher. Prävention und Rehabilitation 2003; 3: 117–126. http://www.dustri.de/zd/pr/15pr0303.htm#pr15_117

20. www.medvip.uni-goettingen.de

21. Schmitz TG, Goldbeck L: Validation of a new CF-specific quality of life module (FLZ-CF) for adolescent and adult patients. Journal of Cystic Fibrosis, Abstracts of the 24th European Cystic Fibrosis Conference 6–9 June 2001 Vienna, 327 (2001)

22. Kleef R: Hyperthermia for specially complicated advanced cases (case reports). Congress paper, 26th Congress of the International Clinic Hyperthermia Society, Schenzen, China, 2004.

8 Cancer and Nutrition

Heide Jonik and Rudolf van Leendert

Introduction

Many components of our diet either protect against cancer or cause cancer themselves. There is now compelling scientific evidence of a causal relationship between many nutritional factors and certain types of cancer. So far, about 700 chemical compounds are known to induce cancer in animal experiments (16).

Despite recent advances, the options for cancer treatment remain quite limited. Hence, prevention plays an important role—especially in the context of nutrition.

In a joint effort, the World Cancer Research Fund (WCRF) and the American Institute for Cancer Research (AICR) have compiled a report entitled "*Food, Nutrition, and the Prevention of Cancer: a Global Perspective*," in which they reviewed and

Table 8.1 Nutritional factors that increase or reduce the cancer risk

	Mouth, larynx, esophagus	Stomach	Colon	Pancreas	Lung	Breast	Ovary	Endo-metrium	Prostate
+++	Smoking, alcohol			Smoking	Smoking			Obesity	
++		Brine curing	Red meat, alcohol		High doses of synthetic β-carotene in smokers	Alcohol, obesity			
+		Barbecuing, heavy roasting	Total fat, animal fat, meat products, eggs, sugar, barbecuing, roasting		Total fat, saturated fattyacids animal fat, alcohol	Red meat	Meat, animal fat	Saturated animal fat	Total fat, animal fat, saturated fatty acids, red meat, alcohol
–	Vitamin C, carotenoids in the diet	Carotenoids in the diet, whole grains, green tea	Fiber, tomatoes, carotenoids, omega-3 fatty acids, fish	Choles-terol, meat	Vitamin C, vitamin E in the diet	Carotenoids, vitamin C in the diet, fiber	Fruits, vege-tables		
– –		Vitamin C in the diet		Fibers, vitamin C in the diet	Caro-tenoids, β-carotene in the diet	Fruits		Fruits, vege-tables	
– – –	Fruits, vegetables	Fruits, vegetables, kitchen hygiene, cool storage	Vegetables, physical activity	Fruits, vege-tables	Fruits, vegetables	Vegetables			
0		Nitros-amines, pickled or smoked food; synthetic β-carotene and vitamin E may increase the risk in smokers	Selenium, calcium, mono-unsaturated and polyunsaturated fatty acids		Vitamin E, synthetic vitamin A	Total fat, *trans*-fatty acids, saturated fatty acids, animal fat, linolic acid, polyunsatura-ted fatty acids, vitamin E, phyto-estrogens			Monounsaturated and polyunsatu-rated fatty acids, linolic acid, selenium, milk, lycopene

Summary of the WCRF report "*Food, Nutrition and the Prevention of Cancer: a Global Perspective.*"
Increased risk: + + +, convincing; + +, plausible; +, possible. Reduced risk: – – –, convincing; – –, plausible; –, possible. 0, effect not clear.

analyzed the available scientific evidence on the topic of nutrition and the prevention of cancer in the mid-1990s (107). They have concluded that a healthy nutrition combined with physical exercise and avoiding becoming overweight may reduce the incidence of cancer by 30–40 %. This amounts to three to four million individuals with cancer every year worldwide.

The nutritional state of the patient plays a major role in cancer treatment, both for the patient's well-being and for the course of the disease and its treatment. Malnutrition hampers metabolism and immune defenses, thus causing organ dysfunction, delayed wound healing, and increased susceptibility to infections. For cancer patients, this means a lower quality of life and higher morbidity and mortality.

Table 8.**1** provides an overview of the assessment of the correlation between certain nutritional factors and specific types of cancer. It is striking to see that both fruits and vegetables play a prominent role in the prevention of cancer. For almost every type of cancer, there is evidence of protective nutritional factors. Among the cancer-promoting factors, obesity plays a major role in addition to smoking and alcohol. The role of animal fats as a carcinogenic factor remains unclear. Although fats are considered to increase the risk of cancer, there is neither compelling evidence from epidemiological studies nor any other indication that a causal relationship exists. This statement does not address the role of fats as energy source or their possible role in the development of obesity.

▬ Carcinogens and Cocarcinogens in the Food

Carcinogens and cocarcinogens occur in our food naturally, but they are also generated during processing, storage, and preservation. Natural ingredients with mutagenic activity include, for example, hydrogen cyanide-containing glycosides in bitter almonds and kernels of stone fruits, and solanine in potatoes (28).

It is still not clear what role additives and residues play in carcinogenesis, but they seem to play a minor role as compared with other factors of nutrition (61).

Alcohol

Alcohol is a risk factor for carcinogenesis in the upper respiratory and digestive tracts, in particular (45). In most epidemiological studies examining this relationship, a direct correlation has been demonstrated—and the risk rises with increasing consumption (26). Alcohol itself does not have a carcinogenic effect, but it acts as a **cocarcinogen** and thus promotes the development of cancer through various mechanisms. In addition, carcinogenic compounds have been detected in various alcoholic beverages, such as polycyclic aromatic hydrocarbons and nitrosamines (61). Alcohol also influences eating habits, metabolism, and adsorption, thus resulting in a poor supply of protective substances (20).

High-proof alcoholic beverages significantly increase the risk of cancer, more so than beer or wine. A dose–effect relationship has also been observed with tobacco use, which often accompanies chronic alcohol consumption. Both factors multiply each other's effect (74).

Fats

A diet rich in fat is thought to promote the development of various types of cancer. There are clear indications that the levels and types of fat consumed correlate with the risk of colon cancer, while a connection between fat intake and cancer of the breast, prostate, endometrium, and ovaries is still being debated (97).

Epidemiological and experimental studies indicate that, especially with colon cancer, it is not only the level of total fat intake that plays a decisive role but also the pattern of fatty acids. Foods with a high proportion of saturated fatty acids (SFAs) seem to increase the risk of colon cancer. The same is true for a high intake of omega-6 fatty acids, whereas omega-3 fatty acids—primarily present in fish oil—have a protective effect (1). According to the new reference values for nutrient intake used in the United States (29) and in Germany, Austria, and Switzerland (DACH reference values, 22), consumption of fat should not exceed 30 % of the total energy intake, and the ratio of omega-3 fatty acids to omega-6 fatty acids should be raised to at least 5 : 1.

Studies examining the influence of the amount of fat intake on the development of breast cancer yielded contradictory results. Experimental findings that fats may promote carcinogenesis have not been confirmed by prospective cohort studies.

It is now increasingly debated whether it is really the amount of fat that plays the decisive role, or whether it is actually the total energy content of the diet—and the obesity associated with it—that increases the risk of breast cancer in women (100).

Recent findings indicate a close relationship between the levels of estrogen and insulin circulating in the blood. It has been demonstrated that insulin resistance can raise the level of free estrogen available to cells, either by lowering the level of estrogen-binding globulins in the plasma or by increasing androgen production in the ovaries. Insulin resistance, on the other hand, is closely related to eating habits: a diet rich in fat leads to a higher proportion of free fatty acids in the plasma, thus causing an increase in the fasting glucose level by means of various metabolic steps. Like a diet with a high glycemic index, this leads to hyperinsulinemia—which, in turn, promotes the development of insulin resistance. Based on these mechanisms, a diet rich in fat may be a potential risk factor for breast cancer by contributing to both intra-abdominal accumulation of fat and insulin resistance (20).

Meat

Some meats and meat products contain a high portion of fat. A diet rich in meat therefore often leads to a high intake of energy, fat, and protein. The iron intake associated with the consumption of meat may also play a role as iron promotes the formation of radicals. In addition, a diet rich in meat is often associated with low consumption of fruits and vegetables.

Increased protein intake results in an increased production of urea, which is broken down in the colon to ammonia. Ammonia causes a rise in cellular metabolism, an increased susceptibility of the cells to viral infections, and an enhanced effect of mutagens. Hence, ammonia is generally regarded as a cocarcinogen (88).

The usual methods of food preparation, such as frying and grilling, may give rise to heterocyclic amines and polycyclic aromatic hydrocarbons, which have been shown to be carcinogenic in animal experiments (20).

Nitrosamines

Of over 300 known N-nitroso compounds, about 90% proved carcinogenic for various organs when tested in animal experiments. Therefore, their role in carcinogenesis in humans has been investigated for many years (26).

Nitrosamines are produced from nitrate and secondary amines through bacterial activity. A major source of nitrate is a diet rich in vegetables. Certain vegetables—such as red beet, spinach, and leaf lettuce—may contain considerable amounts of nitrate, especially when grown in a hot house and when treated heavily with fertilizers. Even drinking water may be rich in nitrate, particularly when nitrate-containing fertilizers get into the water. In meat processing, the nitrate present in pickling solutions is used to redden and cure the meat (19).

Nitrosamines formed in the stomach play a major role in the development of gastric cancer. Their effect is favored by the hypoacidic state of the stomach caused by chronic inflammation. Hypoacidity stimulates bacterial growth, thus speeding up the reduction of nitrate to nitrite. Sodium chloride promotes the development of atrophic gastritis and thus acts as a cocarcinogen. Improved methods of preservation have considerably lowered the risk factors for gastric cancer; it is far less common today that it has been in the past (31).

Mycotoxins

Mycotoxins are produced by molds developing primarily due to improper storage. They are widespread in tropical and subtropical countries, the biggest problem being aflatoxin. Above all, mycotoxins may contaminate peanuts, other types of nuts and seeds, rice, and other grains. Moldy bread should not be eaten because of its aflatoxin content. Just removing the moldy parts is not sufficient because aflatoxin quickly penetrates into deeper layers of the bread without being visible from the surface (81).

Other toxins occur in fruits and vegetables and in products prepared from them. Of special importance is **patulin** generated in fruits affected by blight (61).

Some mycotoxins proved to be highly carcinogenic in animal experiments and are thought to induce cancer in humans as well (20). There is convincing evidence that they may cause liver cancer.

Polycyclic Aromatic Hydrocarbons (PAHs)

PAHs are generated during incomplete combustion and during flash pasteurization of organic matter. PAHs are widespread because such processes are very common not only in domestic settings but also in the food industry. Traces are also found in unprocessed foods. The indicator compound of PAHs is the highly carcinogenic benzopyrene. It is found in foods derived from both plants and animals, and its content may vary with the location. The main source, however, is cigarette smoke. Benzopyrene is therefore thought to be primarily a carcinogen of the respiratory tract, although it seems to have an effect on the development of gastric cancer and intestinal cancer as well.

In the case of animal products, especially food processing plays a major role—apart from environmental pollution—because benzopyrene is also produced during broiling and smoking. High concentrations of PAHs are generated when meat is barbecued over an open fire, particularly when fat is dripping into the fire (23, 24, 85).

Heterocyclic Aromatic Amines (HAAs)

HAAs are produced when food—mainly meat and fish—is heated at temperatures commonly used in the kitchen. Especially the crust is heavily loaded with HAAs, and the content mainly depends on the temperature and the duration of heating. In fact, the small amounts taken in with food are not regarded as harmless because of their mutagenic and carcinogenic properties. Possibly, the HAA content—rather than the meat itself—is responsible for the well-established correlation between meat consumption and cancer risk. As a preventive measure, it is recommended that meat and fish be prepared by more gentle methods, such as stewing. Unnecessarily high temperatures and long preparation times should be avoided when frying, roasting, or barbecuing. Using the juice from heavily roasted meat for the preparation of gravy is not recommended (39).

Obesity

It has been observed for many years that there is a correlation between a high body mass index (BMI, body weight in kg/square of the height in m) and physical inactivity, on the one hand, and an increased risk of certain types of cancer, on the other. Perhaps this can be explained by elevated levels of insulin and other hormones known as growth factors. Consistently elevated insulin levels, favored by insulin resistance at the cellular level, may increase the rate of cell division and thus raise the risk of mutations (105).

Elevated levels of sex hormones and reduced concentrations of sex hormone-binding globulins have been found to be associated with an increase in body mass. Enzymatic conversion of androgens into estrogens can take place in fatty tissue, which again leads to elevated estrogen levels. Estrogens represent a major factor in the development of mammary and cervical carcinomas. The correlation between obesity and the risk of breast cancer has been observed primarily in postmenopausal women (20). In the case of endometrial carcinoma, studies have demonstrated a twofold to tenfold higher risk associated with postmenopausal obesity. Especially at an advanced age, being obese or gaining weight seems to have unfavorable consequences (26).

▬ Dietary Components Effective in Prevention

Diet can influence the process of carcinogenesis at various stages: first, by affecting the initial stages of carcinogenesis (primary prevention), by preventing the malignant transformation of precursor cells (secondary prevention), and by preventing the recurrence of the disease following a recovery (tertiary prevention) (51).

No form of a diet can prevent cancer with certainty, and epidemiological evidence of a correlation between diet and cancer is still incomplete; yet it is possible to establish dietary recommendations that might reduce the risk of developing cancer (26).

The positive health benefits of a diet rich in fruits and vegetables are now common knowledge. However, the question of what the underlying mechanisms may be is still the subject of ongoing research. Experimental research, in particular, has shown that there are many biologically plausible explanations for the anticancer properties of plant-derived food. However, the protective effect cannot be traced back to individual ingredients. According to currently available scientific findings, it is rather the food pattern—the selection, preparation, and amount of food—that seems to be essential for influencing the risk of cancer and other chronic diseases. It seems as if the effects associated with individual food ingredients are adding up and thus determine the risk of developing cancer. However, it is still not clear which mechanisms of action are relevant in humans (20).

A great number of substances that occur naturally in foods are regarded as **protective factors against the development of cancer**. These include antioxidants (e. g., β-carotene, and the vitamins A, C, and E), calcium, selenium, zinc, fiber, secondary plant metabolites, and lactic acid. Also considered are riboflavin and folic acid (61).

When considering individual nutrients in our food, we should be aware of the fact that they always exist in a close relationship with other nutrients. For example, a low intake of fat is correlated with a reduced risk of breast cancer, on the one hand, but associated with a reduced level of fat-soluble vitamins, on the other. We need to gather results that can be properly interpreted. When assessing certain types of diet, it makes sense to define specific indicator substances (markers) that, either alone or integrated, are known to have a preventive effect against the development of cancer. These markers should be detectable in human blood and tissues and be correlated in a quantifiable manner with the respective food items. The following indicator substances are often used:

- in vegetables: β-carotene (as well as vitamin A)
- in vegetable oils: vitamin E
- in fruits, especially citrus fruits: vitamin C.

These markers can be used for interpreting epidemiological studies as well as for analyzing direct interactions in animal experiments and in-vitro assays. A final proof of their isolated mechanisms of action, however, is only possible through targeted dietary intervention studies (6).

Antioxidants

Antioxidants protect DNA and cell membranes from damage caused by oxidation and thus contribute to protecting the organism from mutations and maintaining the cell's integrity. This protective effect is based on the ability of antioxidants to prevent the formation of free radicals by capturing reactive oxygen compounds, or to make an electron available to existing radicals without becoming a reactive radical itself. The so-called exogenous or nonenzymatic antioxidants (vitamins C and E, β-carotene, and some other carotenoids) together with the endogenous or enzymatic antioxidants (superoxide dismutase, glutathione peroxidase, catalase, and others) form an effective protective shield against aggressive oxygen compounds (53).

The balance between free radicals and antioxidants can be disturbed by a number of exogenous and endogenous processes; as a result, the protective antioxidant potential may soon become exhausted. Exogenous tumor initiators include smoke, ionizing radiation, ultraviolet light, ozone, as well as dietary factors and deficits. In addition, highly reactive oxygen compounds are generated endogenously as by-products of the cytochrome system and also in activated leukocytes and macrophages (26).

Oxidative processes contribute to the production of free radicals or other reactive oxygen species. Oxygen radicals can modify deoxyribose or DNA bases and thereby trigger mutations. In addition, they can cause severe changes in the biological activity of proteins. In addition, lipids, especially the highly unsaturated fatty acids in membranes, are often subjected to oxidative damages (63). Free radicals are involved at every stage of carcinogenesis (55).

Based on their different properties of solubility, antioxidants are active either in the hydrophilic or lipophilic phase. Selenium is an essential component of the two endogenous antioxidant enzyme systems, glutathione peroxidase (GSH-Px) and phospholipid-hydroperoxide–glutathione peroxidase (PH–GSH-Px), and zinc plays an important role in superoxide dismutase. The hydrophilic vitamin C and GSH–Px are active in the aqueous environment of the cell, whereas lipophilic antioxidants—such as vitamin E, β-carotene, and PH–GSH-Px—are active within the membranes. The various protective systems act synergistically; they can regenerate each other but cannot replace one another (26).

In addition to essential nutrients that possess antioxidant activity, secondary plant metabolites with proved antioxidant activities are becoming the focal point of research (26).

In terms of primary prevention, the statistical analysis of epidemiological data has led us to the conclusion that regular and ample consumption of vegetables, fruits, and whole-grain products can reduce the risk of cancer (17). This can be explained primarily by the intake of natural antioxidants that are associated with this type of diet, for example, β-carotene, vitamin C, vitamin E, and selenium. However, this does not prove a causal

Table 8.2	Reference values for plasma levels considered optimal for cancer prevention (22)
Vitamin E	> 30 µmol/L
Vitamin C	> 50 µmol/L
β-Carotene	> 0.4 µmol/L
Selenium	> 50 µg/L

relationship between individual antioxidants and the protection from cancer (22).

Based on epidemiological data, plasma concentrations of antioxidants have been established as reference values for the primary prevention of cancer in healthy adults. These values have been derived from the results of prospective studies and case studies and also from comparisons between various countries (Table 8.2).

To reach the established plasma concentrations, a daily intake of 75–150 mg of vitamin C, 15–30 mg of vitamin E (α-tocopherol equivalents), and 2–4 mg of β-carotene in the diet has been recommended at a consensus conference in 1995 (4). However, these recommendations are only valid for healthy persons who are not exposed to special oxidative stress. According to the VERA Study analyzing the relationship between nutrition and risk factors in Germany, the reference values for plasma concentrations can be achieved by just eating a normal diet (43). It should be taken into account, however, that the target concentrations may not be reached in some individuals despite a wholesome diet. Underlying causes may include a variable relationship between intake and plasma concentrations as well as increased requirements due to oxidative stress. Upon consultation with a physician, additional intake of antioxidants in the form of dietary supplements may be indicated. Under no circumstances, however, should this be used to offset an unhealthy diet and/or lifestyle (22). Current knowledge on the mutual supplementation and enhancement of antioxidant substances suggests that eating a wholesome diet should always be preferred to substituting individual active substances by dietary supplements.

To ensure the intake of antioxidant vitamins in the amounts required for prevention, the National Academy of Science has recommended that Americans eat fruits and vegetables five times a day (18). The German Society of Nutrition has developed a similar concept ("five a day") to promote the intake of fruits and vegetables. The major arguments for the intake of vitamins through an appropriate diet rather than through dietary supplements are:

- Consuming lots of fruits and vegetables makes it easier to follow the recommendations for a healthy diet, especially with regard to a reduced intake of energy, fat, and sodium chloride.
- Consuming lots of fruits and vegetables increases the intake of fiber, especially of water-soluble fiber, which is broken down by bacteria in the colon. The short-chain fatty acids generated hereby inhibit the development of colon cancer.
- Fruits and vegetables contain also other carotenoids, such as canthaxanthin, lutein, or lycopene, which also possess anticarcinogenic properties and promote cell communication. In addition, these foods are rich in folic acid, which is thought to reduce the risk of cancer further (34).
- Secondary plant metabolites contained in fruits and vegetables have not yet been sufficiently studied, but they most likely possess anticarcinogenic properties (53).

Clinical Studies

During recent years, several intervention studies involving antioxidants have been carried out, and they yielded contradictory results. Basically, the studies have raised the question of whether the often-confirmed negative correlation between the serum concentration of β-carotene and the risk of bronchial carcinoma is indeed causally connected. High concentrations of β-carotene in the serum seem to be rather an indicator of a diet rich in fruits and vegetables—a diet that contributes to cancer prevention through a multitude of protective substances. Other studies also speak against the use of supplements and for a balanced diet with a high proportion of fruits and vegetables in order to prevent cancer (26, 15).

- A positive result was obtained in a cancer prevention study carried out in China (Province of Linxian), a region known for its above—average incidence of gastric and esophageal carcinomas and insufficient or borderline intake of macronutrients and micronutrients. Within five years, the combined supplementation of **β-carotene** (15 mg/day), **vitamin E** (30 mg/day), and **selenium** (50 µg/day) resulted in a significant reduction in cancer mortality by 13 %. The mortality from stomach cancer even dropped by 21% as compared with the control group (18). The fact that also the total mortality dropped by 9% and the mortality from cardiovascular diseases by 10%, showed that the study was dealing with a population carrying a high risk due to poor living conditions (53).

- In the **Physicians Health Study (PHS)**, which was completed in 1995 and involved 22000 healthy, well-nourished American physicians, the risk of cancer was not affected by supplementation with **β-carotene**. Over a period of 12 years, the study examined whether the intake of 50 mg of β-carotene every second day would reduce the risk of cancer, as compared with a placebo. There was no evidence for a protective effect of β-carotene. There was no difference in the frequency of malignant tumors between the group receiving β-carotene and the placebo group (41).
- The Finnish **ATBC Lung Cancer Prevention Study** yielded a different result. It was carried out with long-time heavy smokers who took vitamin E (50 mg/day) or β-carotene (20 mg/day) as a supplement. Contrary to expectations, there was no change in the incidence of lung cancer associated with vitamin E, and the death rate increased by 18% with β-carotene (40). Largely due to high media coverage in the lay press, this negative outcome caused a feeling of unease in the population with respect to foods rich in antioxidants. After detailed analysis, however, the negative result turned out to be due to errors in the design of the study (53). One critical aspect was that one could hardly expect to find a preventive effect in the study's participants after long-time exposure to cigarette smoke. Most likely, the process of tumor development had already been initiated in a large number of participants. At this stage of carcinogenesis, β-carotene can no longer have an effect (36, 26).
- In the **CARET Study**, smokers and workers exposed to asbestos took β-carotene and vitamin A in order to reduce the risk of bronchial carcinoma. However, the study was terminated prematurely when it was noticed that supplementation was associated with an increased incidence of lung cancer (73).

The results of the Finnish ATBC study and of the two American studies (CARET and PHS) give cause for warning against an uncontrolled intake of pharmacological doses of β-carotene—this is true particularly for groups with an increased risk.

Vitamin A and β-Carotene

Vitamin A is taken up as a provitamin (carotenoids) from vegetable sources or in the form of its ester from animal sources. It regulates the expression of many factors—such as growth hormone receptors, oncogenes, and interleukins—which play a special role in the growth and differentiation of cells and tissues (6).

β-Carotene is the main representative of a large family of carotenoids, some of which can be converted into vitamin A by our body. However, β-carotene is not only a provitamin but has an antioxidant effect on its own and should be regarded as being essential to humans (6). β-Carotene is able to capture singlet oxygen generated primarily through UV irradiation. The mechanisms discussed include its function as a physical filter (protection from light), quenching properties (emission of energy as heat), and incorporation as a membrane component (replacement of oxidation-sensitive parts). Apart from this, β-carotene is also effective as a chain-interrupting antioxidant by forming stable radicals, particularly at a low partial pressure of oxygen (6). In animal experiments, β-carotene increases the activity of T and B cells and enhances the cellular immune response (20).

- In vitro, retinoic acid (vitamin A acid) inhibits the proliferation of neoplastic cells while promoting their differentiation into normal cells. It has been clearly demonstrated in animal experiments that this vitamin controls, in particular, the differentiation of respiratory mucosa and skin (91). Deficiency in vitamin A typically leads to disturbed differentiation of rapidly growing epithelia, especially of mucosal epithelia (6).
- Numerous epidemiological studies have shown that persons who eat a lot of fruits and vegetables rich in carotenoids have a lower risk of developing certain types of cancer (e. g., carcinomas of the lung, stomach, esophagus, cervix) (22). An inverse relationship was found, in particular, between the incidence of bronchial carcinoma and the intake of β-carotene in the form of fruits and vegetables (102). Lower blood levels of β-carotene carry a higher risk of bronchial carcinoma, in particular (25). In 1991, these findings have prompted the German Society for Nutrition (DGE) to establish a recommended

daily intake (RDI) of 2 mg of β-carotene. At the Hohenheim Consensus Conference in 1995, the desirable intake was set to 2–4 mg/day, in order to achieve plasma levels that are considered optimal in preventive medicine. According to the National Consumption Study (NCS) and the VERA Study, these values are generally reached in the average German population. Nonetheless, dietary supplements have become wide spread.

- **Requirement**. Based on the unfavorable findings of the large intervention studies (ATBC, CARET) involving synthetic β-carotene, the World Health Organization (WHO)-founded International Agency for Research on Cancer advised in a press release on 12 January 1998, against the use of β-carotene and other carotenoids for tumor prevention. The German Federal Institute for Health Consumer Protection and Veterinary Medicine (BgVV) followed suit by issuing an urgent warning against the uncontrolled intake of β-carotene through dietary supplements and enriched foods. A recommendation for the maximal amount of synthetic β-carotene is in effect since 31 January 2001. According to the BgVV, the daily intake should not exceed 2 mg of synthetic β-carotene because a daily intake of 20 mg/day can cause health problems in heavy smokers and other risk groups (32).

- **Sources** β-Carotene is only found in fruits and vegetables, and the amount varies widely depending on variety, degree of ripeness, and the season. Bioavailability depends to a large extent on how the food is prepared. Only about 1 % of β-carotene can be absorbed from raw carrots; mashed carrots or carrot juice can provide much more. The same is true for lycopene from tomatoes.

Vitamin C (Ascorbic Acid)

L-Ascorbic acid reduces water-soluble peroxide radicals as well as other reactive prooxidants and is therefore thought to be an effective antioxidant. It captures radicals in the aqueous phase before they can induce lipid peroxidation. Like vitamin E, vitamin C thus inhibits the peroxidation of cell membranes. It is also capable of regenerating both vitamin E and glutathione. Vitamin C inhibits the formation of nitrosamines both in foods and in the intestinal tract (7). In addition, microsomal hydroxylation reactions in the liver are involved in the metabolism and inactivation of drugs and toxic metabolites (6). The mechanism of some activities—such as the regulation of gene transcription and protein translation—and the significance of accumulation of ascorbate in various immunocompetent cells have not yet been elucidated (22).

Several studies have revealed an inverse relationship between the estimated vitamin C intake and the development of various types of cancer, such as gastric, esophageal, and laryngeal carcinomas (76).

In the 12-year follow-up of the Basel Study, an inverse relationship was found between the consumption of vitamin C-rich foods and the development of stomach cancer. In the 17-year follow-up, however, this effect was no longer statistically significant (26).

A statistically significant inverse relationship has also been observed between vitamin C intake with the diet and breast cancer (46).

- In older persons with low plasma levels of vitamin C, the risk of stomach cancer and cancer of the gastrointestinal tract is increased (96).
- There have also been studies in which no correlation was observed between vitamin C intake and various types of cancer, especially stomach cancer and cancer of the gastrointestinal tract (27).
- Evaluation of all known epidemiological studies up to 1998 revealed that a reduction in the risk of chronic diseases—especially with respect to the morbidity and mortality of cancer and cardiovascular diseases in nonsmokers—is best achieved with plasma levels of more than 50 μmol/L and a daily intake of 90–100 mg of vitamin C (17). Intake of 100 mg ensured optimal saturation of immunocompetent cells. At higher dosages, the renal threshold set in and increased dramatically after intake of more than 200 mg. At the same time, reabsorption of ascorbic acid became less effective.
- **Requirement** Vitamin C requirement is increased in times of physical stress and with certain diseases, such as diabetes or infections. Based on current knowledge, it is not yet possible to provide a precise figure for these increased needs. Because smoking decreases the absorption and increases the consumption of vitamin C, it is recommended that heavy smokers take 150 mg/day (22).

In 2001, the research of pharmacologists in Philadelphia caused quite a stir when the results were published in the scientific magazine *Science* (59). According to this study, vitamin C—which acts as an antioxidant within the cells and neutralizes free radicals—may promote the in-vitro production of DNA-damaging compounds. In the experiment, vitamin C and lipid hydroperoxide were combined in a test tube. After two hours, it was observed that so-called genotoxins, which are known to damage DNA, had formed—one of the prerequisites of cell degeneration and, possibly, carcinogenesis. According to the researchers, these findings might explain why vitamin C proved less effective in the fight against cancer than had been expected. However, it would be wrong to conclude from this study that vitamin C would cause cancer and would not contribute to a healthy diet. The results of experiments in vitro cannot easily be applied to the human body. In addition, the notion that vitamin C is essential for human health has been confirmed by other studies.

Vitamin E (Tocopherols)

Numerous retrospective and prospective studies have established a relationship between plasma levels of vitamin E and the risk of cancer in humans. However, the results have not been unambiguously confirmed (80). Other studies have demonstrated that the administration of vitamin E in nontoxic doses has been successful in preventing colon carcinoma and cancer of the mouth and throat as well as esophageal carcinoma (6). Different mechanisms of action are discussed, including the effects of antioxidants in connection with increased cellular immunity. Whereas β-carotene can hardly be discussed separately from foods, this is possible with vitamin E. There is evidence that vitamin E is active also in isolated (synthetic) form (6).

Naturally occurring tocopherols are only produced by plants. Here, as in animals, they act as a protective system against radicals, thus preventing primarily the peroxidation of polyunsaturated fatty acids (PUFA) in membrane lipids, lipoproteins, and depot fats. The fat-soluble vitamin E acts as one of the most important protective systems against lipid peroxidation in vivo (22). The tocopheroxyl radical formed in this way is probably regenerated to tocopherol in the aqueous phase by the antioxidants ascorbic acid and glutathione. Thus, various antioxidants act synergistically to protect cell membranes against lipid peroxidation. Peroxidation of lipids causes membrane changes and lesions that affect membrane properties (7).

Source. The content of vitamin E is expressed as tocopherol equivalents (TE) to reflect the different biological activities of individual tocopherol compounds. In nature, α-tocopherol is the compound with the highest vitamin E activity (79). Wheat germ oil, sunflower oil, and olive oil are particularly rich sources. The much less active χ-tocopherol constitutes the main portion of vitamin E in soy bean oil, oil of maize, and palm oil (Table 8.3) (91).

Unsaturated fatty acids are especially sensitive to oxidative attack at their double bonds. The higher the content in polyunsaturated fatty acids, the higher should be the vitamin E content of the oil in order to protect the fat from oxidative damage. Fatty acids from oils are part of the structure of cell

Table 8.3 Assessment of individual foods as a source of vitamin E (8)

Type of food	Monounsaturated fatty acids (g/100 g)	Vitamin E mg/100 g	Assessment of fatty acid/vitamin E ratio
Wheat germ oil	65	215	+ + + + +
Hazelnuts	6	25	+ +
Sunflower oil	63	50	+ +
Olive oil	9	13	+
Butter	3	2	0
Oil of maize	53	31	0
Herring	7	1	–
Mackerel	3	1	–
Thistle oil	75	35	–
Walnuts	40	6	– –

membranes. A high proportion of omega-6 fatty acids seems to promote colorectal and mammary carcinomas, whereas omega-3 fatty acids have a protective effect (6).

Considering that 0.3 mg of vitamin E per gram double bonds of unsaturated fatty acids are required for the protection from oxidation, there are only few foods that contain an excess of vitamin E. Wheat germ oil is the best source, though it is not widely used because it is too expensive. However, vitamin E is often added to vegetable oils for preservation.

According to the German Society of Nutrition, it is possible to take in sufficient amounts of vitamin E without resorting to supplements. When selecting vegetable oils though, one should pay attention to the vitamin E content and to the ratio of fatty acids to vitamin E (22).

Vegetable oils with a high content of polyunsaturated fatty acids are not suitable for cooking and frying because they decompose easily at high temperatures. Because of the adequate fatty acid/vitamin E ratio and the high content of monounsaturated fatty acids (MUFA), olive oil plays a special role in the prevention of cancer.

Folic Acid

Folate is the generic term for various B vitamins having folic acid activity. The report on Dietary Reference Intakes (DRI) in the United States (29) uses a new definition, which has also been adopted for the new DACH reference values in Germany, Austria, and Switzerland (22):

1 μg of dietary folate equivalent (DFE) = 1 μg of food folate = 0.5 μg of synthetic folic acid = 0.6 μg of folic acid from fortified food or as a supplement taken with meals = 0.5 μg of a supplement taken on an empty stomach.

As an intermediary metabolite, folic acid is mainly involved in cell division and, hence, in the formation of new cells. Folate deficiency manifests itself primarily in cell systems that have a high rate of cell division, for example, in the intestinal mucosa (22). Insufficient supply of folate may therefore be associated with an increased risk of colon carcinoma. Numerous studies demonstrated an inverse correlation between the folate state and the incidence of colorectal carcinoma and, less prominently, other tumors (29).

Requirement and source Folic acid is considered to be a critical nutrient. Almost all age groups in Germany fail to reach the recommended daily intake of 400 μg. Although this rarely creates an actual deficiency, one should nevertheless pay attention to the amount of folic acid in the diet (7). Good sources are green vegetables, oranges, grapes, whole-wheat bread, and other baked goods made of whole grains, as well as potatoes. Especially rich in folate are wheat germ and soy beans (22).

Selenium

Selenium is an essential trace element and, as a constituent of a number of functional proteins, necessary to maintain metabolism and organ functions. As a constituent of glutathione peroxidase, it plays an important role in the protective system of endogenous antioxidants (94). There is also evidence for an immunomodulating effect of selenium. With respect to the protection of lipids from oxidation, there is a synergistic relationship between selenium and vitamin E (5). Epidemiological studies indicate that selenium might play a role in the prevention of cancer.

- In Japan, where mammary carcinoma is comparatively rare, selenium levels in the blood of the population are roughly twice as high as in European countries or in the United States because the diet is rich in selenium.

- In the cancer prevention study in China mentioned earlier, selenium was a component of the supplements that resulted in reduced cancer mortality. However, the study group had extremely low selenium intakes prior to the study, and it is not clear what preventive effects would have been observed in a population already supplied with sufficient selenium in the diet. Based on these findings, one can only speculate on the positive effect of selenium. A clear statement is impossible because a combination of supplements was administered (61).

- **Requirement and source**. Animal and plant proteins are the main source of selenium, but the content and availability of selenium vary depending on the heavy metal load of the ground. In Central Europe, for example, the soils are depleted of selenium through leaching of nutrients, intensive agricultural use, and increasing environmental pollution. Although selenium intake just covers the requirement, it is suboptimal with respect to prevention. For example, the average person in Germany gets only 35 μg of selenium a day—which is extremely low when compared internationally (56). However, there is no direct evidence of selenium deficiency given the eating habits common in Germany (22). Nevertheless, intake values are in the lower range of the recommended values. Since many diseases are correlated with a reduced selenium level, and since incidence and mortality of certain diseases are obviously influenced by the selenium level, dietary supplementation may be indicated. A long series of studies has shown that cancer patients exhibit low selenium levels in serum, plasma, and whole blood. Numerous large prospective epidemiological studies in several countries revealed that low selenium levels often existed long before the disease flared up. Low selenium levels should therefore be considered a risk factor.

- In 1983, a study published in the *Lancet* received a lot of attention. It showed for the first time that low prediagnostic selenium levels promote the development of cancer, particularly carcinomas of the gastrointestinal tract and prostate (94).
- The organic selenium compounds available on the market as nutritional supplements (selenocysteine, selenomethionine) contain 50–100 µg/unit, which is the amount established as additional daily requirement of a healthy person; these compounds are available over the counter. In this form, however, selenium is not sufficiently bioavailable. Preparations containing selenium in the form of an inorganic compound—usually sodium selenite—are much more effective; they are available by prescription only because of their classification as a drug (94). Hence, supplementation should be in the hands of a physician. One reason for restricting intake to naturally occurring selenium is that iodine deficiency is still a problem in some areas. An increased intake of isolated selenium might activate deiodases and thus lead to increased conversion of thyroxine (T_4) to triiodothyronine (T_3) and may cause hypothyroidism by inhibiting TSH release (22).
- Vitamin C and sodium selenite interfere with each other with respect to uptake and function. If both substances are to be taken, it is recommended to take sodium selenite in the morning on an empty stomach and wait at least for one hour before taking vitamin C or vitamin C-containing foods and drinks (94).

Zinc

Zinc is a constituent, or cofactor, of over 200 enzymes and metalloproteins, for example, superoxide dismutase and DNA and RNA polymerases; it therefore has an effect on transcription and translation, that is, gene expression (8). Zinc deficiency reduces T and B cell-dependent immune reactions, thus interfering with the body's defenses. As a constituent of the enzyme superoxide dismutase, which is responsible for the detoxification of highly reactive, cytotoxic superoxide radicals, zinc also has an indirect antioxidant effect. In the case of zinc deficiency, the associated loss in superoxide dismutase activity can lead to oxidative damages (8).

Since the body cannot store large amounts of zinc, which may be mobilized in case of dietary deficiency, it relies on the continuous supply of zinc. Severe zinc deficiency may cause a diminished sense of taste (gustatory hypoesthesia), loss of appetite, dermatitis, loss of hair, diarrhea, and neuropsychological disorders. Delayed wound healing and increased susceptibility to infections are also observed, reflecting an impaired immune system (22).

Requirement and source According to the VERA Study, the average zinc intake in Germany is 10.5 mg/day and thus corresponds to the zinc intake recommended by the German Society of Nutrition (22). Zinc is taken up largely from meat and meat products, where it is highly bioavailable (8). Vegetarians must therefore pay attention to what they eat and should include plenty of whole-grain products in order to get sufficient amounts of zinc with their diet.

Calcium

Calcium plays a role in the prevention of colon cancer, in particular. Its effect is based on the reduction of cell proliferation in the mucosa of the colon, thus lowering the risk of cancer. In addition, calcium binds secondary bile acids, which are considered cocarcinogenic.

One study revealed that, in patients with a high familial risk of colon carcinoma, the rate of cell proliferation in the colon was as high as in patients with colon carcinoma. After calcium supplementation the rate of cell proliferation clearly declined, even reaching levels observed in persons with a low risk of colon cancer (62).

Bioactive Substances

Bioactive substances are currently studied extensively for their health-promoting effects. The increased interest is mainly due to their potential in preventing chronic diseases, particularly cancer and cardiovascular diseases. Numerous epidemiological studies have demonstrated the protective effect of a diet rich in vegetables, fruits, legumes, and whole-grain products. However, an unambiguous assignment and identification of specific components—including known vitamins, minerals, trace elements, and fiber—has not been possible (80, 81). Health-promoting effects have so far been demonstrated only for foods but not for isolated components.

While bioactive substances are health-promoting food components, they do not possess nutritional properties in the narrow sense. Formerly known as nonnutritive components, they largely include secondary plant metabolites, fiber, and substances present in fermented foods. Based on their chemical structures and functions, they can be divided into various groups (Table 8.**4**).

Though low in concentration, plant-derived bioactive substances have multiple activities. They may have protective effects at all stages of carcinogenesis (initiation, promotion, and progression). Secondary plant metabolites with anticancer activity include the following substances (103):

- β-carotene
- other carotenoids (such as canthaxanthin, lutein, and lycopene)
- phytosterols
- saponins
- glucosinolates
- flavonoids
- phenolic acids
- protease inhibitors
- terpenes
- phytoestrogens
- sulfides.

Our knowledge of bioactive substances has clearly increased during recent years. The data presented here (Table 8.**4**) are largely derived from invitro studies and from animal experiments that have been supported, in part, by epidemiological studies.

According to current knowledge, it is fair to assume that all bioactive substances consumed become biologically active. This supports the general recommendation of a diet rich in fruits and vegetables ("five-a-day" campaign). Artificial supply through supplementation, however, should be discouraged in order to avoid negative effects until more detailed data are available (33).

Secondary Plant Metabolites

So far, there is no standard definition for the term "secondary plant metabolites." They are also called "phytochemicals" or "phytoprotectants" because of their biological effects (103). Unlike primary plant metabolites (e. g., carbohydrates, proteins, and fats), which are involved in energy metabolism and the structure of plants, secondary plant metabolites occur only in small quantities but ex-

Table 8.4 Bioactive substances: possible activities (103)					
Bioactive substances	**Anticarcinogenic**	**Antimicrobial**	**Antioxidant**	**Immunomodulation**	**Peptic**
Secondary plant metabolites					
Carotenoids	×		×	×	
Phytosterols	×				
Saponins	×	×		×	
Glucosinolates	×	×			
Flavonoids	×		×	×	
Phenolic acids	×	×	×		
Protease inhibitors	×		×		
Terpenes	×	×			
Phytoestrogens	×		×		
Sulfides	×	×	×	×	
Phytic acids	×		×	×	×
Fiber	×			×	×
Substances in fermented food	×	×			

hibit a wide variety. They usually possess pharmacological activities and are produced by plants as a defense against pests and diseases. In addition, they act as growth regulators, pigments, flavors, and scents (23). Depending on agricultural methods, growing conditions, storage, and processing, the content of secondary plant metabolites in fruits and vegetables may vary greatly. Up to now, there are hardly any data available on their absorption and metabolism in the human body (37).

The total number of secondary plant metabolites occurring in nature is currently unknown. It is assumed that approximately 60 000 to 100 000 of them exist. Up to now, however, only 5 % of plants have been chemically analyzed for their content.

The daily intake of secondary plant metabolites through a normal, mixed diet is about 1.5 g, whereas intake is clearly higher with a vegetarian diet (53). Numerous health-promoting effects have been attributed to these substances (see Table 8.**4**). Particular attention has been paid to their anticarcinogenic potential. The mechanisms of action may include:
- regulation of enzyme activities (inhibition of phase I enzymes, induction of phase II enzymes)
- restriction of cell proliferation by enhancing intercellular communication
- increase in apoptosis
- effects on estrogen metabolism (37).

In the past, the consideration of toxic properties of secondary components has predominated, for example, the toxicity of protease inhibitors, hydrogen cyanide, and solanine. Today, research is focused primarily on the protective properties. Based on common eating habits, secondary plant metabolites are considered to be nontoxic while promoting health (23). Regular intake of certain secondary plant metabolites may play an important role in staying healthy in the long term. They are therefore regarded as semiessential nutrients, even though they are not essential in the classic sense (57). Hence, modern assessments of food components should also consider—in addition to the essential functions of nutrients—biological activities of components that may have a variety of protective effects (103).

So far, no prominent preventive effect of individual types of fruits and vegetables has been found. Epidemiological studies revealed that neither the well-studied broccoli nor the quercetin-rich onions proved to be more effective than all vegetables as a whole. In experimental studies, individual components of fruits and vegetables were systematically examined for their potential of protecting against cancer. They confirmed that many components clearly had an inhibitory effect on carcinogenesis (20).

The potential role of secondary plant metabolites in the prevention of tumor development has raised the question of establishing reference values for dietary intakes. So far, the current state of information supports only a recommendation for β-carotene (22). For most secondary plant metabolites, nutritional science is still at the stage of basic research and in the experimental phase. Although there is a large body of knowledge on various physiological, biochemical, or toxicological activities, there are no scientific data to support any recommendations. In particular, there have been no long-term studies involving humans. Questions regarding absorption, metabolism, and toxicity still remain largely unanswered (82, 83, 85). Some advertisements promote health benefits that have not been scientifically demonstrated through controlled nutritional studies in humans (42). The negative findings of the intervention studies involving β-carotene should be a warning. Based on current knowledge, the administration of plant extracts, undefined mixtures of secondary plant metabolites, or isolated active components as dietary supplements is not recommended. Rather, the notion is still valid that a diet rich in fruits and vegetables largely meets the guidelines for a preventive diet (37).

It can be expected that future research will clearly demonstrate which of the secondary plant metabolites play an important role in the prevention of cancer. Nevertheless, this research—as the one dealing with antioxidant vitamins—will be confronted with the difficult problem of confounding by other food components, which may distort the results of case–control and cohort studies (26).

Carotenoids

Carotenoids are very common in plant foods. They give fruits and vegetables their characteristic yellow, orange, or green coloring. Their most important function, however, is the absorption of light and the transmission of energy to chlorophyll (15, 45).

Independently of their provitamin A activity, carotenoids have antioxidant properties as well. In addition to β-carotene, it is mainly lycopene that has the ability to deactivate singlet oxygen. In addition, carotenoids activate certain genes that control the production of a protein integral to gap junctions, the specific structures of cell communication. Carotenoids also have an effect on cell differentiation.

Numerous epidemiological studies have shown that the concentration of carotenoids in the serum is negatively correlated with the prevalence of carcinomas of the lung, prostate, esophagus, cervix, stomach, and colon. Human serum contains primarily the carotenoids lycopene, α-carotene, and β-carotene, and also the xanthophylls lutein, zeaxanthin, and β-cryptoxanthin (23). Especially β-carotene has been well documented. However, the findings of various intervention studies suggest that the correlation observed is not necessarily of a causal nature. It rather appears that β-carotene should be regarded as an indicator of a healthy diet rich in fruits and vegetables, while the cancer-preventing effect of such a diet is based on its content of secondary plant metabolites, vitamins, and minerals (103).

Phytosterols

Phytosterols occur predominantly in the fat-containing parts of plants. Particularly rich sources are sunflower and sesame seeds and their cold-pressed oils, as well as native soy bean oil. Phytosterols can lower cholesterol levels because their chemical structure resembles that of cholesterol. In animal experiments, they have anticancer activity with respect to colon carcinoma. They are thought to inhibit cell proliferation in the colon by limiting the generation of cholesterol degradation products and secondary bile acids (45, 48).

Saponins

Saponins are wide-spread in plant foods, above all in legumes. They have a very bitter taste and have been regarded as harmful in the past as they may damage erythrocytes. However, they are poorly absorbed and therefore primarily active in the intestine. Saponins are thought to reduce the risk of colon cancer by inhibiting the rate of cell proliferation in the colon as well as growth and DNA synthesis in various types of cancer. Their mechanism of action seems to be related to their ability to bind primary bile acids and cholesterol, thus reducing the amount of mutagenic secondary bile acids formed. Saponins also stimulate the immune system, which might contribute to their anticancer activity (61).

Glucosinolates

Glucosinolates are spicy flavoring agents that give mustard, horseradish, cabbage, and kohlrabi their characteristic tastes. The aromatic compounds are only released when the vegetables are chopped up. Their health-promoting effects, especially on the urinary tract, were already known in the Ancient World. Excessive consumption of glucosinolates may stimulate goiter formation.

In many animal experiments, isocyanates and thiocyanates were shown to prevent neoplastic diseases, such as gastric, mammary, hepatic, and bronchial carcinomas. Various mechanisms of action have been discussed, such as the inhibition of phase I enzymes and the induction of phase II enzymes.

- Clinical studies showed that indoles influence the metabolism of endogenous estrogens. It is therefore possible that they protect from estrogen-sensitive types of cancer (103).

Flavonoids

Flavonoids are pigments that are present in many types of fruits and vegetables and protect these from oxidative spoilage. They are located primarily in the outer layers and are therefore largely lost when the skin is peeled off.

Flavonoids include various plant pigments—flavonols, flagons, anthocyanins—that are responsible for the yellow, red, blue, or purple coloring of flowers and plants. Quercetin, an effective antioxidant flavonol, has been especially well studied. Among the beverages, juices and particularly red wine and black tea contain flavonoids (13). There are numerous indications that flavonoids are anticarcinogenic. Further studies, above all in vivo, are needed since immunosuppressive effects have been observed in addition to immunostimulating ones (104).

Phenolic Acids

Phenolic acids—caffeic acid and ferulic acid—occur in coffee and in the outer layers of various types of vegetables and grains. In various animal experiments, they proved to be an effective protection against carcinomas of the stomach, esophagus, skin, and lung. Their mechanism of action is based on the induction of detoxification enzymes that bind carcinogens and thus prevent them from coming into contact with DNA. In addition, phenolic acids are strong antioxidants, and this may contribute to their anticarcinogenic potential (103). Fruit juices are often protected from microbial spoilage because they contain phenolic acids.

Protease Inhibitors

As the name indicates, protease inhibitors limit the activity of proteases, such as trypsin, chymotrypsin, plasmin, and elastase. They are present in soy beans, legumes, and grains, making sure that protein reserves in the seeds are not degraded before germination. They inhibit human proteases only to a minor extent and do not interfere with the digestion of food. In the past, it has been recommended that these enzyme activities be reduced by heating foods prior to consumption.

Experimental studies using animals have demonstrated anticancer activity with respect to carcinomas of the liver, stomach, intestine, and oral cavity. Possible mechanisms of action include inhibition of tumor-specific proteases, reduced availability of amino acids, and antioxidant activity (45, 103).

Terpenes

Terpenes play an important role as food flavors, e. g., menthol from peppermint, D-carvone in caraway seeds, and citrus oil from limes. They have shown anticancer activity in animal experiments, presumably because they contain alkyl groups. Limonene leads to an increase in the activity of detoxification enzymes in the liver and small intestine, thus possibly playing a major role in the prevention of cancer (103).

Phytoestrogens

Phytoestrogens are found only in a few plant species. The most important representatives occur in soy beans (genistein) and flax seeds (lignans). They resemble human estrogens in structure, though their activity is much lower (0.1 %). Depending on their concentration and the amount of the body's own estrogens, they may act as week estrogens or, through competitive inhibition of endogenous estrogens, also as antiestrogens (26). By stimulating the synthesis of SHBG (sex hormone-binding globulin) in the serum, phytoestrogens may contribute to the inhibition of carcinogenesis during the phases of promotion and progression (37).

Various epidemiological studies and animal experiments have demonstrated that, by influencing the hormone metabolism, phytoestrogens protect from hormone-related cancer, such as mammary, uterine, and prostate carcinomas, as well as from nonhormone-related ones, such as colon carcinoma (103).

Sulfides

Sulfides are sulfur-containing compounds that are responsible for the typical odor of garlic and onions. They have a long history as medicinal remedies, and their antimicrobial activity was demonstrated by Louis Pasteur in 1858. In animal experiments and epidemiological studies, a protective effect was observed against various types of cancer, above all, gastric carcinoma. Presumably, the antioxidant and immunostimulating properties of sulfides contribute to their anticancer activity (103).

Phytic Acid

Phytic acid occurs in grains, nuts, seeds, and legumes; for a long time, it has been played down as an undesirable food component. It binds minerals, such as iron, zinc, and magnesium, and thus reduces their absorption. However, studies have shown that, as a component of a balanced diet, phytic acid does not affect mineral metabolism. In animal experiments, phytic acid exhibited cancer-preventing activity, presumably because of its ability to capture iron radicals (103).

Fiber

In addition to secondary plant metabolites, bioactive substances include also dietary fiber. The term fiber relates to those components in plant food that cannot be digested by the human body's own enzymes in the small intestine. They contribute to normal intestinal function and have an effect on cholesterol metabolism, glucose tolerance, development of cardiovascular diseases, and metabolic activity of the intestinal flora (103).

Those segments of the populations that consume relatively larger amounts of fiber with their food are less often affected by colon carcinoma than other persons. This has led to the conclusion that fiber prevents carcinogenesis in the intestine. Several mechanisms of action have been discussed for the protective effect of dietary fiber.

Nonabsorbed food components are degraded through microbial activity into short-chain fatty acids, e. g., butyrate. This lowers the pH of the intestinal content and thus interferes with the formation of secondary bile acids, which are known to promote carcinogenesis. In addition, low pH stimulates apoptosis. A diet rich in fats and cholesterol raises the amount of bile acids in the intestine and, therefore, also the risk of cancer (Table 8.**5**) (20).

The Nurses Health Study in the United States caused quite a stir when it called into question the protective effect of dietary fiber. In the subsequent analysis, no effect of fiber intake on the development of tumors was observed (30). However, the interpretation of these results did not take into account that even the study group with the highest fiber intake consumed only an average of 24.9 g/day, which is clearly below the recommended minimum intake of 30 g/day. Hence, one cannot draw the conclusion that sufficient amounts of fiber intake had no protective effect (61).

Substances in Fermented Foods

Lactic acid fermentation is an old method of preservation, in which foods are altered through the activity of various microorganisms. Currently, we are witnessing a rising trend to dairy products containing lactic acid bacteria (probiotics), which are believed to have a health-promoting effect.

The major metabolite of food fermentation is lactic acid. It is found in large quantities in fermented vegetable products (e.g., sauerkraut) and in fermented dairy products (e.g., yogurt, cheese).

- Lactic acid bacteria have a direct tumor-inhibiting effect. It has been demonstrated in animal experiments that yogurt inhibits tumor growth (93). Lactic acid-fermented foods play a major role particularly in the prevention of colon carcinoma because they change the human intestinal flora in a positive way. They inhibit the production of several bacterial enzymes in the stool which promote the conversion of procarcinogens into carcinogens (50, 51).

Dietary Recommendations for the Prevention of Cancer

It is assumed that compliance with dietary recommendations will lead to the largest possible decrease in the incidence of cancer within the population. In addition, dietary recommendations give each and everyone the chance to lower the personal risk of cancer. Adhering to these recommendations does not ensure definitive protection; it only reduces the average probability of developing the disease. On the other hand, even the most severe violations will not necessarily result in cancer.

The recommendations have been compiled by the World Cancer Research Fund International (WCRF International) in such a way that they take into consideration all important dietary risk factors for cancer worldwide. They largely agree with the recommendations for the prevention of other chronic diseases, and most of them are identical to the recommendations of the German Society of Nutrition (Table 8.**6**).

▬ The Role of Nutrition in Cancer Treatment

One should distinguish between the nutritional advice for preventing cancer and the nutrition therapy for patients already affected by cancer, even though nutrition therapy will always contribute also to secondary and tertiary prevention. One should take into account that a cure is not possible just by means of a special diet. However, there is no phase in which nutrition therapy cannot contribute to improving the overall situation of the body, thus strengthening the regenerative forces and preventing a potential relapse. The starting

Table 8.5   Fibers: mechanisms of preventing colon carcinoma (8)
• Increased stool volume results in low proportion of carcinogens per total stool volume, reduced contact of potential carcinogens with the intestinal wall, and rapid passage through the intestines.
• Binding of potential carcinogens
• Promotion of a healthy intestinal flora that performs numerous metabolic, immunological, and protective functions
• Immunomodulation by influencing the intestinal flora
• Bacterial degradation of soluble fiber to short-chain fatty acids (acetate, propionate, butyrate); butyrate is the main energy source for the colon epithelium, and it regulates cell proliferation and differentiation
• Reduced pH due to generation of short-chain fatty acids inhibits production of cancer-promoting secondary bile acids
• Removal of ammonia from the intestinal lumen; ammonia increases the pH in the colon, thus increasing the risk of cancer

condition for medical treatment can be improved, and side effects of toxic therapies can be reduced.

Unintended loss of weight is often the first indication that a carcinoma already exists. Malnutrition, no matter what its cause, results in severe metabolic and immunological impairments, which will worsen the prognosis of cancer patients:

- reduced response to a specific treatment
- increase in complications (e.g., during surgery)
- increased morbidity and mortality
- reduced life expectancy
- reduced quality of life (56, 64–68).

Cancer cachexia is the second most common cause of death after sepsis, and it is the direct cause in about 20% of cancer patients (59–61).

The nutritional requirements of the cancer patient are increased due to tumor growth and its treatment. In addition to the direct effect of tumor consumption, there is a reduction in the uptake of energy and nutrients. The possible causes include:

- loss of appetite
- early satiety
- pain
- altered gustatory and olfactory sensations
- obstruction
- treatment-induced side effects
- emotional factors
- hormone-induced and cytokine-induced metabolic processes.

In some patients, the metabolic rate at rest is increased considerably. Essential preliminary examinations as well as surgery further prevent adequate intake and utilization of nutrients. Prior to such examinations, patients frequently must fast for a prolonged period or have their food intake restricted. In addition, major surgery leads to a catabolic state (postaggression syndrome) (77).

Cancer Cachexia and Anorexia

The most common problems are cancer cachexia and anorexia, particularly when the tumor is already in a progressive stage. In a large study, DeWrys and co-workers reported that more than 50% of patients suffered from weight loss (21). About 15% lost more than 10% of their weight during the course of the disease.

Cancer cachexia interferes with the patient's physical and emotional well-being. Patients not only have to cope with their life-threatening disease, they also change in appearance due to severe loss of weight. This leads to a significant increase in morbidity, mortality, and prolonged hospitalization, thus representing a major cost factor (67).

Signs of cancer cachexia are anemia, anorexia, lack of energy, and increasing weight loss. The latter is caused by a decrease in body fat and muscle mass (56–58). There is no clear correlation between the extent of malnutrition, the tumor's size,

---

Table 8.6   Dietary recommendations for the prevention of cancer (20)

Life style
- Eat mostly plant foods derived from various types of fruits, vegetables, and legumes, while avoiding processed starchy foods
- Avoid obesity and underweight; any increase in weight during adulthood should not exceed 5 kg
- Exercise for a minimum of one hour per day, with intense physical activity for a minimum of one hour per week

Food
- Eat five or more servings of fruits and vegetables per day (approximately 400–500 g per day)
- Eat more than seven servings of grain products, legumes, potatoes, or other plant food per day (approxi-mately 600–800 g per day); avoid highly processed foods
- Avoid alcohol; a maximum of two alcoholic beverages per day for men, and one per day for women
- Limit the consumption of meat to an average of 80 g per day; prefer fish, poultry, or game
- Limit the consumption of fatty foods; avoid fat of animal origin, prefer vegetable oils
- Avoid heavily salted foods and those preserved by salt

Handling
- Do not eat moldy or spoiled food
- Store food in fridge or freezer, or use another suitable form of preservation (boiling, pickling)
- Do not eat burnt food; limit your consumption of barbecued, pickled, and smoked meat
- Nutritional supplements, such as vitamin tablets, are usually not required for cancer prevention; uncontrolled intake of high doses may be harmful under certain circumstances

expansion, or degree of differentiation, and the duration of the disease. Hence, it is hard to predict in the individual case whether cancer cachexia will develop (109).

Cancer cachexia is a multifactorial process that is still poorly understood (59). It is a combination of exogenous and endogenous starvation, but substrate metabolism in a cancer patient differs considerably from that of a hungry person because adaptive processes fail to take place (56–58, 62, 63). It seems as if the contributing factors depend on both the tumor itself and the metabolic response of the cancer patient. Cytokines are currently discussed as major mediators of cancer cachexia—in addition to hormones, such as corticosteroids, glucagon, or somatotrophic hormone. Above all, TNF-α, which is also called cachectin, seems to play an important role (108).

Metabolism in a cachectic cancer patient is characterized by increased protein turnover and degradation of muscles proteins, associated with reduced protein synthesis in peripheral muscles. Simultaneously, there is a loss of body fat caused by the high rates of lipolysis and fat oxidation—and not even glucose intake can interrupt this.

Glucose metabolism in a cancer patient is characterized by increased glucose turnover as well as increased gluconeogenesis from amino acids and lactate, with simultaneous reduction of glucose oxidation and elevated lactate production (56–58, 62, 63). Metabolic abnormalities are one of the reasons why it is so difficult to overcome malnutrition and to achieve a build-up of body mass (91). Hence, the best results with nutrition therapy can be expected when the measures are initiated as soon as possible to prevent the onset of cancer cachexia (52, 53).

It has been discussed repeatedly whether or not high caloric feeding will benefit the cancer patient or, rather, promote tumor growth. Such considerations were based on results from animal experiments, but similar findings have not been confirmed in humans. Since tumors take essential nutrients away from the rest of the body—irrespective of food intake and nutritional state of the patient—nutrition therapy benefits first the patient and not the tumor; in particular, it improves the patient's defense mechanisms. In the case of chemotherapy and radiotherapy, stimulation of tumor growth would be even advantageous because it increases the blood supply and the rate of mitosis (44).

Table 8.7 Various ways of alleviating treatment-induced eating problems (109)

Loss of appetite	Nausea/ vomiting	Problems with chewing/ swallowing	Dry mouth	Diarrhea	Constipation
• Eat several small meals (also at night) • Avoid strong-smelling food • Drink only between meals • Prepare food in an appetizing way (including mashed food) • Drink appetizing beverages • Eat what you like, not just what is healthy	• Avoid strong-smelling food • Eat and drink slowly • Chew thoroughly • Eat many small meals • Avoid fatty and sweet foods • Eat dry foods (toast, crackers, biscuits), especially in the morning when getting up • Make sure your upper body is upright when eating • Clean your teeth or drink peppermint tea after each meal • Replenish any loss of fluid and electrolytes	• Fat cold foods to alleviate pain • Avoid crumbly food or soak it • Soft, mild foods are best suited (creamy soups, yogurt) • Butter or cream in the food makes swallowing easier • Avoid bitter and sour foods • Pass foods through a sieve • Avoid carbonated beverages	• Prefer water-containing foods (fruits, soups, dairy products) • Drink often and take many small sips • Peppermint tea and lemon tea stimulate the flow of saliva • Eat sour candies or citrus fruits between meals	• Drink plenty of fluids (2.5–3 L) • Avoid fatty and bloating meals • Eat fruits rich in pectin (apples, bananas, carrots) • Eat rice or oat gruel, or drink black tea (let stand for 5 min) • Eat foods rich in potassium (bananas) • Drink sour milk rather than fresh milk • Use soy milk in case of lactose intolerance • Avoid alcohol, coffee, and carbonated beverages	• Drink plenty of fluids • Prefer foods rich in fiber • Make sure to drink lots of fluids when eating isolated fiber (bran, flax seeds) • Physical exercise • Gentle massage of the abdomen

Table 8.8 Nutritional consultation for cancer patients
• Record the actual symptoms (loss of appetite, pain, intolerance)
• Develop a menu ("favorite diet," considering aversions and preferences)
• Pay attention to food preparation (size of the meal, appearance, consistency)
• Monitor nutritional parameters (amount of food taken in, nutritional condition)
• Involve and educate caretakers (family, friends, family doctor, nurses)

Nutritional care of cancer patients plays an essential role in the therapeutic concept because the nutritional state of a patient can be improved by adequate supply of nutrients. Cancer patients depend on nutritional advice because they are especially susceptible to self-proclaimed healers or to impressive, but unfortunately often health-threatening cancer diets (77).

The main goal of nutrition therapy for cancer patients is to maintain or achieve an adequate nutritional state. This strengthens the immune system, improves the physical and emotional state, increases the patient's tolerance to treatment, and enhances the quality of life. Early nutritional intervention might also prolong life expectancy—a goal that has not been achieved so far (56, 64, 66, 70, 71).

Table 8.7 shows how treatment-induced eating problems may be alleviated.

The diet should be adjusted to the situation and fine-tuned to the individual needs of the patient. A "favorite diet" may contribute to improving the quality of life, independently of whether or not it represents "healthy" food. There is no use in providing a balanced, healthy diet when the patient

cannot eat it because of pain or loss of appetite, or does not like or tolerate it.

When giving advice to patients, it is important to take a detailed nutritional history and to determine any individual intolerance as well as the nutritional state. If sufficient nutrients cannot be taken in with an oral diet, supplementation with vitamins, minerals, and trace elements is needed (23). Possible ways of nutrition support include special drink mixes and additional enteral or parenteral feeding.

Proper education of patient, relatives, and nursing staff often makes it possible to discharge the patient earlier. This is of major importance for the patient's quality of life, and it saves costs. An interdisciplinary nutritional team would be ideal, and outpatients should have access to it. Timely and adequate nutrition therapy does avoid follow-up costs arising from treatment of malnutrition, and it improves the quality of life for severely sick patients.

Physicians, dietitians, hospital administration, nursing staff, and politicians should collaborate to ensure financial and personal conditions for a high-quality nutrition therapy of cancer patients (Table 8.**8**) (77).

Determination of the Nutritional State

Nutrition therapy should be based on the accurate determination of the patient's nutritional state (72, 73). The simplest parameter is weight control under standardized conditions (weighing in the morning, with an empty stomach and after having been to the bathroom). It should be taken into account that about 50 % of people are overweight at the beginning of their disease. Even with these pa-

Table 8.9 Diagnostic parameters of malnutrition (68, 106)	
Parameter	**Normal values**
Body mass index (BMI)	20–25 kg/m^2
Triceps crease *	Men: 13.7–11.3 mm; women: 18.1–14.9 mm
Circumference of upper arm *	Men: 27.8–22.8 cm; women: 25.5–20.9 cm
Creatinine height index (g creatinine × kg body weight **/height in cm)	Men: 0.5–0.8; women: 0.2–0.4
Lymphocytes	
Serum albumin	> 1500/μL
Serum transferrin	> 35 g/L
	> 200 mg/100 mL

* In the middle of the upper arm; ** ideal body weight.

tients, an unintended weight loss of more than 5% of the starting weight within three months suggests an inadequate supply with nutrients. Fluid retention may obscure a loss of weight. Table 8.9 provides an overview of further easy-to-record diagnostic parameters of malnutrition.

Nutritional Recommendations for Cancer Patients

Cancer patients do not require a diet of special composition. In most cases, it is sufficient to offer a mixed, varied diet that is easy to digest and takes into account any aversions and preferences the patient may have (54, 56, 64, 70). On principle, patients should be informed that sufficient intake of food is important for their nutritional state and well-being and that a targeted diet is possible.

Dietary recommendations for cancer patients are currently based on reference values for the diet of a healthy person, like those established by the German Society of Nutrition (22). As there is evidence that certain nutrients (e.g., omega-3 fatty acids) influence the growth and metabolism of cells, the condition and regeneration of tissues, and also the modulation of immune defenses, attempts have been made to improve the nutritional state of cancer patients by means of such substances (77, 78). However, clear recommendations are not yet available.

The nutrition of cancer patients should be as physiological and free of complications as possible; hence, oral nutrition should be maintained as long as possible (Table 8.**10**). This is also important for normal function of the gastrointestinal tract.

Proper digestion and absorption are essential, and so is the mental willingness to eat (87).

If, for an extended period, adequate food intake is no longer possible, dietary drink mixes and supplements may be added to the diet. (An energy intake of less than 1200 kcal/day no longer guarantees adequate intake of essential nutrients.) Individual needs of the patient can be addressed by a special composition of the diet (rich in energy and proteins, with or without fiber, with fats containing medium-chain triglycerides, without lactose). Formula diets are well suited, especially for patients who live on their own and, due to their disease, may not have the possibility, energy, or desire to cook a meal adjusted to their individual needs (77).

Only when all options for oral nutrition have been exhausted, or when the patient feels too much put under pressure, enteral or parenteral feeding is indicated. Both forms of artificial nutrition support can be performed at home. Basically, enteral feeding harbors fewer complications and stimulates normal digestion. Whenever possible, it should be preferred over parenteral feeding as long as the gastrointestinal tract is intact (52, 53).

Preoperative Nutrition Therapy

- Prolonged phases of fasting can be compensated by shifting the time of eating or by changing the composition of a meal. High-calorific drinks and soups with little fiber are often allowed until a few hours before the scheduled examination. The patient should be allowed to eat a high-quality meal immediately after the exam-

---

Table 8.10 Types of diets for cancer patients (106)

Oral nutrition
- Full diet, or a light full diet, in the form of a varied "favorite diet," considering any aversions and preferences
- Adapted full diet, using special methods of preparation (e.g., mashed food, liquid food)
- Special composition of diet (e.g., lactose free, fats with medium-chain triglycerides)
- Full diet with nutrients added (balanced nutritional drink mixes, dietary supplements)

Artificial nutrition support
- Enteral nutrition (also as semienteral nutrition)
  - tubes (nasogastral, nasoduodenal)
  - percutaneous endoscopic gastrostomy (PEG) and jejunostomy (PEJ)
  - percutaneous sonographic gastrostomy (PSG)
  - fine needle catheter jejunostomy (FNCJ)
- Parenteral nutrition
  - injection into peripheral vein (short-term to supplement oral or enteral nutrition)
  - injection into central vein ("total parenteral nutrition", TPN) (also as parenteral nutrition at home)

ination rather than having to wait until the next regular mealtime (109).

- In malnourished patients, enteral or parenteral nutrition therapy should be applied for at least seven days before surgery. This can lower the number of postoperative complications.
- The benefits of parenteral nutrition have also been documented in patients undergoing bone marrow transplantation (59, 76).

Postoperative Nutrition Therapy

Professional dietary care during the first weeks and months after surgery is of utmost importance for the future course of the disease. Following a phase of adaptation, the body weight will stabilize, and most of the patients will be able to eat all kinds of food again, depending on the type of the disease.

- In patients who have lost all appetite, or in palliative patients, it is recommended that additional enteral or parenteral nutrition be provided at night for an extended period; this applies also to outpatients. Application of a tube or catheter during surgery is desirable. It facilitates postoperative nutrition therapy in a timely fashion.
- In case of side effects and loss of appetite due to cancer treatment, the patient can be supplied with additional nutrients (101).
- A significant reduction in postoperative complications and less time spent in the hospital can be achieved through special immunonutrition (19). Such diets usually contain several immunomodulating substrates, such as arginine, glutamine, and omega-3 fatty acids. However, appropriate indications are still being discussed (106).

Adjuvant Nutrition Therapy

Patients who cannot eat enough should receive enteral or parenteral nutrition in a timely fashion, in addition to their normal diet. This makes it possible to supply sufficient nutrients and fluids, thus preventing the progression of malnutrition. Enteral and parenteral substitution of nutrients can relieve the patient from major stress. In an effort not to get weaker, many patients force themselves to eat. Because of their disease and/or due to side effects from the treatment, they often fail to eat suf-

ficient amounts, thus promoting depressive mood and confrontations. Hence, it is important that artificial nutrition support is initiated in a timely fashion, preferably in the least invasive and most natural form.

To prevent additional reduction of oral food intake due to the intake of nutrient solutions, nutrient substitution during the night makes sense

▬ Benefits of Nutritional Consultation— Conclusions

The demands on evidence-based medicine, together with economical problems of health care, have lead to critical questions regarding nutrition therapy. For both patient and therapist, the goal of nutrition therapy lies in preventing the nutritional state from getting worse (22), whereas others generally demand a significant effect on the outcome together with a reduction in costs (105).

Is nutrition therapy not an allocation that is equivalent to basic human needs? Is it important to measure its effect in terms of efficacy, effectiveness, and efficiency? Is it ethical to analyze artificial nutrition in terms of economic efficiency when a patient is extremely ill?

A consensus conference in the United States in 1997 concluded that parenteral nutrition is indicated in postoperative patients if oral or enteral nutrition cannot be initiated within days (105). When immunonutrition is used for therapeutic goals—such as improving the nutritional state or influencing the disease favorably—proof of economic profitability by criteria of evidence-based medicine is mandatory. In the case of palliative patients, therapy is focused on stopping weight loss and improving the quality of life. Here, the form of therapy has to be adjusted to the wishes of patient and family.

In conclusion, it becomes clear that evidence for a therapeutic indication of nutrition therapy must be presented and that the economic profitability should be discussed. In the case of nutrient substitution and palliative nutrition, it seems ethically problematic to argue with parameters like outcome, effectivity, efficiency, and cost–benefit ratio (105).

Professional dietary care ensures that nutritional problems can be recognized and alleviated. The patient's uncertainty and the dangers of a lopsided cancer diet can be avoided. It is a fact that a clear improvement in the nutritional state is rarely achieved when an advanced carcinoma is associated with prominent malnutrition. Nevertheless, nutrition therapy improves the patient's emotional state and quality of life, especially if offered to outpatients.

▬ References

1. Bartram HP, Kasper H: Bedeutung mehrfach ungesättigter Fettsäuren bei der Kolonkarzinogenese. Akt Ernähr Med. 1995; 20: 31–35.
2. Belitz HD, Grosch W: Lehrbuch der Lebensmittelchemie. 4th ed., Berlin, Springer Verlag, 1992.
3. Bendich A: Carotenoids and the immune response. Am J Nutr. 1991; 136:112–114.
4. Biesalski HK: Antioxidative Vitamine in der Prävention. Dt Ärzteblatt. 1995; 92:1316–1321.
5. Biesalski HK et al: Kenntnisstand Selen–Ergebnisse des Hohenheimer Konsensusmeetings. Akt Ernähr Med. 1997; 22:224–231.
6. Biesalski HK et al. (eds): Vitamine. Stuttgart, Georg Thieme Verlag, 1997.
7. Biesalski HK: Vitamine. In: Biesalski, HK et al. (eds): Ernährungsmedizin. 2nd ed., Stuttgart, Georg Thieme Verlag, 1999.
8. Biesalski HK et al. (eds): Ernährungsmedizin. 2nd ed., Stuttgart, Georg Thieme Verlag, 1999.
9. Block G et al.: Fruit, vegetables and cancer prevention: a review of the epidemiological evidence. Nutr Cancer. 1992; 18:1–29.
10. Blot WJ et al.: Nutrition intervention trials in Linxian, China: supplementation with specific vitamin/mineral combinations, cancer incidence and disease-specific mortality in the general population. J Natl Cancer Inst. 1993; 85:1483–1491.
11. Bode C, Parlesak A: Ernährung und Krebs–Welche Ernährungsweisen begünstigen die Krebsentstehung? Akt Ernähr Med. 2001; 26:121–129.
12. Boeing H: Kalzium und Anitoxidanzien als Supplemente in der Krebsprophylaxe–Statusbericht zu den Interventionsstudien. Akt Ernähr Med. 2001; 26:130–136.
13. Böhm H et al.: Flavonole, Flavone und Anthocyane als natürliche Antioxidanzien der Nahrung und ihre mögliche Rolle bei der Prävention chronischer Erkrankungen. Z Ernähr-Wiss. 1998; 37:147–163.
14. Bozzetti F et al.: Artificial nutrition in cancer patients: which route, what composition? World J Surg. 1999; 23:577–583.
15. Bürger B, Ollenschläger G: Ernährungsberatung des Tumorpatienten. Akt Ernähr Med. 1992; 17:293–299.
16. Canzler H, Brodersen H: Ernährung und Tumorhäufigkeit. In: Schauder P (eds): Ernährung und Tumorerkrankungen. Basel, Karger Verlag, 1991, pp. 28–56.
17. Carr AC, Frei B: Toward a new recommended dietary allowance for vitamin C based on antioxidant and health effects in humans. Am J Clin Nutr. 1999; 69:1086–1107.
18. Committee on Dietary Guidelines Implementation, National Academy of Sciences, Improving America's Diet and Health. Washington DC, National Academy Press, 1991.
19. Daly JM et al.: Enteral nutrition with supplemental arginine, RNA, and omega-3-fatty acids in patients after operation: Immunologic, metabolic and clinical outcome. Surgery; 1992. 112: 56–67.
20. Deutsches Institut für Enährungsforschung (DifE) (ed.): Krebsprävention durch Ernährung. www.dife.de, Bergholz-Rehbrücke 1999.
21. DeWys WD et al.: Prognostic effect of weight loss prior to chemotherapy in cancer patients. Am J Med. 1994; 69:491–497
22. DGE: Referenzwerte für die Nährstoffzufuhr. Deutsche Gesellschaft für Ernährung (DGE). Frankfurt am Main, Umschau/Brauss-Verlagsgesellschaft, 2000.
23. Dittrich K, Leitzmann C: Bioaktive Substanzen, Stuttgart, Georg Thieme Verlag, 1996.
24. Doll R, Peto R: The causes of cancer: quantitative estimates of avoidable risks of cancer in the United States today. J Nat Cancer Institute. 1981; 66:1191–308.
25. Eichholzer M, Stähelin HB: Antioxidative Vitamine und Krebs–eine Übersicht. Akt Ernähr Med. 1994; 19:2–11.
26. Eichholzer M et al. (eds): Ernährung und Krebs: epidemiologische Beweislage. Bern, Schweizerische Krebsliga, Schweizerische Vereinigung für Ernährung, 1998.
27. Elmadfa I, König JS: Vitamine in der Ernährung des Tumorkranken, Akt Ernähr Med. 1992; 17:320–325.
28. Fink-Gremmels J, Leistner L: Mutagene in der Nahrung. In: Schauder, P. (ed.): Ernährung und Tumorerkrankungen. Basel; Karger Verlag, 1991, pp. 168–184.
29. Food and Nutrition Board, Institute of Medicine: dietary reference intakes for thiamine, riboflavin, niacin, vitamin B6, folate, vitamin B12, pantothenic acid, biotin and choline. Washington DC; National Academy Press, 1998.
30. Fuchs CS et al.: Dietary fiber and the risk of colorectal cancer and adenoma in women. N Engl J Med. 1999; 340:169–176.
31. Gärtner U, Seitz HK: Krebsentstehung–ernährungsbedingt? Klinikarzt. 1993; 22:114–124.
32. Gaßmann B: β-Carotin–Mythos und Dilemma der Nahrungsergänzung. Ernährungsumschau. 1998; 45:79.

33. Gerhäuser C: Flavonoide und andere pflanzliche Wirkstoffe. Akt Ernähr Med. 2001; 26:137–143.

34. Glynn SA, Albanes D: Folate and cancer: a review of the literature. Nutr Cancer. 1994; 22:101–119.

35. Gröber U: Orthomolekulare Medizin. Stuttgart; Wissenschaftliche Verlagsgesellschaft, 2000.

36. Großklaus R: Functional Food–Lebensmittel oder Arzneimittel? Ernährungsumschau. 1998; 45:70–73.

37. Großklaus R: Sekundäre Pflanzenstoffe–Was ist beim Menschen wissenschaftlich hinreichend gesichert? Akt Ernähr Med. 2000; 25:227–237.

38. Haas O et al.: Bilanzierte Diät mit hohem Fettgehalt versus Normalkost bei Patienten mit gastrointestinalen Karzinomen. Eine prospektive, randomiesierte Studie. Akt Ernähr Med. 1995; 20:60.

39. Hapke HJ: Toxikologische Aspekte der Ernährung. In: Deutsche Gesellschaft für Ernährung (ed.): Ernährungsbericht 1996. Commissioned by: Bundesministerium für Gesundheit und des Bundesministeriums für Ernährung, Landwirtschaft und Forsten, Frankfurt a. M. 1996.

40. Heinonen OP, Albanes D: The effect of vitamin E and beta carotene on the incidence of lung cancer and other cancers in male smokers. N Engl J Med. 1994; 330:1029–1035.

41. Hennekes CH et al.: Lack of effect of long-term supplementation with beta carotene on the incidence of malignant neoplasms and cardiovascular disease. N Engl J Med. 1996; 334:1145–1149.

42. Henning KJ, Großklaus R: Schutz des Verbrauchers vor ungesicherten Wirkungsangaben bei Lebensmitteln. Lebensmittel & Recht. 2000; 4:38–48.

43. Heseker H et al.: Vitaminversorgung in der Bundesrepublik Deutschland. In: Kübler W et al. (eds): VERA-Schriftenreihe, vol. 4, Niederkleen, Wissenschaftlicher Fachverlag Dr. Fleck, 1992.

44. Holm E: Ernährungstherapie bei Tumorerkrankungen: Wird der Tumor gefüttert? In: Schauder P (ed.): Ernährung und Tumorerkrankungen. Basel, Karger Verlag 1991.

45. Homann N, Seitz NK: Alkohol und Krebs. Klinikarzt. 1996; 25:216–219.

46. Howe GR et al.: Dietary factors and risk of breast cancer: combined analysis of 12 case–control studies. J Nat Cancer Inst. 1990; 82:561–569.

47. Hunter DJ et al.: A prospective study of the intake of vitamins C, E and A and the risk of breast cancer. N Engl J Med. 1993; 329:234–240.

48. Imoberdorf R: Sinn und Unsinn von Krebsdiäten. Akt Ernähr Med. 2001; 26:164–166.

49. Jordan A, Stein J: Ernährung von Tumorpatienten: neue diätetische Strategien. Ernährungsumschau. 1997; 44:289–293.

50. Jordan A et al.: Enterale Ernährung tumorkranker Patienten. Ergebnisse einer 4-jährigen retrospektiven Studie. Akt Ernähr Med. 1997; 22:4–8.

51. Jungi WF: Diätetische Möglichkeiten zur Krebsverhütung. Forum Deutsche Krebsgesellschaft e.V. 1997; 12:209–216.

52. Jungi WF: Kachexie als eigenständiger Prognosefaktor bei Tumorleiden. In: Schauder P (ed.): Ernährung und Tumorerkrankungen. Basel, Karger Verlag, 1991.

53. Kaspar H: Tumorentstehung–hemmende und fördernde Effekte von Ernährungsfaktoren. In: Deutsche Gesellschaft für Ernährung (ed.): Ernährungsbericht 1996. Commissioned by: Bundesministeriums für Gesundheit und des Bundesministeriums für Ernährung, Landwirtschaft und Forsten, Frankfurt a. M. 1996.

54. Konhorst ML: Ernährungsberatung versus Produktempfehlungen–Definitionen, Möglichkeiten und Grenzen. Ernährungsumschau. 1997; 44:380–383.

55. Krämer K: Antioxidanzien in der Onkologie. Dtsch Z Onkol. 1994; 26:76–83.

56. Krämer K et al.: Selen und Tumorerkrankungen. Akt Ernähr Med. 1996; 21:103–113.

57. Kühnau J: Unterschiede in der ernährungsphysiologischen Bedeutung pflanzlicher und tierischer Lebensmittel für den Menschen. Ernährungsumschau. 1976; 23:43–48.

58. Laviano A: From laboratory to bedside: new strategies in the treatment of malnutrition in cancer patients. Nutrition. 1996; 12:112–122.

59. Lee SH et al.: Vitamin C-induced decomposition of lipid hydroperoxides to endogenous genotoxins. Science. 2001; 292:2083–2086.

60. Leitzmann C et al.: Ernährung bei Krebs. München, Gräfe und Unzer, 1996.

61. Leitzmann C et al.: Ernährung in Prävention und Therapie. Stuttgart, Hippokrates Verlag, 2001.

62. Lipkin M, Newmark H: Effect of added dietary calcium on colonic epithelial-cell proliferation in subjects at high risk for familial colonic cancer. N Engl J Med. 1985; 313:1381–1384.

63. Löffler G, Petrides PE: Biochemie und Pathobiochemie. 6th ed., Berlin, Springer Verlag, 1998.

64. Lordan A, Stein J: Ernährung von Tumorpatienten: neue diätetische Strategien. Ernährungsumschau. 1997; 44:289–293.

65. Milner JA: Functional foods and health promotion. J Nutr. 1999; 129:1395–1397.

66. Müller C et al.: Der Einfluss von Sauerkraut und Kimchi auf bakterielle Enzymaktivitäten und den pH-Wert im Stuhl des Menschen. Akt Ernähr Med. 1993; 18:351–356.

67. Müller JM et al.: Preoperative parenteral feeding in patients with gastrointestinal carcinoma. Lancet. 1982;1:68–71.

68. Müller MJ: Strategien der Ernährungsmedizin. Akt Ernähr Med. 1993; 18:87–96.

69. Müller MJ et al.: Tumorkachexie: Pathophysiologische Grundlagen und ernährungsmedizinische Aufgaben. Akt Ernähr Med. 1991;16:1–6.

70. Ollenschläger G et al.: Orale Ernährungstherapie des internistischen Tumorpatienten–ein integraler Bestandteil der supportiven Behandlungsmaßnahmen. Akt Ernähr Med. 1990; 15:66–71.

71. Ollenschläger G: Orale Ernährungstherapie bei Tumorerkrankungen. In: Schauder P (ed.): Ernährung und Tumorerkrankungen. Basel, Karger Verlag, 1991.

72. Ollenschläger G, Bürger B: Die Bedeutung der natürlichen Ernährung für den Tumorpatienten. Akt Ernähr Med. 1992; 17:278–284.

73. Omenn GS et al.: Effects of a combination of beta carotene and Vitamin A on lung cancer and cardiovascular disease. N Engl J Med. 1996; 334:1150–1155.

74. Osswald B et al.: Krebsrisiko durch Alkohol. Akt Ernähr Med. 1991;16:33–40.

75. Ovesen L et al.: The interrelationship of weight loss, dietary intake and quality of life in ambulatory patients with cancer of the lung, breast and ovary. Nutrition and Cancer. 1993; 19:159–167.

76. Palmer S, Bakshi K: Diet, nutrition and cancer: interim dietary guidelines. J Nat Cancer Inst. 1983; 70:1151–1170.

77. Paul C: Ernährung und Krebs–Was kann die Diätberatung leisten? Akt Ernähr Med. 2001; 26:153–159.

78. Pirlich M et al.: Mangelernährung bei Klinikpatienten: Diagnostik und klinische Bedeutung. Akt Ernähr Med. 1999; 24: 260–266.

79. Prasad KN: Vitamins in cancer prevention and treatment: a practical guide. Rochester, Healing Arts Press, 1994.

80. Prasad KN, Edwards-Prasad J: Vitamin E and cancer prevention: recent advances and future potentials. J Am Coll Nutr. 1992; 11:487–500.

81. Rabast U: Ernährungseinflüsse in der Entstehung und Prävention von Tumorerkrankungen. Akt Ernähr Med. 1992; 17:215–222.

82. Rayman MP: The importance of selenium to human health. Lancet; 356: 233–241 2000.

83. Rechkemmer G: Beeinflussung der Darmflora durch Ernährung. In: Deutsche Gesellschaft für Ernährung (ed.): Ernährungsbericht 1996. Commissioned by: Bundesministeriums für Gesundheit und des Bundesministeriums für Ernährung, Landwirtschaft und Forsten, Frankfurt a. M. 2000.

84. Richter G: Enterale Ernährung von Tumorpatienten. Aktuel Ernähr Med. 1996; 17:69–78.

85. Roth E: Besonderheiten des Intermediärstoffwechsels tumorkranker Patienten und ihre Bedeutung für die Ernährungstherapie. In: Schauder P (ed.): Ernährung und Tumorerkrankungen. Basel, Karger Verlag, 1991.

86. Sailer D: Ernährung und Lebenserwartung bei onkologischen Patienten. In: Schauder P (ed.): Ernährung und Tumorerkrankungen. Basel, Karger Verlag, 1991.

87. Schauder P: Ernährung und Tumorerkrankungen: Prinzipien und Standortbestimmung. In: Schauder P (ed.): Ernährung und Tumorerkrankungen, Karger Verlag, Basel 1991.

88. Scheppach W: Ernährung und Tumorerkrankungen. Ergebnisse klinisch-experimenteller Studien. Akt Ernähr Med. 1992; 15:139–143.

89. Schrauzer GN: Selen–essenzielles Spurenelement und Krebsschutzfaktor. Münch Med Wschr. 1985; 127:731–734.

90. Schutz Y: Bestimmung des Ernährungszustandes. In: Biesalski, H.K. (ed.): Ernährungsmedizin. 2nd ed., Georg Thieme Verlag, Stuttgart 1999.

91. Selberg O et al.: Genese der Tumorkachexie. In: Schauder P (ed.): Ernährung und Tumorerkrankungen, Karger Verlag, Basel 1991.

92. Selberg O, Müller MJ: Ursachen der Tumorkachexie. Akt Ernähr Med. 1992; 17:274–277.

93. Shahani KM, Ayebo AD: Role of dietary lactobacilli in gastrointestinal microecology. Am J Clin Nutr. 1980; 33:2448–2457.

94. Sill-Steffens R: Die Bedeutung von Selen in der Therapie. In: curriculum oncologicum; Zeitschrift der Österreichischen Gesellschaft für Onkolgie. 2001; 2:12–19.

95. Spittler A et al.: Immunologie und Ernährung. In: Biesalski HK (ed.): Ernährungsmedizin. Stuttgart, Georg Thieme Verlag, 1999.

96. Stähelin HB et al.: Plasma antioxidant vitamins and subsequent cancer mortality in the 12-year follow-up of the prospective Basel Study. Am J Epidemiol. 1991; 133:766–775.

97. Stangl G: Zur Wirkung des Nahrungsfettes auf das Krebsgeschehen. Ernährungsumschau. 1999; 46: 4–9.

98. Tavani A et al: Fruit and vegetable consumption and cancer risk in Mediterranean population. Am J Clin Nutr. 1995; 61:1374–1377.

99. Thomas W, Ollenschläger G: Ernährung und subjektives Wohlbefinden. In: Schauder, P. (ed.): Ernährung und Tumorerkrankungen. Basel, Karger Verlag, 1991.

100. Trentham-Dietz A et al.: Body size and risk of breast cancer. Am J Epidemiol. 1990; 145:1011–1019.

101. Vestweber KH et al.: Postoperative enterale Ernährung. In: Bünte H et al.: Jahrbuch der Chirurgie. Biermann. 1990; 201–212.

102. Watzl B, Bub A: Carotinoide. Ernährungsumschau. 2001; 48:71–74.

103. Watzl B, Leitzmann C: Bioaktive Substanzen in Lebensmittel. 2nd ed., Stuttgart, Hippokrates Verlag, 1999.

104. Watzl B: Gesundheitliche Bedeutung sekundärer Pflanzenstoffe. In: Deutsche Gesellschaft für Ernährung (ed.): Ernährungsbericht 1996. Commissioned by: Bundesministeriums für Gesundheit und des Bundesministeriums für Ernährung, Landwirtschaft und Forsten, Frankfurt a. M. 1996.

105. Weimann A: Sinnvolle Ziele für eine Ernährungstherapie beim Tumorpatienten. Akt Ernähr Med. 2001; 26:167–169.

106. Weimann A, Bischoff SC: Künstliche Ernährung. München/Jena, Urban und Fischer Verlag, 2001.

107. World Cancer Research Fund, American Institute for Cancer Research (ed.): Food, Nutrition and the Prevention of Cancer: a global perspective. Washington DC, 1997.

108. Zürcher G: Ernährung bei Tumorerkrankungen. In: Ambulante Onkologie. Balingen, Spitta Verlag, November 1999.

109. Zürcher G: Tumoren. In: Kluthe R (ed.): Ernährungsmedizin in der Praxis: Aktuelles Handbuch zu Prophylaxe und Therapie ernährungsabhängiger Erkrankungen. Balingen, Spitta Verlag, 2001.

9 Exercise in Cancer Prevention and Follow-up

Gerhard Uhlenbruck and Ilse Ledvina

Introduction

When we recommend exercise to cancer patients, we assume that there is a close correlation between cancer, physical activity, and the immune defense system. These interrelationships are clearly shown in Table 9.**1**.

Cancer imposes an enormously burdensome strain on those afflicted, weakening the immune defenses. Exercise, in contrast, ensures a certain tolerance or resistance to stress, which can be developed particularly through **endurance training**.

In this context, it is important to consider that stabilization of the patient's mental state has a positive effect on the body's immune defense mechanisms. The diagnosis of cancer exerts a maximum of stress that is processed in a variety of ways. Stress entails an adaptation syndrome of neurovegetative and psychoimmunological regulatory circuits as a result of an acute or chronic challenge to the physical and psychological capabilities of a person. The patient can be trained to successfully adapt to this burden by means of a coping strategy commensurate with the circumstances.

Therapies that follow the diagnosis (surgery, chemotherapy, radiotherapy, hormonal therapy) present an additional physiological and psychological burden, further weakening the immune defense system. Exercise creates stress resistance and has a beneficial effect on the psyche, thereby strengthening the immune defenses.

The topic of sports and cancer was first taken up by the German rural doctor Ernst Van Aaken in 1967. He claimed to have statistically proved that an endurance-training regimen designed by him led to a protective effect against cancer. He attributed a vital role to the increase in oxygen supply brought about by exercise. The role of exercise in this context was first indicated in 1973 (15), but it was only as of 1980 that exercise became an accepted rehabilitative procedure in cancer patients (6, 7, 10, 14).

Effect of Exercise

Exercise in the form of **moderate endurance training** strengthens the immune system mentally through fun, joy, and success on the one hand,

Table 9.1 Cancer, exercise, and the immune system	
Exercise as a cancer-triggering or cancer-promoting factor	• Is lymphogranulomatosis more frequently found in young, achievement-driven sports people? • Does an immune system that is weakened by high-level physical exertion promote the development of cancer? • How does psychological stress during physical exertion effect the immune defense, e.g., increased sufferance, overexertion, and excessive demands?
Exercise as a cancer preventive life style	• By strengthening the immune system, training immune defense • By development of a certain resistance to stress • Through reduction of fears and increase in well-being combined with experiencing success • Through changes in life style: changes in diet, avoidance of excess weight, improvement in sleep
Exercise in the cancer follow-up period	• Improvement in the immune defense, specifically activation of natural killer cells (NK cells), but also of T lymphocytes and macrophages • Through psychosocial effects within the group: contacts, talks, concerted undertakings • Improved acceptance of the body: increase in self-esteem, sex life is possible once again, feeling of fitness develops

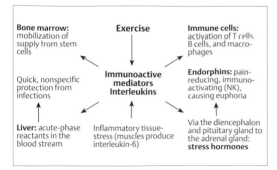

Fig. 9.1 Exercise as inflammatory tissue-stress with immunologic consequences.

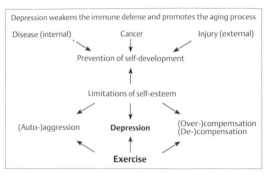

Fig. 9.2 Psychoneuroimmunological aspects of exercise.

and physiologically by inducing moderate inflammatory reactions on the other (Fig. 9.**1**).

Diseases, injuries, losses, and handicaps often lead to chronic loss of self-esteem that can be effectively compensated for by physical activity.

It is important to achieve **muscular tissue stress**, be it by functional gymnastics, sports, and play or specific endurance training as set forth by the guidelines of national sport societies (NRM). The tissue trauma after an operation is also a stress for the immune system, which—in contrast to exercise—exerts a negative effect on the immune functions (Fig. 9.**3**).

The following immunological phenomena can be observed during exercise in the context of cancer follow-up, and are scientifically proved:
- activation of natural killer cells (NK), whose destructive effects on cancer cells are significantly improved (5, 10, 14)
- activation of macrophages (14)
- psychoneuroimmunologically exercise has an anti-depression effect (Fig. 9.**2**).

- improvement of antibacterial characteristics of neutrophilic granulocytes, reducing susceptibility to infections
- overall, the condition of the immune system is improved, which has been demonstrated by functionality tests of the various immune cells, in particular T lymphocytes.
- all rules of exercise immunology have been proved. Initially a mass of undifferentiated immune cells is mobilized, after which smaller groups of immune cells with a specific functional ability are produced. One can trace the cancer-protective effect of exercise back to this phenomenon in retrospective studies. The same seems to hold true for exercise within follow-up for cancer patients. However, too much exercise is not healthy, and too much training can harm the immune system (4, 6, 7).
- the immune fitness of patients who are exercising can be determined and followed with the help of a simple immunology skin test (11). Psychooncological effects of exercise in cancer survivors are listed in Table 9.**2** and Table 9.**3**; the latter also summarizes an optimistic perspective.

Table 9.2 Effect of exercise on the psyche durng cancer follow-up
• Mobilization of self-healing powers: support for self-help and finding of one's self
• Reduced feeling of isolation and loneliness: the psychosocial net catches the soul's needs and bodily discomforts
• Exchange of information: therapy, regimens, physicians, clinics, diet, complementary medicine
• Fewer fears and depressions: saving of medication for pain, sleep, and anxiety
• Mental fitness and strength for a new, intense life of one's own responsibility and with realizable perspectives increase
• Chronic fatigue is reduced

Table 9.3 Psycho-oncology effects of exercise as an enhanced measure in the follow-up of cancer
• Individual fitness: exercise and physical activity three times a week for one hour
• Hobbies: mental training, arts and culture
• Change in diet: fresh fruit and vegetables; fish instead of meats
• Ecoimmunology: family, friends, sexuality (more sense of comfort and love and security)
• Meaningful duty requirements, reachable goals in the job and family or, for example, also volunteer work

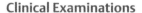

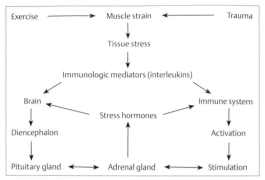

Fig. 9.3 Exercise as muscle tissue stress with effects on the central nervous system and the immune system. Since the immune system as the sixth perceptive sense is derived from the brain, mediator substances from the brain are also "understood" by the cells of the immune system and vice versa ("concerted action").

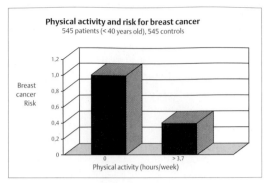

Fig. 9.4 Four hours of physical exercise per week suffice to drastically reduce the risk of breast cancer (7).

Clinical Examinations

- Statistical investigations have shown, that with respect to prevention regular endurance training significantly reduces the risk for individual types of cancer including breast (see Fig 9.**4**) and colorectal cancer (see Fig. 9.**5**). It probably offers some protection against prostate, testicular, and lung cancer, as well as endometrial and ovarian cancer (9) and also other forms of cancer (4, 6, 7, 12).
- Not merely animal experiments (13), but also clinical experience and studies (which have not yet been scientifically evaluated on the topic of remission prophylaxis through moderate endurance training) indicate a postoperative can-

cer-protective effect, mediated by activation of immunological and psychoimmunological circuits. Further research in this direction is highly recommended. Informal studies done so far indicate that this will be a fruitful area of investigation.
- For some types of tumors, the protective effect of regular exercise has been demonstrated. This is true for breast cancer (Fig. 9.**4**), colorectal cancer (Fig. 9.**5**), but also for prostate cancer seminal (testicular) and lung cancer (9).
- Regular physical exertion in the form of endurance training not only activates NK cells but also improves the psychological state as well as the stress resistance, even in the elderly age groups (Fig. 9.**6**) (7, 10, 14).

There are also other **forms of well-being** that can be enhanced through sports, vacation, successes,

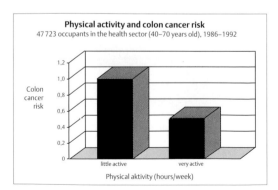

Fig. 9.5 People who are physically active reduce markedly their risk of developing colon cancer (7).

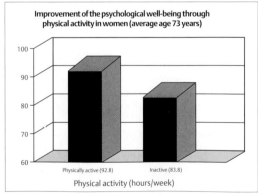

Fig. 9.6 Comparison of women exercising (average age 73 years) and women that are not physically active (7).

> Training signifies daily repetitive physical exercise, as well as physiological and mental exertion with the goal of improving the physical and intellectual capabilities, in order to achieve a meaningful and fulfilled life through adaptation.

and rehabilitation. the term "**training**" should be explained in this context.

Training in the form of moderate exercise and endurance brings all bodily functions back to a healthy stable middle ground: poorly performing systems are restored to normal function (immune system), malfunctions are corrected (blood fats, blood pressure), and excessive overload of physical and psychological stress (stress hormones) are down-regulated.

The sick patient has limitations that he must learn to recognize, since disease results in restricted physical and mental well-being through reduced or impaired biological and ecological conditions. Achieving a positive sense of self is not only realized through free development of genetically predetermined dispositions within the constraints imposed by the disease, but can also be achieved via completely new possibilities. This range of new possibilities includes not only exercise, but also activities such as music, art, literature, painting, reading, and writing, in other words activities that are mentally stimulating and that result in an individual and highly creative healing process.

Regarded in this way, the immune system can be stabilized in multiple ways, as demonstrated in the following figures (Figs 9.**7** and 9.**8**), in which psychological and immunological factors are integrated, while co-stimulating and influencing each other.

The immune system should be regarded today as the sixth organ of perception; see current overview under (9). When we strengthen our senses by "exerting" them, we are also strengthening our immune system. Exercise has a positive effect on the psychological and physical defense mechanisms and promotes stress resistance. Such defenses, however, depend on the **autonomic nervous system**. It is therefore an important question whether a person has inherited a vagotonic or a sympathetic nervous system dominance. **Vagotonic** persons have a higher stress resistance, while sympathetic persons react more sensitively to stress. Through exercise, stress resistance can be positively influenced. The sympathetic system is particularly heavily activated during cancer. Stress hormones are released and the immune system is weakened. An immune system that is markedly weakened, not only because of disease but also by unnecessary and intrusive therapeutic procedures (see Fig. 9.**3**), requires stabilization. In this respect, the development of stress resistance through exercise is particularly important.

There are exceptions for exercising during cancer follow-up. These are the **contraindications** (2):

- metastases of the bone
- disease that puts heavy strain on the cardiovascular system (e. g., cardiac insufficiency)
- strongly weakened immune system creating danger of infection.

For the training of the immune system, it is sufficient to continually exert oneself for one hour

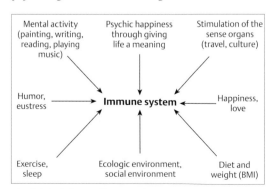

Fig. 9.7 Stabilizing effects on the immune defense mechanisms in cancer patients.

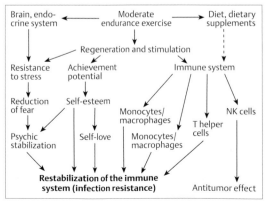

Fig. 9.8 Influence of endurance training on the immune system and the psyche.

(heart rate: 180 – age) or 4×45 minutes. One should choose the type of exertion that one enjoys most (walking, jogging, hiking, swimming, bicycling, tennis, inline skating, and so on). A suggested regime for cancer follow-up would be 1–1.5 hours once a week to start with, leaving more extensive regimens (at least two more training entities) up to the individual after consultation and discussion.

In total, about 2000 calories are to be consumed through exercise each week (one minute of jogging consumes 10 calories). Emphasis should be placed on regularity and endurance of exertion. Certain courses given by licensed trainers in weekend seminars or sports institutes are normally offered. Functional gymnastics, endurance training, sports, and fun activities, as well as relaxation exercises can be included. It would be good before starting such a complementary measure to consult the family practitioner in order to ensure fitness for performing sports (stress ECG).

Exercise regimens for cancer follow-up can reduce the need for anxiety-reducing, sleeping, and pain medication. At the same time, mental agility is increased and reintegration into work or family circles is facilitated.

With increasing customization to a training program, patients are motivated to exercise more continuously. In addition, one should make it clear to the patient that exercise not only helps to prevent a cancer recurrence, but also lowers the risk for other diseases:
- cardiovascular diseases (heart attack, stroke)
- infections and aging processes (there are close correlations between the two)
- metabolic disturbances (type II diabetes)
- osteoporosis.

At the center of all these diseases is the process of inflammation. Inflammation also plays a pivotal role in aging as well as arteriosclerosis. In contrast to that, slight infections and moderate endurance exercise strengthen our immune system. Paradoxically, this can also be seen as a beneficial effect of the inflammatory process. With heavy and chronic infections the immune system is overburdened, however. The **correlations between cancer and infections** are interesting: while smaller infections strengthen the immune defenses, chronic infections seem to promote the development and growth of cancer (e.g., prostate cancer).

Also, **metabolic disturbances**, such as overweight and metabolic syndrome, can exert a nega-

tive influence on cancer: on the one hand insulin and related growth hormones stimulate cancer cells (breast cancer) to increased multiplication, on the other hand fat-soluble carcinogens can be stored or produced (estrones) in fatty tissues.

The diabetic patient poorly supplies a newly developing tumor with blood, due to pathological vessels and new vessel growths (diabetic microangiopathy). In a professional athlete the exact opposite would be expected. Calcium antagonists reduce the blood pressure and the number of adhesion molecules in endothelial cells. These, however, are necessary for the metastases of cancer cells. It can be demonstrated that various diseases are correlated with each other and are able to influence one another.

We must passively endure diseases. However, moderate exercise gives us an active strategy to combat it, that is even fun. Exercise can prolong our lives, and it is even more certain that exercise improves our quality of life. It is precisely this aspect that should be emphasized for cancer patients. Exercise is of great value when the family and work environment of the patient shows understanding for the "change in lifestyle" and lends support in this matter.

▬ Organization of Sport Groups

At all times, depending on their individual capabilities, athletic people have continued to engage in physical activity, both individually and in groups, after a diagnosis of cancer. Whether this has always been uneventful and has not incurred undue complications has never been studied, but positive experiences have consistently been reported.

It is certain that cancer primarily affects middle-aged people and the elderly, groups that typically have less inclination to indulge in physical activity and sports, since their exercise-related experiences often lie decades in the past.

Slowly, the fact that exercise and physical activity can have positive aspects particularly for their age group has increased in the consciousness of elderly people: for example, cardiovascular diseases and osteoporosis can be prevented, and the risk for diabetes and obesity reduced.

It can be assumed that a large proportion of elderly cancer patients have been unaccustomed to exercising for long periods of time and fail to see any direct correlation between cancer, exercise, well-being, and the health benefits of regular physical activity.

For almost two decades, cancer patients have been offered the opportunity to take part in special events for their disease group organized by regional sport clubs, much as has been done, for example, for cardiac patients. In Germany, there are currently roughly 500 groups of which 250 are in the region of Northern Palatinate.

Generally, affected women or men following respective diagnosis, therapy, and follow-up treatment (rehabilitation) go to a sports group that is close to their hometown. Many of the participants have received information on the programs offered by rehabilitative clinics, or they have been informed by physicians, daily newspapers or through public relations efforts conducted by local groups.

Some of the newcomers have pre-existing experience in sports and may indicate that they would like to get to know their body afresh, and that they want to return to the same kind of sport or sports group after an introductory period of strengthening. This is not a problem if the type of sport does not adversely affect the altered physical status of the patient. (For example, a breast cancer patient should not take part in sports that may aggravate brachial lymphedema.) Some types of sport such as gymnastics, water gymnastics, long-distance running, or swimming can usually be taken up again without difficulties or problems. It is not advisable to engage in types of sport that entail prolonged and unforeseeable periods of strain, such as handball, basketball, volleyball, and martial arts, especially when they are conducted in a competitive manner.

Some patients who are newcomers to cancer follow-up sports groups may not have taken part in any type of special exercise for a considerable length of time—often as much as a decade or even more. The exercise programs offered to such patients must be tailored according to the following considerations:

- disease
- different pre-exposure
- different age groups
- needs and preferences of the group.

The qualifications and the general outlook of the teacher determine what the key aspects of the activities will be. From the developmental history of "exercise in cancer follow-up," which at the begin-

ning was targeted primarily toward breast cancer patients, we have developed a concept that has stood up well to expectations in practice and is constantly being developed further.

All trainers that lead a cancer follow-up sports group appear in the list of respective national sports leagues. All have received and effectively passed a specialty education and are required to regularly take part in continuing education programs. Only in this way can new insights in cancer research and sports science be passed along through trainers to participants, in order to maintain a consistent standard of quality.

Entrance Examination

Before a patient is permitted to take part in an official sports group in cancer follow-up, a complete physical examination is required by the treating physician in order to exclude any possible contraindications regarding physical activity.

- The trainers are given support in designing the content of their exercise regimens, taking into account the individual patient's ability to tolerate stress. They are informed in advance by the physician of any accompanying disease or special considerations. Of special interest to the cancer patient are the following:
  - duration of disease
  - classification of the tumor and eventual metastases
  - prior therapies.
- The physician notes down any accompanying diseases that relate to physical activity:
  - metabolic disorders such as diabetes or arthritis
  - cardiovascular diseases such as high blood pressure, infarcts, heart rhythm irregularities
  - musculoskeletal diseases such as arthrosis, invertebral disc damages
  - tumor-relevant diseases such as bone metastases, implants, stomas.
- It is essential that all medical data are stored securely by the group's director and that third parties are not given any access to these data.
- Exercise is prescribed in cancer follow-up on a special document for rehabilitative exercise, which can be received in the doctor's practice or is handed out to the participants by the group trainer. Every group has the opportunity

to receive an advance payment on the account of the (sport club) society by their respective health insurance. The only prerequisite is that the health insurance confirms responsibility for the costs through a signature/stamp of approval on the document.

- Generally, exercise is recommended once to twice a week for at least half a year.

Preparation

- Most of the sports groups in cancer follow-up meet once a week for 1–1.5 hours in an exercise room, a gym, or a swimming pool.
- Besides comfortable clothing, participants bring with them into the gym a prescription filled out by the treating physician, on which "exercise in cancer follow-up" has been prescribed as a rehabilitative measure, and on which the health insurance has agreed to take over the costs for half a year.
- Before the first exercise class begins, the trainer conducts an interview with each new participant to the group, in which it is clarified, for example, whether other physical limitations besides cancer might influence the participation in physical activity.

Exemplary Exercise Units

A typical exercise unit in the gym is divided into the following parts:

Preparation for the Main Focus of the Class
This includes notification of the content of the class and questions to the group, whether everybody is able to take part in the planed exercises or whether some individual variations in positions or exercises must be offered. The exercise machines and techniques are explained and potentially perilous points and how to avoid them are pointed out.

Warm-up follows in the form of movement variations, gymnastic, small games, coordination exercises, and light stretching exercises. Classical hand equipment used in gymnastics (ball, rope, pole, wedge) or even everyday devices such as towels, newspapers, and neckties may be employed. Music as a motivational support is generally a helpful tool.

Functional Gymnastics
Strengthening and stretching exercises are the mainstay of this part of the exercise class. These are predominantly exercises intended for the large muscle groups of the extremities and the torso. The overwhelming majority of participants we have studied were treated for breast tumors and showed limitations as to how far they were able to move their shoulders and arms, at least on the operated side, so this part of the exercise takes up the greater proportion of the hour.

Exercises intended to improve lymphatic drainage are also included in this part of the class, or whenever it is optimal. Movements that simulate pumping and loosening up activate the lymphatic pumps to redirect lymphatic fluid from the tissues into the venous bloodstream. In order to enlist the help of gravity to this end, exercises to loosen up the arms are always performed above the head.

Main Focus of the Class
In this part of the class a clearly defined area will be taught, improved, tried out, or experienced. This can be, for example, an introduction into endurance training, or the training and practice of walking. Subtopics include the delivery of techniques, functional training, for instance, lymphedema prophylaxis, teaching of time and distance units, and working on interval-training or endurance-training methods. Depending on the ability of the group, various different exercise entities are required.

Further focus areas of the main part were:
- introduction to volleyball (beach ball or softball as a training device)
- introduction to racket games (family tennis, badminton, table tennis), whereby the respective techniques should always be rehearsed on both sides
- breathing exercises, relaxation techniques, tai chi
- endurance training (walking, jogging, low-impact aerobics)
- introduction into popular sports (step aerobic, aqua-jogging)
- circuit training (focus: improvement of regional muscle strength, endurance, dexterity, agility etc.)
- dancing (folk dance, dance gymnastics, modern dance)
- perception exercises.

Conclusion of the Class

The conclusion of each class should offer a complementing or contrasting item to the main topic of the exercise class. In this way a quiet movement such as stretching or massage (with brightly coloured spiky plastic massage balls) can be experienced as soothing. In contrast, exercise classes that have focused a lot on high concentration or relaxation may profit from a finale that is a bit more movement intensive, such as a group dance or a little game such as "ball over the line" (i.e. throwing a ball over the rope).

The Group Discussion

There is a distinct difference between exercise in cancer follow-up and other sport groups. Because of the intrusive experience of an operation for cancer and the ensuing therapies, there is often a desire to exchange experiences with other cancer patients. Common themes include:

- Rehabilitation, specifically questions concerning the best clinics and doctors.
- Problems in the professional environment and in the family.
- How can I best help my body and mind to heal?
- How can I vent my fears or give voice to my newly gained self-esteem?

Obviously the group supports those who must return to cancer therapy or who are unable to continue participation in the exercises due to a progression of their disease. Whether a group discussion takes place at every exercise session or only every so often depends on the individual participants of the group and the trainer of the group. The group indicates how often and whether there is a need for discussion. The trainer is responsible for moderating the group in such a way as to ensure that all-important topics are sufficiently covered and discussed. Exercise itself should not be forgone because of this. If there is a high individual need for discussion or a serious problem, it makes sense to refer to self-help groups and cancer advisory agencies.

In this part of the class the possibility exists for referral to areas that lie outside of the realm of exercise, such as disease-coping strategies or to combine some of these creative areas with movement or **dance**. In some groups there is experimentation with free dance-like movements. In others, creative self-expression through **painting** can motivate participants to translate inner feelings into movement.

Recreational Activities

Leisurely activities can also be performed with the entire group or with interested individuals. The entire group is always addressed when "social events" are concerned such as summer festivities or the end of a course, or Christmas parties and the like. In other activities those individuals that are interested get together. Hiking expeditions, museum or concert excursions, or visiting a medical presentation are a few examples that vary from group to group. An advantage of these gatherings is that discussions can take place between the individual group members without time limit and totally unconstrained, so that more time remains during the exercise hour for actual exercising.

The individual construction of the exercise class and also the overall content of the group concept is naturally dependent on the following fixed factors:

- qualifications and exercise focus of the trainer of the group
- facilities for space and time
- range of ages of the members of the group
- group size and ratio of sexes
- active disease states of the participants and their general health condition
- preferences of the participants
- season and weather.

The focus of each class of "exercise in postcancer follow-up" should be on physical and mental well-being. The participants should feel individually addressed and challenged according to their general status in terms of health and motivation. An open atmosphere conducive to constructive criticism in which questions and topics can be discussed that are felt to be stressful or burdensome, should be encouraged. Since new patients continuously join the group, many of whom are still in the first stages of coming to terms with their disease, it is important to create ample room for communication during the exercise sessions, in which private or informal talk is made possible. The exchange of experiences is always honored during the exercise sessions next to the pure exercise time in the groups. In contrast to discussion groups, it is possible to talk to other patients about the disease, but no one is forced to do so. The main emphasis is on the communally experienced exercise, which reduces stress and dissolves fears. For some participants it is only possible to engage in a discussion on the topic of cancer and to bring forth their own experiences following such an hour of exercise.

Contraindications and Application Restrictions

New participants are advised to be careful in the first training sessions and to slowly approach and test their individual capabilities. Generally, it is advised not to take part in an outpatient exercise group if cancer therapy has not yet been completed.

- In **radiation therapy** the area of skin that received radiation should not be exposed to additional mechanical strain. In addition, it would also lead to problems concerning hygiene, since the radiated area is not allowed to come into contact with water.
- During **chemotherapy** the prerequisites for participation are less clearly defined. Individuals who are receiving chemotherapy for the first time should wait until the end of therapy before starting an exercise program. Patients who have been active for a longer period of time in an exercise group and must undergo renewed chemotherapy once again usually know instinctively whether they would benefit from exercise or not. They decide which training modules increase their well-being and on which days to participate. These are usually the less intense units of the program, such as breathing exercises, relaxation techniques, functional gymnastics, or perception exercises.
- In the clinical area, possibilities are being tested through moderate endurance training on a bicycle ergometer in order to support treatment success as well as to reduce the side effects of therapy.
- Women who suffer from manifest **brachial lymphedema** participate in the exercises using a compression stocking.
- Stimulation of the immune system is also possible with **diseases of the lymphatic system or bone marrow**, however extreme exercise training should be avoided.
- There are no objections to exercising after a **bone marrow transplantation**.
- Increased blood flow and increased oxygenation of muscle and tissues achieved during exercise can lead to acute and sometimes life-threatening exacerbations of certain conditions. It is therefore of the utmost importance

Table 9.4   Contraindication for exercise
• Bone metastases in the spine (aqua-jogging, swimming, ergometric-bicycling are possible)
• Current allergic reactions (bad bronchial status)
• All fever diseases and infections (flu-like infection, also tooth decay)
• Poorly adjusted diabetes
• Antibiotic therapy

to only participate in an exercise program if one is physically healthy enough to do so, as shown in Table 9.**4**.

Exercise for the Cancer Patient Outside of Specialized Types of Sport

Despite several official exercise groups in cancer follow-up there are still some "white spots" on the map. Many cancer patients who are interested in special sport programs are unable to find adequate offerings in their nearby surroundings. These patients can only be advised to join a group that offers an individually appropriate and physically noninjurious type of activity, or to take up their own physical activity.

When choosing an appropriate type of activity, persons interested in exercising should discuss their medical history and preferred activity with the program director. In the course of mutual conversation critical exercises will quickly become apparent. Well-educated trainers, regardless of which sport, will at least attempt to offer adequate exercises and point out any harmful ones. The trainer should always be aware, for example, of the possibility that an affected arm in women after breast cancer may be overstrained, overstretched, or in any other way injured.

Enterostomy patients are advised against lying on the stomach and performing backward stretching of the torso. When doing abdominal exercises this can lead to problems. Affected individuals should also avoid games in which exercise machines could hit the stoma with uncontrolled force and velocity.

Water Gymnastics

Besides "exercise in cancer follow-up," another recommended physical group activity is water gymnastics. In contrast to movements on land, specific physical laws govern in water. This is predominantly due to the higher density of the medium. Through buoyancy, body weight is reduced to one seventh of the weight on land: this is a beneficial phenomenon, since the strain on joints is low, which is also helpful for obese people during training.

Due to water resistance, movements in water are notably more difficult than on land. The more dynamically an exercise is conducted, the more difficult it is to see it through. The pressure present in the water results in a mild drainage of the skin and its underlying tissues. This leads to an effect similar to lymph drainage that is perceived by women as being particularly soothing after a breast cancer surgery. Additionally, water slows down each movement through its specific characteristics, so that sweeping movements that push the blood and lymphatic fluid into the extremities on land are impossible to conduct in water.

The **risk of injury** is very low in water, since falls are practically excluded. Nonetheless, movement in the water allows the improvement of fundamental motor qualities of the human body, such as strength, endurance, flexibility, and dexterity. Besides manifold organizational forms such as single, partner, and group training sessions, there are various specific exercise programs, so that training can have a wide breadth of variation.

A large number of exercise devices developed specifically for work in the water, such as swimming boards, balls, water noodles (made of highly buoyant soft plastic foam), dumbbells, and a large choice of equipment from the area of aqua-fitness guarantee a diversified exercise program.

Relaxation techniques can also be done in the water, if the water temperature allows this. Exercises in which one partner lies on the back while being tugged or pushed through the water by the other partner are especially popular. The integration of music is obligatory in aqua-fitness training.

One training unit should last between 30 and 60 minutes. A water temperature between 28–30 °C is optimal. Providers are swimming clubs, the lifeguard associations, cities and communities with public pools in addition to independent providers.

Swimming

Swimming puts strain on the entire body and can also be seen as recommended physical exercise. As was mentioned for water exercises, the element of water supports lymph drainage through its hydrostatic pressure. Risk of injury is practically zero.

When swimming is conducted as endurance training over a long period of time, a lot of positive health effects set in:

- strengthening of the muscles of the torso and extremities (depending on the posture while swimming, different areas are specifically trained)
- beneficial effects on the cardiovascular system and blood pressure regulation
- improvement of breathing and respiratory volume
- through the partial abolition of gravity, less strain is placed on the joints
- increase in resistance toward infections through the cold stimulus of the water.

Swimming has especially beneficial effects for the **tracheostomy patient**. The humid and relatively dust-free air in the swimming pool, the arm movements specifically trained during swimming as well as the shoulder and arm movements required are ideal training stimuli. Technically, swimming for those without a larynx is only possible with a special **snorkeling device** (aqua-mat). The laryngectomy associations give information on where to find instruction and introduction into snorkeling techniques. Swimming with a snorkel should only be performed in chest-deep water, in order to enable quick contact with the ground in the event of choking or tiring.

The swimming technique that is probably the most commonly mastered is **breaststroke**, which has a beneficial effect on the chest muscles. Since movements are conducted symmetrically with the left and right half of the body, this type of swimming puts an even strain on the breast and arm muscles. **Women after breast cancer surgery** profit even when parts or all of the big breast muscles have been removed through a radical operation method.

Unfortunately, many lay people swim with their heads upraised during breaststroke, resulting in a prolonged duration of strain on the neck and head muscles. When the head is dipped into the water during the pulling movement of the arms, air is breathed out under water and the head is lifted only to inhale, such tensions do not occur. By dipping the head into the water, an improved flat positioning in the water ensues, allowing the arms and legs to initiate stronger propulsion. To avoid **red eyes due to chlorine** the wearing of well-fitted swimming goggles (sold by specialty stores) is encouraged.

Freestyle front crawl is a way of moving in which the arms are alternately dipped into the water in front of the head to propel the body ahead under water. A phase of relaxation is created each time the arm is brought to the front above the water, and a phase of tension, when the arm pulls underneath the water.

The legs also move alternately in small up and down movements and support forward propulsion. Exhalation takes place under water (as in breaststroke), and inhalation occurs to the side underneath the elevated elbow of the right or the left arm. This quite advanced and challenging swim technique is well suited to endurance swimming and can be used as an alternative to breaststroke, as can the following swim styles.

On the back there are commonly two ways of movement. During **backstroke** swimming, the legs are symmetrically pulled close to the body, similar as in the breast position, and then swung together from the outside to the inside, resulting in a stretching of the entire body. The arms support the propelling movement by opening symmetrically alongside the body and pulling sideways through the water up to the thighs. This technique is very gentle on the back, and is relatively easy to learn.

The **freestyle backstroke** is similar to freestyle front crawl in the alternative arm movements, with one arm above and one below the water, and the alternating leg thrust. The advantage of the back position is that the breath can flow with less hindrance. The disadvantage in all types of swimming that are conducted backward is the limited view.

Due to its demanding technique, the necessary high energy consumption, and the required large shoulder–arm flexibility, **dolphin butterfly stroke** is not appropriate for participants in cancer follow-up.

Aqua-Jogging

Aqua-jogging with a suspension aid (aqua-jogging belt) is a relatively new form of movement and training in deep water. The person exercising wears a buoyancy belt wound tightly around the waist.

With the help of this belt, walking and gymnastic exercises are enabled in deep water, where it is impossible for the patient to touch the ground. This type of movement is very gentle on the joints, so that even overweight persons, poor swimmers, or those with an **artificial hip or knee replacement** are able to participate in the sport.

In persons with an **enterostoma** the belt may result in pressure pain. In this event the belt should patiently be tried on land. Belt buckle pressure on the stoma must be avoided at all costs. Soft, original aqua-jogging belts are usually well tolerated.

Gymnastics

The term gymnastics includes a variety of types of movement:
- classical gymnastics while standing and in movement, with or without hand devices (such as a pole, tire, ball, rope, and clubs)
- stretching gymnastics
- so-called problem-zone gymnastics (callanetics)
- spinal column gymnastics
- functional gymnastics
- dancelike gymnastics.
- trend gymnastics with a Pezzi ball, tubes, or Thera-band.

Most of these types of gymnastics can be taken up again or newly begun after a cancer operation without major difficulties. **Women after breast cancer surgery** should be very careful to avoid any swinging movements with the arms, because the blood and lymph can move to the extremities, increasing the risk of developing a lymphedema.

Exercises that require strong overstretching should also be avoided, since the skin and scars that have been predamaged due to radiation may be injured in this way.

Men or women who wear an **ileo stoma** often have difficulties with exercises that strengthen the abdominal muscles and with exercises that are performed while lying down on the stomach. This problem should be discussed with the course teacher before beginning training, in order to look for alternative exercises.

Aerobic and step-aerobic exercises are especially popular with young women. These exercises, usually offered by fitness studios and other health-oriented sports clubs, are exercises that are principally also suited for women after a breast cancer operation. It is very important that the movements are not conducted too hastily (low-impact course) and that the important loosening exercises are individually and independently performed as often as possible. This is not easy for women with little previous experience in physical activity. Thus, this form of training is usually preferred for women that are more experienced athletes.

Many sports groups in cancer follow-up offer modified aerobic programs in their training sessions.

Ball Games

The ball games known to our culture such as handball, basketball, volleyball, and soccer are only appropriate in a limited way for the area of cancer follow-up. An intense dynamic and emphasis on the body are features of all these games. It cannot be ruled out that some movements will be performed that may extend personal stretching limitations, and injuries to the operated region may occur through physical contact with other players.

In an altered form, these games can be employed for cancer follow-up. In the exercise groups of cancer follow-up, volleyball played with a light foam ball or a beach ball, is very popular.

Racket Games

In racket games, such as tennis, table tennis, or badminton, the racket is usually only held in one hand (exception is the backstroke and forehand stroke with both hands in tennis).
For **breast cancer patients** it is logically very important whether the hand that is used to guide the racket is the side that was operated on, since this may lead to pain and excess strain. If the "healthy" side is the one being used, then this type of exercise is well tolerated. Due to its easily learnable

technique, badminton is highly recommended and very popular. However, breast cancer patients must be cautious and test whether the movements cause any problems in the shoulder–arm area.

Martial Arts

Judo, jujutzu, karate, tae kwan do, and others, are body-oriented types of exercise in which strong, quickly mastered techniques are aimed at overpowering one's opponent with the aid of exercise-specific handholds and steps, shots, and strokes. These types of sports are inappropriate for stoma carriers or women after breast cancer.

Tai Chi

Also known as **Chinese shadow boxing**, tai chi is a gentle, calm and flowing set of movements. Bodily procedures such as breathing are harmonized, the sense of balance is enhanced and the joints gently moved. Tai chi and also the remotely related **qi gong** are especially well suited for introduction into cancer follow-up. Such courses are offered at local sports clubs, adult education centers, or private clubs.

Winter Sports

Alpine skiing harbors two main dangers for women after breast cancer: interlocking of ski poles can result in pain and injury in the shoulder–arm area. The same holds true for falls, and these cannot always be prevented.

Cross-country skiing, by contrast, is much better tolerated. Forward movements should mainly stem from the legs, while the arms are only used subordinately. A good walking, as well as braking, technique can be learned in any cross-country skiing school.

Tight, constrictive clothing should be avoided in order to prevent lymphedema of the arm. **Backpacks** are only suitable when they are not too heavily packed and have comfortable, broad straps. Since hypothermia can also promote the development of lymphedema, special safety measures should be met to avoid these complications.

Hiking

Hiking is recommended without constraints, since it does not place too much strain on the joints, does not harbor too many dangers, and appeals to the elderly. In addition, hiking can be an adventurous undertaking, since all senses are stimulated in a beautiful landscape. Also, the gregarious aspect of this type of sport can be beneficial.

Women after breast cancer surgery are recommended to avoid tight constrictive clothing including tight cuffs at the wrists. Backpacks are suitable when they are small and not too heavily packed and have comfortable, well-padded broad straps for insertion of the thumbs while walking. This will prevent the collection of lymph in the lower arm and the hands.

Besides wearing comfortable shoes and adequate clothing, it is particularly important for this type of sport that a protective sunscreen is provided. Not only women after breast cancer surgery should protect the affected arm and side from too much UV light; an excess of sun suppresses the immune system and promotes the development of aggressive skin tumors. This is why headgear and sunglasses should not be missing during long hikes.

Walking

Walking is a special type of endurance exercise. Due to its low-impact strain on the joints walking is excellent endurance training for older people and for people with preimpairments in the joints of the lower extremities and the spinal column.

In contrast to **long-distance running**, there is always a leg on the ground in walking, which explains why there is a reduced compression of the spinal column. The intensity of training is determined by the length and the increased frequency of the steps. When the intensity is high for the individual and when the hands hold additional weights in the form of small dumbbells, this form of exercise is referred to as **power walking**.

Table 9.5 Overview of the types of sports that are suitable or unsuitable for cancer patients

	Breast cancer	Laryngeal cancer/ stoma patient	Colon cancer/ stoma patient	Elderly/out-of-practice
Water gymnastics	Yes	No	Yes	Yes
Breaststroke	Yes	Only with a snorkel	Yes	Yes
Freestyle front crawl	Yes	Only with a snorkel	Yes	No
Freestyle backstroke	Yes	Yes	Yes	No
Backstroke	Yes	Yes	Yes	Yes
Aqua-jogging	Yes	No	Within limits	Yes
Large ball games: handball, basketball, soccer, volleyball	No	No	No	No
	However, all ball games can be changed and adapted to smaller playing fields, with lighter balls, with changed rules etc.			
Racket games	Only popular sports			
Martial arts	No	No	No	No
Tai chi, qi gong	Yes	Yes	Yes	Yes
Hiking	Yes	With adequate distance	Yes	Yes
Walking	Yes	Yes	Yes	Yes
Long-distance running	Yes	No	Yes	Within limits
Cross-country skiing	Yes	No	Yes	Yes
Gymnastics	Yes	Yes	Yes	Yes
Aerobics	Only popular sports			

Long-Distance Running

Long-distance running is an effective and simple form of endurance training that achieves cardio-pulmonary training effects and boosts the immune system. The running can be learned most easily when interested people join a sports club. Different group levels exist as well as teachers that give tips on the correct running style and shoes, and conduct the exercise.

Whoever chooses to do **long-distance running** by themselves is advised to start at a very slow pace, a pace at which a conversation can be held without strain (i.e., a pace that does not induce breathlessness). Primarily, one can alternate long-distance running phases with phases of walking. With increasing endurance the practicing individual can shorten the walking phases and prolong the time actually running.

The **training intensity** can be determined through the **training pulse**. This is the pulse per minute that is reached at the end of the period of strain. While exercising this should be around 180 beats per minute minus the age. If this value is 10 beats short, the training intensity is too low.

If the value is clearly exceeded, the endurance strain is too high, and this can result in a number of undesirable factors. For all types of endurance sports two, or better even three, training units of 30–60 minutes should be performed a week.

Gymnastic exercises used for training at home.
- For breast cancer patients:
  - exercises for support of lymph drainage
  - exercises for stretching of shoulder and arm muscles
  - exercises for strengthening of shoulder and arm muscles.
- For laryngeal cancer patients:
  - exercises for stretching of the neck and shoulder muscles
  - exercises for the strengthening of the neck and shoulder muscles.
- For colon cancer patients (stoma patients)
  - exercises for loosening the trunk muscles
  - exercises for strengthening of all straight and oblique abdominal muscles.

▬ References

1. van Aaken E: Kann man durch Sport dem Krebs vorbeugen? Turnen, 1967; issue 26, Dec. 21.
2. Autoren der AG des LSB: Bewegung und Sport in der Krebsnachsorge. Schriftwerke des LSB in Duisburg, 1997.
3. Friedenreich CM: Physical Activity and Cancer Prevention: From Observational to Intervention Research. Cancer Epidemiol Biomarkers Prev. 2001; 10:287–301.
4. Lötzereich H, Uhlenbruck G: Präventive Wirkung von Sport im Hinblick auf die Entstehung maligner Tumore? Dtsch Z Sportmed. 1995; 46:86–94.
5. Lötzerich H, Peters C: Krebs und Sport. Cologne, Germany: Verlag Sport und Buch Strauss; 1997.
6. Mackinnon IT: Advances in Exercise Immunology. Human Kinetics, 1999.
7. Nieman DC: The Exercise–Health Connection. Champaign, Il, Human Kinetics, 1998.
8. Pape D, Schwarz R, Gillessen H, Uhlenbruck G, Mader A: Gesund, vital, schlank. Deutscher Ärzteverlag, Cologne, Germany; 2001.
9. Parkin J, Cohen B: An overview of the immune system. Lancet. 2001; 357:1777–1789.
10. Peters C, Lötzerich H, Niemeier B, Schüle K, Uhlenbruck G: Influence of a moderate exercise training on natural killer cytotoxicity and personality traits in cancer patients. Anticancer Research. 1994; 14:1033–1036.
11. Sommer P, Uhlenbruck G: Immunfit forever. Arsnova Publ. Bad Sobernheim, 2003.
12. Thune I, Furberg AS: Physical activity and cancer risk: dose–response and cancer, all sites and site-specific. Med Sci Sports Exercise. 2001; 33:530–550.
13. Uhlenbruck G, Order U: Can endurance sport stimulate immune mechanisms against cancer and metastasis? Dtsch Z Sportmed. 1987; 38:40–47.
14. Uhlenbruck G, Peters C, Schüle K, Lötzerich H: Sport in der Krebsnachsorge: Rolle der natürlichen Killerzellen und Monozyten. Gynäkol Prax. 1998; 22: 403–407.
15. Uhlenbruck G: Lieber Laufen-lernen, lerne Laufen lieben. Condition. 1973; 14:32–36.

10 Psycho-oncology

Karl Friedrich Klippel

Introduction

Psycho-oncology is not a self-contained medical subject. It attempts to offer a concept of coping with disease through therapeutic conversation and psychotherapies, in order to elicit a change in the meaning of life through an integration of the disease. The treating physician must recognize the reactive psychogenic processes in the patient and also within himself or herself.

It is not only the patient who needs psycho-oncological support; the assisting therapist also needs to possess the knowledge-based tools. The therapist needs supervision to prevent himself or herself from losing sight of the healing mission in the face of the demands placed on him or her through burnout.

According to a poll, 72% of the German population believes that physical illnesses, such as cancer, can have psychological causes and 83% of people desire an increased use of complementary–alternative and naturopathic healing methods.

The majority of the medical profession rejects complementary cancer therapy and sometimes even acts with open hostility toward it—at least when it comes to their own patients. They only open themselves up to the possibility of alternative therapies if the physician himself or herself, or a family member is affected by cancer.

The theoretical and practical basic instructional principles are the same in the conventional as in complementary medicine. Medical education is generally based on the rational scientific insights of accepted conventional medicine. Despite sharing a common foundation of knowledge, two schools of thought have developed in the field of oncology that are not only oriented according to different interests, but also represent different and occasionally opposing points of view in terms of philosophy.

The field of psycho-oncology can help patients, doctors, and therapists to overcome conflicts and crises by employing cognitive processes, self-reflection, and psychosomatic insights. It describes psychological phenomena in persons with malignant diseases as well as the interactions with the therapist and the social environment.

In many medical fields catalogued knowledge is organized and offered in a very dogmatic manner. This may be appropriate for technical issues, but it is unsuitable for the purpose of describing the psyche, since psychological processes cannot be classified into subject areas and fields of reference. Mental events display framework and textural characteristics. A specific dynamic of processes exists that is directed intrapersonally as well as interpersonally toward the conditions of the environment.

The necessary scientific analysis of singular phenomena, as we know from broad areas of medicine, is required for didactic reasons, but must not lead to the loss of awareness for the interrelatedness and uncontrollable interactions of psychological processes. The subdivision into various areas and subject areas suggests an underlying order to the psychological system. The completeness and simultaneousness of psychological issues are analyzed into their one-dimensional components, where a multidimensional approach within the time axis of anteprojection and retroprojection would be appropriate. Psychological events do not take place in the abstract realm, but in concrete persons in concrete situations (50).

The Term "Health"

The term "health" as defined by the World Health Organization (WHO) does not only mean the absence of disease, but also denotes health as the condition of complete physical, psychological, and social well-being.

This contentious definition allows normal deviations and places the power of decision on the subjective level of the individual. Freud similarly defined the goal of psychoanalysis as having been achieved once a patient attained a full ability for love, pleasure, and work. In psychoanalysis one does not differentiate between norm and neurosis in a quantitative fashion, since a conflict-free normality does not correlate with reality or real-life experiences. **Psychological health** equates to the competence to lead one's life and an ability to deal with life's daily conflicts, fears, and troubles. A conflict-free life is considered an illusion, and not the norm.

Disease is ever present. In 25 years of adult life, the human being is afflicted, on average, by one life-threatening disease, 20 serious, about 200 moderate-to-serious and roughly 1000 trivial diseases.

In the world of employment, the **health standard** is defined as the fulfillment of a function, while society, through peer pressure, subliminally demands a willingness to adapt and perform as the norm.

In the natural sciences the distribution of the norm is simply determined by quantifiable values (for example through Gaussian normal distribution curves). Psychosocial data, such as intensity of fear, pain, depressive mood, or ability to perceive enjoyment, are, in contrast, difficult to measure and always require a frame of reference as well as an interpretation. The fear of cancer can be pathological in the sense of hypochondria, but fear can also be adequate, rational, and functionally correct when cancer is actually suspected.

The Cancer Diagnosis as Psychological Trauma

The classic, reductionist world perception of conventional medicine observes the patient only as a carrier of symptoms with organic disturbances, and not as a person who suffers from a disease (26).

Kreibich-Fischer (39) showed that the reactions of the doctors, patients, and nurses to the disease entity "cancer" was responsible for disrupting the therapeutic relationship itself. Doctors and patients know about the possibility of death as a likely outcome, but find themselves bound within a therapeutic community of fate, that extends beyond the normal communication relationship between doctor and patient. The imbalance between the demands of the medical community and the powerlessness of the patient occasionally makes this relationship unbearably strenuous.

Every physician who treats cancer patients must be aware of the psychological processes that humans have at their disposal when **coping with crises**. Processes for overcoming crises are dependent on the concentrated life experiences of the individual and his or her level of maturity, so that each oncology patient brings his or her own strategies for coping with disease.

The direct confrontation with the often deadly disease and the not infrequently crippling therapies generally present a **psychological trauma** for patients. The diagnosis of cancer is experienced as a personal catastrophe and immediate threat to the patient's existence. The patient is fundamentally and effectively rendered insecure in his psychological and social identity, and these fears become conscious. Social relationships and the patient's orientation toward life are often newly evaluated, and future perspectives are questioned.

Every physician knows that feelings and physical functions are inextricably linked. The interactions between a mental crisis and physical reactive well-being are caused by the simultaneousness of mental–physical experience: humans cry when they are sad, and shiver when they are scared, not the other way around. The physical processes are not an expression of an individual organ, but are triggered and influenced through experience, sadness, or fear. Experienced affects of emotion are inextricably linked with concurrent physical events (44).

Coping Mechanisms and Defense Mechanisms

Defense mechanisms should not be seen as pathological but should be considered as a means of self-protection. They can be life saving and are utilized subconsciously by most people. A life without a defense system, be it on a physical, immunological, or psychological level, is plainly inconceivable. This defense system must, however, be adapted to the real situation.

Oncology patients do not want to accept the reality of their cancer and the threat to life, and they often repress this. The denial of a malignant disease can initially protect from a flood of affect that could lead to panic reaction. In order to develop targeted coping strategies, it is necessary to accept the diagnosis of cancer over the course of time, in order to be able to achieve the capacity to make therapeutic choices.

The treating physician must recognize and take into account the defense mechanisms of the patient vs. the diagnosis with respect to his diagnostic and therapeutic approach strategy.

One must differentiate between a whole slew of defense mechanisms (37):

Repression—the Basic Mechanism

The ambivalent "mercy" of an inability to remember can be conscious or unconscious.

Not everything that appears to the conscious mind is stored in the memory, and even what is stored in the memory cannot be entirely recalled over the course of time. Repression protects from traumatic memories that bring out unpleasant feelings. These feelings are neutralized and exposed to the process of forgetting. Freud called these repressions during childhood "**primordial repression**." The contents thereby displaced into the subconscious mind have an effect in the later adult lifetime, not only content—related, but also in terms of repressing similar episodes, situations, and feelings.

Suppression

Suppression is a conscious activity that is closely related to the unconsciously triggered repression.

Modern, legally required informed consent of patients before diagnostic or therapeutic procedures must include statistical reporting of the risk of death before an operative procedure. This can lead to considerable fear and insecurity that are not repressed but consciously suppressed. In this way, the threatening tension of operative risk can be tolerated. The same holds true for daily risks, such as the participation in city traffic with permanent risk suppression.

Case report A 43-year-old physician erroneously misdiagnose a rapidly growing melanoma of his left groin area with lymph node involvement, as a birthmark. Only after appearance of multiple chicken egg-sized metastases did he agree to a biopsy that confirmed melanoma. He did not survive the first chemotherapy cycle. Retrospectively, it has been shown that he was very much aware of the correct diagnosis, but had totally negated and suppressed this.

Introjection and Identification

Introjection refers to the construction of an inner representative of a person, who can desert someone, or whom one decides to keep at a distance.

In contrast to the interaction with actual persons, which are also represented as a notion, the **inner representation** is based upon memories and not the actual experience. During introjection, the internal representation of persons—from whom one is actually separate—can be questioned. "What would dad have to say about that?" Introjection is a normal process. Through introjection, a so-called **object constancy** is preserved, because these persons are represented internally and the relationship with them is upheld.

If the representation with the object is positive, one can speak about an identification with the object. Identification makes the object into an idealized person. The pathological step is characterized when attributes of the idealized person are not only assumed ("I would like to be like Elvis"), but when there is an attempt to actually be the other person ("I am Elvis").

Identification as a defense mechanism ultimately means giving up one's own identity and neglecting the ego functionality.

Case report A patient with a kidney tumor consistently rejected nephrectomy, referring to his father, who, despite a tumor growth (benign cyst) of the left kidney, lived to be over 80 years old. The patient died four years after the diagnosis due to a metastasizing kidney tumor.

Reaction Formation

Under the term "reaction formation" one understands the phenomenon of taking feelings and turning them into their opposite.

Aggressions that are not permitted can turn into feelings of particular affection or strong pity. On the other hand, reaction formation can also hinder a necessary aggressiveness and thus inhibit necessary action, if highly valued life is at stake and needs to be saved or protected, as in an emergency, for instance.

In addition, the aggressive and partially painful tumor therapy often creates aggression in patients, causing them to appear especially submissive in their behavior through reaction formation.

Reaction formation can also be seen in the physician, when affection is presented as narcissistic aggressiveness.

Case report An engaged 40-year-old surgeon greeted his especially attractive patient: "Dear Mrs. Meier, I have both bad and good news for you. First the bad news: You have breast cancer—now the good news: I will personally be operating on you."

The visibly engaged physician taking a liking toward his patient tried to hide his feelings behind the narcissistically inflated message, that he personally takes it upon himself to offer the medical treatment for the patient as a "labor of love." He thereby hoped to play down the "you have breast cancer" again inflating himself.

Negation
Negation—like reaction formation—entails a non-recognition of reality, whereby reaction formation refers to emotion that is reverted to its opposite, while negation actually refuses to recognize the actual situation ("I do not have cancer").

Autoaggression
When aggressions cannot be tolerated in the social environment or in the interpersonal argument, aggression can be applied against oneself as a form of defense mechanism. This can happen through self-accusations, when a person cannot disassociate himself from other aggressive people, since he or she is dependent on these and the loss would be more painful than the self-accusation. The self-accusation of guilt of depressed subjects ("I alone am to blame for everything") simultaneously discloses fantasies of omnipotence, since nobody can possibly be the one to blame for everything (**self-aggrandizement**).

Denial
A fact cannot be refuted, but its meaning can be rejected.

Denial, which is similar to repression or suppression, means that the knowledge of the malignancy of the disease is concealed from oneself and others. Denial implies phenomenological perception and makes the selective derangement of interpretation become apparent. An unwillingness to recognize is often unconscious and protects the patient from the pain of the acknowledgement, for example, the fact that he or she is suffering from an untreatable disease. The occasionally experienced misunderstood therapeutic aim of forced confrontational intervention toward the patient by the therapist may lead to an increase in denial, or the intervention may succeed—albeit with severely destructive potential.

Only an empathetic systematic intervention may offer hope and alternatives and may attempt to establish the necessary correlation to reality as a basis for deciding on therapeutic measures. It is to be noted that denial as a form of defense mechanism acts to stabilize the ego, similarly to other defense mechanisms. The big difference between suppression and denial lies with the fact that suppression is a conscious action while denial is a totally subliminal process. By contrast, repression tampers with the process of forgetting and of not remembering.

Case report A 25-year-old student presented himself to his urologist with a testicular tumor twice the size of an egg. The palpated diagnosis of testicular cancer was supported both by ultrasound and through elevated levels of tumor markers such as β-HCG and PLAP. Family history was reported as negative. Despite being given thorough information on the diagnosis and treatment, the patient rejected surgery on the affected testicle, giving the argument that he banged his testicle and therefore it swelled up. He even strictly rejected an initial impulse chemotherapy (without histology, only marker directed).

Six months later, the clinic was informed of his death and of the fact that his younger brother died six years ago due to a metastasizing chemotherapy-resistant testicular cancer.

Projection
Projection relegates one's own psychological contents, evaluations, and effects to other persons.

One reason for this is to expel something from the internal world that is bothersome and that creates conflicts. Those who do not want to experience themselves as being weak, sick, and helpless, project the moods, affects, and impulses associated with this on to others. With projection, distance is not only initiated, but the opposite can also be encouraged; intimacy and a feeling of closeness can be established. The patient projects his own feelings on to others and thereby seeks a companion in misfortune, a fellow sufferer.

A projection can proceed more unrestricted the more unrealistic and fantastic the cover is, so that it cannot be refuted and endangered by realistic circumstantial evidence.

Case report A 16-year-old woman, who suffered under a strict regime of a compulsive father (a Prussian official), fell in love with a married chief surgeon 40 years older than herself during an inpatient sojourn at a surgical clinic due to an appendectomy. She ordered flowers to her bedside as an indication of apparent gifts from the doctor. Her desire for love and affection lead to self-mutilation requiring multiple operative procedures.

During the course of a few years she was operated on exactly 125 times, lost her right leg, parts of her hip bone, the intestine, and the bladder. Only following the last urology procedure and psychosomatic counseling did she grasp the background story. Since then (over 17 years) she no longer required surgery.

Selective Perception
One does not acknowledge unpleasant things, or through simultaneous denial the significance of the perception changes (for example, skin metastases are explained by a traumatic impact).

Rationalization
Logically deducible explanations are to distract from the emotionally directed decision or action, whereby the actual feelings are subliminal.

Case report A 61-year-old man suffered from obstructive disuria with excessive nocturia. The clinical examination resulted in a 30 g prostate adenoma with slight hardening of the right lobe, upon which a fine-needle biopsy was recommended. The patient rejected the extraction of tissue, since the tumor "would explode" through the entering of air. The patient refused an operation, the radiologist refused radiation therapy without histology. After an immediate therapy with antiandrogens the symptoms improved remarkably, so that the patient only appeared in the clinic after two years, now with PSA values around 40 ng/mL. Bone scintigraphy that was previously negative, now showed multiple metastases.

The pleading of pseudorational reasons for rejection alleviated the patient from the danger to divulge his deep-seated fears. His action appeared to be well-founded to the outsider: the temporarily introduced therapy fatally supported the disease construct, since symptomatic improvement was achieved initially,

Coping
In contrast to the described psychological phenomena, coping is the ability of a human being to come to terms with his or her disease in the sense of an **adaptation**. The disease is overcome or ac-

cepted. The evaluation scales for surveying the "**cancer personality**" measure the coping disposition in order to achieve control with future-oriented data.

A further measurement instrument is the **vulnerability scale** as well as the questioning about stressful situations (losses), risky behavior (alcohol, nicotine etc.), and various other parameters such as, for example, social adaptation, denial, despair, alienation, and dysphoria (74).

▬ Clinical Studies

> "Cancer develops through a palace revolution inside the cell, less by an attack from the outside." (42)

This describes the dilemma of cancer research very well. Healthy and diseased states lie close to one another. In the past decades, an endless amount of information was gathered on cancer, its genetic causes, and the psychological interactions. Cancer cannot be understood as a simple technical problem that can simply be solved with sufficient efforts. The disappointment regarding numerous failed cancer programs has been great, not only for those affected, but also with doctors, scientists, and sponsors.

Cancer Personality

Whether or not there actually is a "type-C patient" (typus carcinomatosus) who projects psychological conflicts within the context of somatic phenomena on to a visible physical level in the form of tumor growths is still debatable.

The term "**cancer personality**" has established itself in the literature to a great extent, but is still a speculative empirical term and not a scientific designation. According to phenomena, he is described as friendly, with an outwardly optimistic, cheerful façade, not complaining, not aggressive, and incapable of dealing with anger in an appropriate fashion (Table 10.1) (2).

A premanifest classification of a person as a type C would entail a considerable psychological strain and stigmatization and equate to a social–medical "preconviction."

Table 10.1 Apparent characteristics of cancer patients—psychological test outcome (64)

	Lung cancer	Breast cancer
Denial and repression	+/+	+/−
Reduced emotional release	+/−	++/−/−/−
Rigid, conventional life-style	+/+	0
Inhibited sexuality	+	++++
Problems of dependency	+	++++ (on the mother)
Anal psychological level	+/−	0
Submissiveness	+/−	+
High level of assertiveness	+/−	+/−
High moral self-concept	+/−	+
Increased fear	+/+	+
Reduced expression of rage	0	++
Readiness to make sacrifices	0	+
Masochistic character structure	+/−	++

+, confirmed; −, not confirmed; 0, no data available.

Genetic influences, environmental conditions, malnutrition, and abuse of nicotine are considered to be more severe criteria for estimation of risk.

While the **psychogenesis of cancer** remains largely in the dark, the defense mechanisms and coping mechanisms are recognized as "self-defense" of the soul. Even though patients occasionally experience their disease in a skewed fashion, depending on their personality, with partially strange accusations and explanations, the psychological defense phenomena are uniform. These can become chronic and display a pathological pattern through unopposed self-enhancement.

Case report A 53-year-old bank manager who was suffering from a prostate carcinoma for eight months, reports that he "contracted" the disease during an accidental homoerotic episode with anal sex while drunk. The single episode had caused much shame and considerable feelings of guilt, so that he experienced the diagnosed prostate cancer six weeks later as a fatalistic penalization and initially rejected further (antiandrogen) treatment. Only after overcoming the pain of feeling lost and the depressive somatization (after eight months), causal therapy (radical prostatectomy) was successfully completed.

- While various authors support the correlation based on individual observations and statistical examinations (3, 4, 38, 41, 67), some authors ac-

cuse the supporters of these theories as lacking scientific rigor in their textbooks (75).

However, epidemiological studies prove a correlation between crisis situations and the frequency or course of disease, not only with respect to cancer (75).

- Kissen (33) tried to prove the following hypothesis: the relation between lung cancer and **emotional suppression**. Using the study of Le Shan (42) as a point of reference, he conducted a double-blinded study. Additionally, he chose an accepted control group, used objective instruments for measurement and put the results through excellent statistical analysis. This procedure, which nowadays is generally accepted, was completely new at that time, especially in the realm of psychosomatics.

Patients with a low **emotionality score** (Maudsley Personality Inventory) as an expression of their suppression of feelings, would, according to the hypothesis, get lung cancer at a higher rate than those in a collective control group with normal emotionality scores. The examiners did not know to which group the participants (healthy vs. diseased) belonged.

The study showed that a much higher emotionality score was achieved in the study group compared with the control group (level of significance $P < 0.01$).

The study was repeated several times with similar results. The probability of a person with a low emotionality score suffering from lung cancer was found to be six times higher than for persons with a normal emotionality score. This estimate, relying as it does on several observed studies, seems to indicate that even a single personality factor (emotional suppression) can demonstrate a strong correlation to lung cancer (15).

- Even though the proportion of smokers was identical in both groups, Kissen detected synergistic relationships between smoking behavior and personality. He wrote (as became evident in his later studies): "the lesser the personal possibilities for emotional release, the greater the chance that even short periods of exposure to nicotine could induce lung cancer."

- Schmähl and Habs (60) proposed using a so-called "cancer equation," a type of operationalization of the construct "cancer personality" (61): Probability of getting cancer = f (disposition, exposure, time/age).

- Additional studies, specifically in reference to **breast cancer**, also showed a positive outcome and supported the hypothesis. The cautious summarization of these studies indicates that there is a substantial connection between the development of cancer and the suppression of emotions (8).

- Tumor patients showed a reduced reaction to evoked potentials at the level of the cortex, whereby the fact that these effects appeared 200 milliseconds after stimulation seems to indicate that suppression of potentials occurred involuntarily (34).

- **Type-C cancer patients** were compared with type-A patients with coronary cardiac disease, who are better able to verbalize anger, aggression, and aggressive behavior as compared with the former. Additionally, a control group with type B persons (healthy) was conducted alongside this study.

The participants were exposed to stressful situations in order to trigger anger, rage, sorrow, fear, and disturbed self-esteem as well as interpersonal stress. At the same time, vegetative reactions were measured.

The participants were asked to what degree they felt disturbed by the testing conditions. The patients were also classified as emotionally repressed if they gave no verbal indication of being affected but showed strong autonomous vegetative reactions. According to the hypothesis, cancer patients displayed emotional repression the most, while coronary heart patients (type A) were the lowest, type B (normal healthy) were found to be between the two groups (35).

- An older study by Schmähl and Habs took up apparent personality characteristics of cancer patients: inability to react appropriately to stressful situations, low endurance tolerance, and the development of helplessness and hopelessness (62).

The group was made up of women who were to undergo conization due to suspicious cervical smears. Of 68 women who received conization, 28 had **cervical cancer**, and 40 were tumor negative. Interviews conducted *before* conization diagnosis were intended to offer a measure of the predictability of pathological results. The objective was to estimate the degree of hopelessness and helplessness experienced at six month before the first suspicions cervical smear.

Of the 28 tumor-positive women (proof through conization) the tumor-positive result was correctly predicted in 19 women, nine were categorized as false-negative, while 31 of the 40 tumor-negative women were correctly predicted as such. Nine women in the group were estimated as false-positive. In conclusion, the outcome was correctly predicted in 50 of 68 women, which corresponds to 74% (level of significance of $P < 0.01$).

Subsequent studies have validated this outcome for the most part with other histological tumor entities as well (59, 76, 21, 28, 30). Nonetheless, these studies are not easy to interpret, since even simple rolling of dice (negative–positive) would have led to a 50% chance of correct predictability. In combination with preselection of the group (suspect cervical smears), for both patients and interviewers an attitude of expectancy was produced—albeit subconsciously—that was essential for evaluation.

This underlines the methodological difficulties in trying to prove the intuitively perceived possibility of a psychogenesis of cancer with statistical methods. The type C, who is at risk for cancer, is more of a retrospective emotional construct, based on the emotional constellation of patients already afflicted with cancer. The truth of the matter is that, independently of any such constructs, everyone may be affected by cancer, but that psychological traumas and life crises, and the resulting changes in behavior, are able to activate a latent tumor and lead to its dissemination.

- The Heidelberg Working Group Schwarz (64) demystified the myth of the type-C cancer personality in **breast and lung cancer**. According to research outcomes the cancer personality is much more plausibly understood as a reaction to the diagnosis and disease. On the other hand, there were correlations between risk behavior, e.g., nicotine abuse, and carcinogenesis. Despite the knowledge of the risk for cancer, nicotine abuse was demonstrated in a high percentage of patients with lung cancer, which must be questioned further as a distinctive feature of behavior. One should possibly take a closer look at characteristics such as self-neglect, reduced attention to symptoms, and depressive deferral of reality.

Cancer Biography

The psychosomatic models for explaining cancer as a regressive somatization serving to defend conflicting urges, are still a burning issue, not only in the sense of psychogenesis of cancer, but also with respect to psychotherapy of cancer (41).

Many theories and hypotheses try to approach the problem of psychogenesis of cancer, and partial results (excluding fashionable theories) in the context of a patchwork hypothesis are currently being tested again.

C.G. Jung was of the belief that during periods of stagnation and loss of personal developmental possibilities and creative growth, cancer presented a new and different way of filling the denied stagnation with life.

In psychogenetic cancer therapy of actual neurosis, the blocked energy of urges is seen as a partially responsible trigger, while the symptoms of neurosis according to the **conversion theory** are the symbolic expression of conflicting urges in the sense of organ language (Table 10.**2**).

- Booth found that **prostate cancer** was especially commonly among those patients that were easily sexually aroused but did not experience the releasing orgasm (10).

Table 10.2 Potential triggers cancer of apostulated by conversion theory	
Breast cancer	Symbolization of the mother conflict of guilt-ridden sexual self-destruction
Stomach cancer	Result of problems in the relationship with the parent of the opposite sex
Cervical cancer	Sin against motherhood and regretted lust (25)
Thyroid cancer	Converted aggressive impulses as a symbol for an unlived freedom and desire for independence
Lung cancer	Converted aggressive impulses as a symbol for an unlived freedom and desire for independence

- Lust, fear, and libido build-up were the basis of carcinogenesis according to **W. Reich** (53). The following psychological findings were supposed to be typical for the psychogenesis of cancer diseases:
  - resigned character
  - feeling of emotional emptiness
  - reduced ability to perceive pleasure in life
  - repressed aggression
  - orgiastic impotence
  - metaphorical subliminal suicide.

These psychological findings may characterize the actual persons afflicted by cancer, but they have not been confirmed co-factors through prospective longitudinal studies.

- In a simplified theory supported by an explanatory optimism, the **cancer metaphor** was regarded as a perversion of the possibility of asexual procreation, which was refuted or put into perspective by scientifically reproducible studies, also partially receiving validation by others.

Overall, a paradigm shift is now becoming visible in medicine, not least due to developments in information technology and gene technology. One-dimensional notions of cause-and-effect relationships have been abandoned. Multiple interrelated, constantly flowing and changing regulatory circuits, and information streams for maintenance of intracellular and extracellular balanced conditions, are now dominating the way of thinking. The

Table 10.3 Hypotheses of the psychogenesis of cancer
• Current neurosis
• Unconscious suicide
• Conversion symptom (organ language)
• Asexual procreation
• Desire for independence and freedom
• Hypothesis of loss (loss of an object: symbolic substitute for broken relationships)
• Syndrome of discouragement
• Defect hypothesis
• Alexithymia (blindness of the soul)
• Stress
• Cancer patients as symptom carriers of a "cancer family"

immune surveillance theory seems to imply that an unbalanced, regulatory-resistant immune system promotes the development of cancer. According to the psychosomatic theory of cancer development, psychogenetic mechanisms (Table 10.3) can influence the diverse regulatory circuits of tumor defense and tumor dissemination (13).

Stress and Cancer

Since H. Seyle defined the phenomenon "stress" and described the pathophysiology, the disease-promoting effects of distress (in contrast to eustress) have been demonstrated. The hypotheses that are derived from this are supported through research approaches in medical sociology that have verified risk and damage factors as well as health-promoting protective phenomena such as social support, loving behavior in relationships, religiousness, and self-conscientious behavior on cognitive and emotional levels. These are individual variables that only exert protective or deleterious effects when acting in a concerted fashion.

It is beyond any doubt that stress can also induce **adaptive processes** and **learning curves** that ultimately increase the resistance to stress through positive accomplishment.

- Some authors believe that chronic stress initiates cancer (3, 58, 69), while other examiners assert more meaning to the single, short acting but profoundly damaging stressful event (46).
- Physiological stress responses to traumatizing and burdensome life events can be demonstrated through determination of hormonal, immunological, and endocrine parameters. A cor-

relation between stress and cancer development is becoming increasingly apparent in the recent literature (5, 27, 64, 65).

- Experimentally, animals carrying tumors were exposed to life-threatening stress with and without escape options (68). Flight hindrance led to significantly increased tumor growth, while successful escape resulted in retarded tumor growth.

Psychosomatic Strain in Cancer

That cancer has psychological implications, is experienced daily (Table 10.4) (7).

The mental processing of cancer occurs in approximately three phases, even though there are huge discrepancies, depending on the personality. Long-term observations have shown that with the help of loved ones and self-help groups as well as active cognitive coming to terms with the disease, the course can be more beneficially influenced than with a withdrawn passive-resigned or accusatory attitude.

- In a study, 86 patients with metastasized breast cancer were randomly assigned to either an intervention group (n = 50) or a control group (n = 36).
- While the intervention group participated at least for a year once weekly in group therapeutic meetings with the goal of controlling symptoms and promoting coping strategies, the control group was merely observed. The median survival time of the intervention group was 36.6 months, while that of the control group was 18.9 months (70).

The scientific explanation for a doubling in survival time is difficult to trace back and is not related to a selective advantage of the intervention group. This has been shown in several instances throughout literature.

The reproducibility of the study also suffered because the special relationships and interactions in the therapeutic group were strongly influenced by the charismatic leadership of the therapist, who had suffered and survived breast cancer herself. The living model was not an abstract entity, no smart advice, no statistics, but a tangible proof of real hope presented to the participants every week, and this was translated into optimism and a will to survive. Ultimately, the study proves the

Table 10.4 Psychosomatic strain in cancer	
Threat through physical symptoms	– esthetic deformation (e. g., loss of hair) – loss of function – reduced efficiency – pain, nausea, vomiting – implants
Changes in social relations	– loss in attractiveness for the partner – fears of separation and loss – reduced value of the role played in family and workplace – loss of job/restrictions in the workplace – dependency on nurses/doctors
Loss of psychoemotional stability	– fear of tumor recurrence, metastases – fear of death, of dying, of wasting away – fear of loneliness, loss of control, and mental disintegration – fear of depression: loss of hope, life perspective and enjoyment of life – despair, hopelessness, anger and aggression over fate, and healthy individuals, loss of dependency – self-degradation through loss of self-esteem, disease as an insult and a defeat

fact once again that people are not mentally motivated by moralistic appeals or abstract statistics, but through human beings who can be seen as role models, similar to the way children learn life and behavior through imitation of parental figures.

Tumor Activation

The psychogenesis of the transformation of benign cells into malignant cells has been discussed repeatedly, and numerous examples have been cited. Nonetheless, the hypothesis has never been verified.

On the other hand, it has been empirically validated through numerous observations that clinically diagnosed cancer can be negatively influenced through psychological factors. That is why it is being speculated whether losses, worries, needs, and fears are capable of activating a latent tumor:

- Emotional, negative stress can increase the serum levels of cortisone (normal about 40 ng/mL) to levels above 700 ng/mL. Thymus involution and T-cell lymphopenia are a result (54).
- Some studies emphasize the tumor-promoting role of life stressor events in women with breast cancer (12, 14, 18), while other authors were unable to find any correlation between stress and the incidence of breast cancer (52). Obviously the psychosocial support that

patients received played a part as a mediator. Since some studies imply a correlation between stress and cancer, psychopathological phenomena that explain such a relationship must be present. Hopelessness has often been assumed to be a possible indicator for cancer (3, 41, 61), partially even as one of many causes (16).

- Losses such as death, divorce, and so forth, do not only appear to reduce the life expectancy, but also seem to be associated with a measurable immune suppression. Several studies reported on a restricted cellular immunity directly after the death of a beloved person (6, 59) with a return to normal values after about six months. Other studies show that sorrow induces a long-standing activation of the hypothalamic–pituitary–adrenal hormonal axis with increased values in cortisone and reduced activity of natural killer cells (29, 31). The psychological and biological stress responses vary a lot from one individual to another. While fearful stress in patients who are about to undergo a big operation, coupled with loneliness, feeling of forsakenness and depression, led to a marked weakening of the immune system, patients with sufficient social support (family, friends) and thereby less emotional stress were normoreactive (9).
- Various animal studies support the hypothesis that emotional stress significantly influences

the emergence and further development of cancer (5, 47, 55, 73). Long-lasting emotional stress in these studies resulted in a significant increase in breast cancer. Using animal studies it was shown that 92 % of the mice that had been infected with the Bittner oncogenic virus for breast cancer, developed a tumor when they were exposed to chronic stress, but only 7 % of animals that grew up in a protected environment developed breast cancer (54). By eliminating the genetic risk (no virus infection in isogenic mice). The explanation lay in the stress-related increase in release of cortisone with involution of the thymus gland and accompanying lymphocytopenia of the T and NK cells.

Case report. T. H. was an attractive woman of 48 years, mother of three children and engaged in the local district life of her small town. She was married to a very busy trauma surgeon who dedicated himself to his very demanding career, also to satisfy her high expectations. Due to a combination of boredom, dissatisfaction, and the fear of dwindling attractiveness, she neglected her family and took up relations haphazardly with (mostly) much younger men. The family tensions that ensued and problems her children had in school were not left unrecognized, and she led an expansive life of "self-realization" causing considerable damage to her family. Desperate and resigned over the resistance of his wife to hear advice, even professionally, the husband filed for divorce. The one family house was auctioned off. During the dramatic three years of the divorce phase that followed, her only grandson died, as did her brother and her dog. Six months after the legal divorce, a uterine cancer was diagnosed, and radical extirpation with ensuing chemotherapy followed.

The case can be looked at from three angles:
1. genetic risk factors
2. stress and environmental factors
3. psychoneuroendocrine and immunological reactions to psychocausal origins.

While most studies support the model of a possible additional pathogenic principle through life stress, negative correlations have also been reported (52).

The widely held unanimous opinion in literature attributes "psychosocial support" as having a major mediator role (22). Despite these insights, there are many unanswered questions. Why does a tumor develop in a person with less psychological trauma and why not in those with considerably more difficult and problematic relations to the internal and external world? Can this variability be explained through biological factors that yet remain unknown? Can social support or other psychosocial conditions influence tumorigenesis in terms of inhibition?

The difficulty lies with the fact that the assessment of a psychosocial trauma can only be individually evaluated. Even the most serious trauma may show relatively few somatic effects under beneficial circumstances, while even relatively small traumas can show catastrophic effects, even suicide.

A considerable mistake in the evaluation of earlier studies has been that the noninvolved observer categorized traumas into serious and less serious, a categorization which did not necessarily correspond to reality. Psychological traumas can be evaluated individually and intrapersonally, but never collectively.

The hypothesis states that individuals who are prone to the same biological risk, increase the overall risk for development of tumors through individually more strongly perceived stress. Stress by itself does not induce cancer. It is possible, however that it is responsible for the activation of latent neoplasms, that could have otherwise never become clinically apparent, e. g., through weakening of the immune defenses during a critical phase.

Latent cancer stages are occasionally diagnosed during **autopsies** that are performed due to other causes of death. Latent prostate cancers are seen in 26–40 %, prostate intraepithelial neoplasms in 80-year-olds in up to 80 %, precancerous adenomas of the colon and rectum in 40 % of autopsies (71). In women between the ages of 20 and 54, latent cancerous areas were found in the breast in 20 % of all autopsies (49).

The idea that psychogenic factors should be regarded as playing only a minor role as possible cofactors in the pathogenesis of certain types of cancer—rather than as etiologically relevant factors—should be the starting point of further trials. Large epidemiological studies on stress, emotional loss, and cancer are necessary, although the critical variable is not stress and loss in itself, but the individual meaning of psychostressors in a critical phase of life. These therapeutically important questions relating to psychosomatic tumorigenesis have not gained much attention within the medical literature (only 1.2 % of all publications on oncology touch upon this subject)—especially in the daily clinical oncology practice, aspects of psychosomatic aspects are rarely given much notice.

Psychotherapeutic Aspects in Oncology

The investigation of psychogenetic causes for cancer not only serves in prevention, but also in coping with the disease, and at best in influencing the course through psychotherapeutic interventions.

All knowledge remains futile, however, if it fails to lead to action. The inability of some excellent oncologists to be able to verbally communicate or comprehend their patients is reflected, for example, by some of the topics of oncology conventions. The suffering, dying patient is no longer represented here: not the level of doctor–patient interaction is important—just the interaction of molecules.

The subordination of psychological aspects of disease to the dominant molecular model of disease makes room for brilliant hypotheses and visions. However, the suffering of patients, the fear and pain they experience daily, remain excluded.

The defense mechanisms previously alluded to are not only instruments of the patient's psyche, but are used in the same way by the therapist's psyche. Both groups require help, supervision, and Balint Group activities for their own mental sanity. The strategies that leading personalities in the industry, administration, and politics have successfully implemented, with the help of mental health measures, as a reaction to the enormous burdens presented to them by their profession, should be a matter of course for physicians practicing in the field of oncology. This is not only because efficacy and utility of psychotherapeutic treatment are undeniable (17, 23, 40), but also because the population is demanding more from its doctors than merely certified specialty knowledge. They request empathy that is convincing and presented in a manner that reveals self-reflection as well as fluency within a social relationship.

Effective Factors in Psycho-oncology Therapy

- Prerequisites for a good **therapeutic relationship** are specific interventions, regular exper-

tise training of the therapist as well as acceptace by the patient.
- Through **open-mindedness** of the treating physician the patient is drawn into an object–subject relationship, in which he is actively involved reinforcing the will to self-healing.
- For **activation of hope and potential for faith** in the patient, the therapist must be convinced of his or her own ability to help the patient, to enable him or her to overcome a fundamental despair engendered by the disease.
- The foundation of the relationship is the **confrontation of the problem**, not the suppression of the problem. In this way the patient gains confidence and the experience that his or her individual problems are taken seriously.
- The problem of the patient is given new meaning and value. The negative and positive aspects are discussed.
- Mutually searching for constructive problem solving, physician and patient comprise a therapeutic team.
- Solutions that have been developed are noted down in a time-event table with definition of goals laid down (problem management). Medical markers can be included as goals (e.g., definition of a certain level of tumor marker as a result of which a change in therapy is laid down).
- Retrospective **analysis of progressions and set backs** are discussed, analyzed and may perhaps lead to the correction of a goal (question: "How was the course so far? Where do we stand now? Are there periods without any fear? How do I behave toward my family? How does my family relate to me?")

Subjective Disease Concept

Each patient generates his or her **own theory** surrounding the disease. The question about the etiology and the reason for discomfort is one that is universal to all of humanity. Humans need an individual value system for discomfort and their unhappiness, in order to be able to meet their life's coordinates. In this way, completely neutral occurrences, such as, for example, rainy weather, can be experienced on the one hand as a refreshing, and on the other as an unpleasant event.

Guilt and sin, warning and also reorientation, often play a large role in these moral concepts.

Subjective disease theories provide a means to cope with the fatalistic disease processes, thereby serving health, since they give a meaning that promotes acceptance of the disease. Subjective disease theories, on the other hand, may also be an unhappy, often failed, way of coming to terms with the disease, and may thereby have an adverse effect.

Subjective disease theories and attempts at explanation should always be taken very seriously by the therapist, who should react in a neutral and tolerant manner when faced by them in order to allow these subjective theories for disease to evolve and become clearer by targeted questioning. It is only through empathic accepting and also modifying additional information from the therapist that inappropriate disease theories can be modified in accordance with an internal logic and acceptable reality.

The Patient–Doctor Relationship in Oncology

There is hardly any other area of research in medicine that has achieved so little with so much financial investment as has the field of oncology. Only 6% of all advanced epithelial cancers are cured (1). The patterns of healing of conventional medicine do not apply to cancer—it is not a disease in the classical sense.

Twenty-five percent of the population in the industrial world will get cancer in the span of their life times, 20% will die due to their disease. This means that only 20% can be cured of cancer, even though the five-year survival time is 30–40%, which does not permit calculation of cancer-free survival with any certainty.

The high ethical demands placed on oncologists occasionally result in disfiguring and risky therapies, with considerable morbidity and subliminal inhumanity. Nagel speaks of "ill medicine" (39, 48).

Whether psychological etiologies play a decisive part in the development of cancer, is still up for debate. However, the insight that psychological influences may be the cause of differences occasionally seen in the course of diseases with identical diagnosis and tumor stage, is gaining traction. The stigmatizing term "cancer patient" is felt as an immense emotional burden that is often combined with strong despair and depression. The psychoso-

cial environment is also part of psycho-oncology, as well as the socioeconomic level of interest.

Psycho-oncology presents the actual situation in a matter-of-fact communicative dialog addressing the disclosure of all levels of access and observation of both cancer patient and therapist, as well as the interactions between the two. This appears to be important for introducing necessary changes and for stimulating self-reflection by the oncologist outside of the traditional ways of thought, in addition to discussing assistance programs for the "**helpless helper**."

In particular, the results of psycho-oncology have shown that the treating physician is at least as important for the patient's well-being as the treatment itself (63).

When conveying the diagnosis "cancer" it is clear to both the conveying physician as his patient that one is dealing with a potentially deadly disease, which must be further mutually fought through a therapeutic communal destiny. The intensity of the doctor–patient relationship carries far more weight than the common communicative relationship between an advice seeker and an advice provider. Not only for the patient, but also for the physician, the burdens of this unique relationship are quite sizeable.

Table 10.5 Weak points in the doctor–patient relationship (20)
• Instead of listening, I spoke
• Because I posed the wrong questions, I did not receive the right answers
• I misunderstood my patient because I did not recognize the various messages of the speaking, or I confused them
• Instead of showing empathy, I behaved "professionally"
• Instead of accepting the patient, I rejected him or her
• The discussions with my patients were unsatisfactory for both parties, due to a lack of a right start, a clear goal and a concrete continuation
• I created time pressure and allowed time pressure to be felt
• I ordered instead of motivating
• I treated the patient as a so-called difficult patient
• I did not acknowledge fears, and triggered fears in the course of conversation
• I did not understand that the reality of my patient and my own reality were not identical
• I did not make it clear to myself that language is the most important tool a physician has

Mutual expectations influence the interaction between patient and doctor quite considerably, and not only on the individual level, but also in terms of questions pertaining to the roles of conventional medicine, alternative medicine, and psycho-oncology in society.

Cancer is a chronic disease that is often ultimately incurable, despite decades of therapy and intense connection to the treating physician. The threat of death during the entirety of the course of the disease is a burden for both the patient and the physician, although this is often not openly discussed.

The self-accusatory insights in Table 10.**5** are important, because the physician must also learn to recognize the patient's subjective reality, since it is only in this way that the physician can understand the patient. It is only through communication, through empathically conveyed information, that it becomes possible to combine the patient's own thought processes and fantasies over the development and etiology of his or her disease with scientific therapeutic possibilities.

Information and Communication: Doctor–Patient
Role allocation and role expectations are barriers to mutual understanding.

A typical role play between patient and physician is the expected devout attitute of the patient, along with the entitlement to omnipotence the doctor receives from the patient together with delegation of responsibility. In this way, the patient transfers his fears and needs on to the physician and places himself into a regressive position (also through actualization of neurotic conflicts).

The **transference of conflicts** on to the physician brings about a **countertransference** that may become apparent through conscious or unconscious attitudes when confronted with the patient. The patient is allocated a role by the doctor, whereby the latter emphasizes those attributes in front of the patient, which he attempts to repress within himself. Mutual role expectations lead to ritualized patient–doctor encounters in the private sessions or during visitations. The verbal and nonverbal messages exchanged can very well be contradictory. Specifically, the law that governs at the bedside may be dominated by gestures of dominance and submissiveness, which the cancer patient often associates with repression and denial of death and suffering.

Typical for the **visitation in the clinic** is not only the lopsided nature of communication, but also personal asymmetry. Many people rush into the patient's room with the physician, and one no longer talks *to* the patient, but *about* the patient. The "pure lecturing" protects the physician from entering a critical dialog with the patient. Rational medicine does not permit perceptions of the patient's well-being, since these can no longer be treated with the system's standard norms. Behind all this, the physician is hiding fears that his therapeutic powerlessness may become all too apparent.

The fixation of the medical world on natural sciences has so far hindered an anthropological concept of medicine. The actual treatment concepts relate to the physical–chemical realities, but not the psychological ones (72).

Treatment Planning

- The disease model and treatment strategy are developed together with the patient:
  - How and why has the patient become sick?
  - How can he or she get well or reduce his or her complaints/pain?
  - How can he/she reduce his/her fears (of death)?
  - How can his or her condition and life satisfaction be increased in a practical way?
- Depending on the required somatic treatment and with respect to the possible morbidities, psycho-oncological treatment goals and steps are determined and laid down in writing.
- Strategies for assessment and their execution are planned. The assessment should be constructed as a process that the patient can experience. Complicated and difficult courses are to be discussed ahead of time in order to allow for early arrangements in the event of bad developments (e. g., loss of weight, increase in tumor markers: emergency planning).
- The assessment of prognosis should be realistic, without destroying hope. Every somatic complaint should be realistically and optimally assessed, and surprising positive developments should be acknowledged and not excluded as a possibility (43).

— Points of Emphasis in the Physician's Conducting of Conversation and the Conversational Setting

The possibility of setting boundaries is important for the therapist so that the circumstantial energies triggering intensive affects can be accepted and overcome. Only then is the therapist able to conduct a structured conversation with the patient. This requires:

- professionalism
- maintenance of the interpretative role
- effort and understanding
- neutrality
- effort for an appropriate relationship
- dependability within the realm of trust
- clear time frame and transparency
- clear, previously defined goals.

The therapist must be able to successfully conduct **crisis interventions** through his or her therapeutic attitude. Crises always represent a regression of the ego, whereby the balance between compensatory regulating ego functions and unhindered impulsive action and emotions is considerably disturbed. Crisis patients present the psycho-oncologist with special challenges.

The **affect-flooding crisis** with uncontrolled impulsive action is contagious. The patient in a panic–chaotic status threatens to pull along everybody else and requires intensive measures of care.

The **muted crisis** of the presuicidal and withdrawn patient, on the other hand, is very different and demands immediate action, while simultaneously rejecting the helper and making the helper appear helpless.

Crises always provoke severe feelings of countertransference. The patient underscores his demands of allowances (of intense immediate procedures) through staging, and often also through presenting "important people" (lawyer, physician, acquaintance, and so on). In order for the therapist to remain true to his or her professional role in these difficult situations, it is important for him or her to set boundaries. This will only be effective if the therapist's own implicit affects (anger, aggression, fears) are accepted and overcome, in order to make the patient a structured offering:

- "We have exactly 15 minutes of time today in order to take a closer look at your problem."

- "In the coming six weeks, we will always be conducting a 15 minute-long talk. This talk will always take place on Thursdays at 1900. Should I be unable to keep this appointment due to an emergency, we will defer the conversation and schedule a new appointment."
- "For me it is very important to obtain a clearer picture of your complaints and their causes. Once I have obtained a better understanding, I will be able to recommend treatment. Should a more protracted therapy be necessary, I will inform you about it."
- Conversation should always be concentrated, clearly defined in content, and ended on time. It should take between 15 and 30 minutes, and be divided into content segments.

Questioning Techniques

- Open-ended questions benefit the guidance of conversation. They aim in no particular direction and allow the other person the option of free speech.
  Examples:
  - "What brings you to me?"
  - "When did your complaints begin?"
  - "What are the situations in which you feel unpleasantly touched?"
- If you would like to receive a clarifying, precise answer, ask a **closed question,** a question, in other words, one that can only be answered by "yes" or "no" or that allows a distinct answer only.
  Examples:
  - "Do you have pain in your joints?"
  - "How often do you need to void at night?"
  - "How many cigarettes do you smoke a day?"
- Questions that delve deeper, **clarifying questions** require precise answers. They challenge the patient to divulge more detailed, more intimate information. These questions complete a story. They clarify the who, what, when, where, how, and why.
  Examples:
  - "When exactly did your complaints start?"
  - "How was the pain precisely?"
  - "In what situation were you back then?"
  - "You stated that you were angry. Please describe your feelings when you were angry."
  - "Please describe what you are feeling in this precise moment."

– "You have mentioned that you have always felt misunderstood by your mother. Please describe the last of these situations that you can recall."
– "What do you believe is the cause of your heart pain?"

- **Circular questions** and the **family conversation** The inclusion of the partner or the family can be reasonable when, in the event of a serious (cancer) disease, not only the patient, but also the partner and the entire family are brought into an emotional crisis.

On the other hand, psychological symptoms of a cancer patient can be an expression of individual or familial disruptions and therefore not only require individual therapy, but also family therapy, or a cautious inclusion of the family, in order to utilize this health-promoting resource.

Circular questioning frequently opens up the entrenched subjective points of view to offer new perspectives and provides new information, allowing differences to be aired, and it may rekindle deadlocked conversation.

Examples:
– "What do you think your wife believes you should do to make you feel better?"
– "What would your daughter say, if I were to ask her, about what she thinks you should do now?"
– "What would your wife say about your daughter's recommendations?"
– "What does your daughter think you would have to do, if you were to feel worse once again?"

Conversation Techniques

- **Positive connotation** The positive connotation underlines an optimal perspective. It elevates self-esteem and self-competency. The doctor–patient relationship is stabilized and simultaneously more open, one's own forces and resources for coping with disease are activated. They give the patient self-confidence and a therapeutic goal.

Example:
– Patient: "My pain is getting worse and worse, my hope is sinking. Even though I have seen six doctors, no one has been able to help me."

– Positive connotation: "All the more respect to you for having the energy to come in to see us here today."
– Patient: "I am a social worker, and the misery and destitution that I see and must endure in my job has begun to upset and depress me."
– Positive connotation: "You have something that other people lack—the ability to sense what others are feeling and to also communicate these feelings."
– Patient: "Yes ... (positively touched) ... you are right, but sometimes I would just like to be able to withdraw myself."
– Positive connotation: "Yes, you have detected one part of your problem. You have this great ability that can become a problem if you are not able to set boundaries, or if others take advantage of this great ability of yours."

- Through **resource activation** (social support) health-inducing factors are strengthened and new levels in healing are opened up with new options for action. The patient's responsibility for his own health is made clear to him and is reinforced, which takes the burden off the doctor.

Examples:
– "What should stay the same in your life?"
– "Which aspects and areas of your life are you satisfied with?"
– "What would you do to make yourself feel less stressed as of tomorrow?"
– "What has particularly helped you in stressful situations so far?"
– "How did you manage, despite your fears and pain, to come to this appointment today?"

- **Explanations** The patient receives new information and can learn to accept new disease models out of these explanations that can be adapted to his situation. The patient is included on the cognitive mental level and gains more control over his disease.

Examples:
– "If you take your problems with you to bed at night, your trouble with falling asleep may be related to your work."
– "Elevated blood pressure has to do with internal tensions and stress."
– "Headaches and stress can lie close together."

– "The value for prostate-specific antigen may increase during inflammations of the prostate as well as during benign increases in size of the prostate."

- **Conclusion** It enables patient and physician to evaluate and summarize previous conversations. It stimulates thought and self-reflection and serves as the foundation of hypothesis generation. A physician working in the field of oncology is not only required to reflect, such as with the question: "What does oncology do to me, what does it evoke in me?," but he or she also requires supervision to complete self-perception as well as object recognition. It is important for the therapist within oncology to be able to recognize the conditions of his or her problem-solving behavior and his or her capacity to create the prerequisites needed for a therapeutic relationship through awareness of his or her feelings during the encounter with the patient.

It is important that he or she is thorough, takes adequate time, not only treading on common pathways, but also allowing himself or herself to listen to his or her own insights, which can also bring about original solutions.

Complementary and enhancing cancer treatment refers to the inclusion of psycho-oncology, the attempt of a new design for treatment options and attending to the fear that dominates everything, and is ultimately the reason for taking new paths.

Example After a tumor conference a colleague reports that he distinctly senses how tensed up and concerned he is. During the conversation, his exaggerated correctness and strictness are verbalized and he is able to understand open and externally visible strictness as a part of his efforts. In the further course of the discussion it becomes evident that the external strictness, correctness, and compulsiveness is actually symbolic of his fear of change.

The danger of a medicine governed by guidelines resides in the stereotypical manner of dealing with patients. The conversation is the most important therapeutic instrument of the psycho-oncologist, and guides the partners in communication toward a continuous process of self-exploration and learning. It is important to always be aware that during the course of a therapeutic conversation energies can be released that can positively stimulate healing forces through hope, joy, and confidence, but that are also able to destroy these positive possibilities.

Example: A 56-year-old physician-in-chief, who has just been informed that he has prostate cancer (pT3, NX, M0, G3, Gleason 7) is seeking a second opinion with a renowned professor at a university clinic. The latter tells him: "In terms of your life's survival time: I give you another two years!" This axelike prognosis turns the next two years into a torturous period of misery for the patient, in which he would have almost died in the sense of a self-fulfilling prophecy. He turned to complementary and also alternative medicine based on acknowledged conventional medical therapies and is now—utterly surprised himself about this—in the fifth year after hearing his prognosis with normalized PSA values.

This example demonstrates the mythical power of the physician, who even takes all hope from a colleague who is fearful and regressive. This abuse in the form of a pseudoprognostic predictive wisdom can be seen throughout all of medicine. Causes include the rejection of one's own fears, insufficient self-awareness and the accompanying lack of empathy for those seeking help.

Obviously, one's own helplessness that one is unwilling to admit—in order to not lessen and interfere with the self-constructed grandiosity—is reflected there. This little example also demonstrates that psycho-oncology does not require large programs, but that one can start with little words in order to be perceived with endless gratitude by those seeking help.

- **Confrontation** The confrontation makes that patient aware of disharmonies. It is comprised of attentive, occasionally aggressive aspects of relationships that require clarification. It acts to stabilize the patient–doctor relationship through poignant definitions. Accusatory "you" messages should not be utilized—"I" messages are always preferred.

Example:
– "In the last conversation we had discussed for you to keep a pain diary. Now you tell me that you did not have time for it. I cannot help you if you do not collaborate and it makes me angry when you do not keep up your part of the agreement."

Table 10.6	Dealing with difficult situations in communication

- Precise listening, understanding the issues of the patient
- Analyze the goals and motives of patient
- Analyze diagnosis and divide course of treatment into individual components
- Analyze the patient–doctor relationship
- Analyze the counter-transference
- Analyze the structural situation in which the patient is situated, e.g., through insufficient resources

Table 10.7	Supportive measures during conversation

- Express understanding and empathy
- Verbally express, reformulate, and name emotions, even if they are unpleasant feelings
- Show where and in what way support can be offered
- Communicate hope
- Offer helpful measures
- Show solutions
- Make problem-solving concrete through single steps
- Define goals and then develop a solution step by step

- "In the last conversation I suggested that you should keep a protocol of your feelings. You have not done this, even though you had agreed to do so. If you only give me such threadbare information about your work situation, I cannot ascertain whether this plays a role in your disease. I would greatly like to know why it is so hard for you to talk about this."
- "Last week you urgently requested an appointment, which I then proceeded to arrange, requiring me to cancel another patient. I have to tell you that it aggravated me a lot that you did not show up then."

— The Power of the Word

Psychotherapy always takes place on the extended linguistic level. While the surgeon utilizes and must master the knife, the radiation specialist the linear accelerator-driven reactor, and the internist chemotherapy as a tool, the **instrument of the psycho-oncologist is the word**—the verbal intervention. This must also be mastered in the same way as the responsible handling of the scalpel.

Synaptic structures of neuronal networks can also be altered through intensely perceived conversation, as soon as the conversation is stored in the memory (32). Just as information or events (e. g., the 11 September 2001) not only change individuals but also human groups, and create a new consciousness, the individual paradoxically uses reason as a means of constructive aid, in order to repress the truth of his mental vulnerability.

With quite a bit of certainty, neuronal networks and cross-links are newly structured in the brain in the course of psychotherapy, similarly to molecular "remodeling" following a period of learning, through structural and biochemical changes in the sense of neuronal plasticity. Learning or memory content is coded in the form of engrams through activation of multiple neurons. Storage occurs in the form of a neuronal mosaic, a so-called "ensemble." These acquired or experienced structures, that ultimately only obey a hierarchical operating system, store ideas, hopes, beliefs, and also pictures, emotions, and facts. These plastic switch operations in the nervous system develop particularly strongly in the early learning stage of childhood, and are also involved in all later psychosocial processes, or rather, react to these. Everything that we absorb from birth onwards and later through the spoken word, what shapes us, what we learn, determines our synaptic interconnections.

Culture and human society can only develop through language. An exchange of information occurs through the empathically spoken word not only on the verbal plane, but a materialized energetic transference ensues that programs the grammatical neuronal networks.

While one still differentiates between hardware and software in computer technology, this difference does not apply to psycho-oncology. The brain, with its neuronal network represents the self-regulating, genetically coded hardware exposed to growth impulses in the sense of an "enamelware" as well as software at the same time, and that optimizes itself through self-programming and continuous processing of information. It is rare that the capacities of the human brain are utilized during a lifetime. All the more reason to employ the incredibly powerful resources of the mental, positive influence through verbal intervention in the framework of a psycho-oncological treatment. This requires mastering the verbal intervention techniques in addition to medical knowledge.

Psycho-oncological therapeutic measures should be an integrative component of every type of tumor therapy, even though not primarily. Although the efficacy and the usefulness of psycho-oncological therapeutic measures has been proved multiple times, the actual mechanisms of efficacy remain unclear for the most part and are being discussed with much controversy (17).

Psycho-oncology, for the most part, entails a great deal of grieving together with the patient, who is marked by a potentially deadly disease. The unavoidability of death becomes tangible for the patient through the diagnosis of cancer. The horror and the fear of the certain end to life is not determined by the fact in and of itself, since everyone knows that he or she will die, but paradoxically, through the painful loss of the illusion of immortality or health until old age and of retaining a youthful appearance.

The "victory over cancer" or also "antiaging" are cultural lies that have been taken from scientific materialism, in order to introduce economic principles into the medical–ethical realm. With the consequent change in terminology, the consciousness can be altered: insurance for sick patients are masked as insurances for the healthy—*health* insurance—the five-year survival rate is defined as a cure. The exclusion of a positive reality of death through organized institutions for the dying such as old age homes, intensive care units of hospitals, hospices, and so forth, lead to mental loss of dealing with the experience of death by the individual as well as by society.

Death has become anonymous, removed and is virtually only administered as a peripheral medical side-event in obituaries. Despite the unavoidable truth that death statistically occurs later in many tumor-therapeutic options (although death is thereby prolonged), the empathic affection, the loving hope, should never be given up. In this way every physician working in the field of oncology is required to also be a psycho-oncologist.

References

1. Abel U: Chemotherapy of advanced epithelial cancer. Stuttgart, Germany: Hippokrates Verlag; 1990.
2. Bacon CL, Rennecker R, Cutler M: A psychosomatic survey of cancer of the breast. Psychosom Med. 1952; 14:443–460.
3. Bahnson CB: Stress and cancer. State of the art Part I. Pyschosomatics. 1980; 21:975–981.
4. Baltrusch HJF, Stangel W, Waltz ME: Cancer from the biobehavioral perspective: The type "C" pattern. Act Nerv Super. 1988; 30:18–21.
5. Bammer K, Newberry BH: Stress and Cancer. Göttingen, Toronto: Hogrefe Verlag: 1981.
6. Bartrop R, Luckhurst E, Lazarus L, Kiloh L, Penny R: Depressed lymphocyte function after bereavement. Lancet. 1977; 1(8016): 834–836.
7. Bauer KH: Das Krebsproblem. Berlin, Germany: Springer Verlag, 1963.
8. Bernd H, Gunther H, Rathe G: Persönlichkeitsstruktur nach Eysenck bei Kranken mit Brustdrüsen- und Bronchialkrebs und Diagnoseverzögerung durch die Patienten. Archiv für Geschwulstforschung. 1980; 40:359–368.
9. Biondi M, Costantini A, Parisi A: Can loss and grief activate latent neoplasia? Psychother Psychosom Med Psychol. 1996; 65:102–105.
10. Booth G: Psychobiological aspects of spontaneous regression of cancer. J Am Acad Psychoanal. 1974; I:303–317.
11. Bräutigam W: Zur Psychosomatik des Krebses. Dtsch Med Wschr. 1981; 106:1563–1565.
12. Bremond A, Kune AG, Bahnson CB: Psychosomate factors in breast cancer patients. Results of a case control study. J Obstet Gynaecol. 1986; 5:127–136.
13. Burnet FM: Immune Surveillance. Elmsford, NY; Sydney: Pergamon Press; 1970.
14. Cooper CL, Faragher EB: Coping strategies and breast cancer. Psychol Med. 1992; 22:447–455.
15. Eysenck HJ: The prediction of death from cancer by means of a personality/stress questionnaire: too good to be true? Percept Motor Skills. 1990; 71: 216–218.
16. Eysenck HJ: Anxiety, learned helplessness and cancer. J Anxiety Disord. 1987; 87–104.
17. Federschmidt H: Wirksamkeit und Nutzen von psychotherapeutischen Behandlungsansätzen. Dtsch. Ärzteblatt. 1996; 93:34–38.
18. Forsen A: Psychosocial stress as a risk for breast cancer. Psychother Psychosom Med Psychol. 1991; 55.176–185.
19. Garfield SL (ed.): Handbook of Psychotherapy and Behaviour Chance. New York, NY: John Wiley and Sons; 1994;143–189.
20. Geißler I: Arzt- und Patientenbegegnung im Gespräch. Frankfurt am Main, Germany: Pharma Verlag; 1987; p. 9.

21. Goodkin K, Antoni MH, Blaney PH: Stress and hopelessness in the promotion of cervical intra-epithelial neoplasia to invasive squamous cell carcinoma of the cervix. J Psychosom Res. 1986; 30:67–76.
22. Grassi L, Nappi G, Susa H, Molinari S: Eventi stress anti, supporto sociale e caratteristiche psicologiche in pazienti affette da carcinoma della mammella. In: Stress, emozioni e cancro. Il Roma, Italy: Pensiero Scientifico; 1987.
23. Grawe K, Donati R, Bernauer F: Psychotherapie im Wandel. Von der Konfession zur Profession. Göttingen, Germany: Hogrefe Verlag; 1994.
24. Greer S, Morris T, Pettingale KW, Haybittle J: Psychological response to breast cancer and 15-year outcome. Lancet. 1990; 335:49–50.
25. Groddek G: Von der psychischen Bedingtheit der Krebserkrankung in Groddeck, G.: Psychoanalytische Schriften zur Psychosomatik. Wiesbaden, Germany: Limes Verlag; 1966.
26. Heim E: Krankheit als Krise und Chance. Munich, Germany: MVG Verlag; 1998.
27. Helmkamp M, Paul H: Psychosomatische Krebsforschung. Bern, Switzerland: Huber Verlag, 1984.
28. Hislop GT, Waxler NE, Goldmann AJ, Elwood JM, Kann L: The prognosic significance of psychosocial factors in women with breast cancer. J Chron Dis. 1987; 40:729–735.
29. Hofer MA, Wolff CT, Friedmann SB, Mason JW: A psychoneuroendocine study of bereavement. Psychosom Med. 1972; 34:481–491.
30. Horne RL, Picard RS: Psychosocial risk factors for lung cancer. Psychosom Med. 1971; 41:503–514.
31. Irwin M, Jones L: Life stress, depression and reduced natural cytotoxicity. In: Stress and Immunity. New York, NY: CRC Press; 1991.
32. Kandel ER, Schwarz ICH, Jessel TM: Principles of Neural Science. New York, NY: Elsevier; 1991: 1009–1030.
33. Kissen DM: Some methodological problems in clinical psychosomatic research with special reference to chest disease. Psychosom Med. 1988; 30:324–335.
34. Kline J, Schwartz G, Fitzpatrick D, Hendricks S: Defensiveness, anxiety and the amplitude/intensity function of auditory-evoked potentials. Int J Psychophysiol. 1993; 15:7–14.
35. Kneier AW, Temoshok L: Repressive coping reaction in patients with malignant melanomas as compared to cardiovascular disease patients. J Psychosomat Med. 1984; 28:145–155.
36. König F: Suizidalität bei Ärzten. Dtsch. Ärzteblatt. 2001; 47:2641–2642.
37. König K: Abwehrmechanismen: Göttingen, Germany: Vandenhoeck and Ruprecht, 1996
38. Kowal SI: Emotions as a cause of cancer 18th and 19th century contrications. Psychoanal Rev. 1955; 42:217–227.
39. Kreibich-Fischer R: Krebsbewältigung und Lebenssinn. Weinheim, Germany: Beltz Verlag; 1994.
40. Lambert MJ, Begen AE: The effectivness use of psychotherapy. In: Bergin AE, Garfield SL (eds): Handbook of Psychotherapy and Behaviour Change. New York, NY: Wiley and Sons; 1994:143–189.
41. Le Shan L: Psychotherapie gegen den Krebs. Stuttgart, Klett-Cotta, 1982.
42. Le Shan L: You can fight for life: emotional factors in the causation of cancer. New York, NY: M. Evans; 1977.
43. Lehrmann C, Kämmerer CB, Hentschel HJ, Lempard W: Weiterbildungskurs psychosomatischer Grundversorgung 8/2000, Hanover, Germany.
44. Mitscherlich A: Krankheit als Konflikt. Studien zur psychosomatischen Medizin. Frankfurt am Main, Germany: Surkamp Verlag; 1967, p. 13.
45. Mölling K: Die Gene und Krebs. Mannheimer Forum. Munich, Germany: Piper Verlag; 1992.
46. Moser KA, Fox AI, Iones DR, Goldblatt PO: Unemployment and mortality: further evidence from the OPCS Longitudinal Study 1971–81 Lancet. 1986; 1(8477):365–367.
47. Newberry BH, Gordon TL, Meehan SM: Animals studies of stress and cancer. In: Cooper CC, Watson M (eds) Cancer and Stress. Chichester: John Wiley and Sons; 1991:27–43.
48. Nagel G: Interview mit Dr. R. Kreibich-Fischer. In: Krebsbewältigung und Lebenssinn. Weinheim, Germany: Beltz Verlag; 1994.
49. Nielsen M, Thomsen JL, Primdahl S, Direborg U, Andersen JA: Breast cancer and atypia among young and middle-aged women: A study of 110 medicolegal autopsies. Brit J Cancer. 1987; 56:814–819.
50. Nolting HP, Paulus P: Psychoonkologie lernen. Weinheim, Germany: Beltz Verlag; 1996.
51. Paget J: Surgical Pathology. London: Longman's Green; 1870.
52. Priestman IJ, Priestman SG, Bradshaw C: Stress and breast cancer. Brit J Cancer. 1985; 5:493–498.
53. Reich W (1948): Die Entdeckung des Orgons Vol 2: Der Krebs. Frankfurt am Main, Germany: Fischer Verlag; 1981.
54. Riley V: Mouse mammary tumors: Alteration of incidence as apparent functions of stress. Science. 1975; 189:465–467.
55. Riley V: Psychoneuroendocrine influences on immunocompetence and neoplasia. Science. 1981; 212:1100–1109.
56. Schafft: Psychische und soziale Probleme krebsranker Frauen. Munich, Germany: Minerva Publications; 1987.
57. Scherg H: Zur Kausalitätsfrage in der psychosozialen Krebsforschung. Psychother Med Psycholog. 1986; 36:98–109.

58. Schleifer SI, Keller SE, Camerino M, Thornton JC, Stein M: Supression of lymphocyte stimulation following bereavement. JAMA. 1983; 250:374–377.

59. Schmähl D, Habs M: Krebs als Funktion von Disposition, Exposition und Alter. Naturwissenschaften. 1982; 69:332–335.

60. Schmale AH, Iker H: The effect of hopelessness and the development of cancer. Psychosom Med. 1966; 714–721.

61. Schmale AH, Iker H: Hopelessness as a predictor of cervical cancer. Soc Sci Med. 1971; 5:99–100.

62. Schwarz R: Die Krebspersönlichkeit: Mythos und klinische Realität. Stuttgart, Germany: Schattauer Verlag, 1994.

63. Schulz KH, Schulz H: Overview of the psychoneuroimmunological stress and intervention studies in humans with emphasis on the use of immunological parameters. Psycho-Oncology. 1992; 1:51–70.

64. Selye H: The physiology and pathology of exposure to stress. Montreal 1950.

65. Simonton OC: Prinzip Mut. Munich, Germany: Wilhelm Heyne Verlag; 1989.

66. Shavit Y, Lewis IW, Temann GW, Gale RD, Liebekind IC: Endogenous opioids may mediate the effects of stress on tumor growth. Proc West Phamacol Soc. 1983; 26:53–56.

67. Smith WIR, Sebastian H: Emotional history and pathogenesis of cancer. J Clin Pathol. 1976; 32:863–866.

68. Spiegel DJR, Bloom, Kraemer HC, Gottheil E: Effect of psychosocial treatment on survival of patients with metastatic breast cancer. Lancet. 1989; 2(8668):888–891.

69. Tullinus H: Latent malignancies and autopsy: a little used source of information on cancer biology. In: Riboli E, Delendi M (eds): Autopsy in Medical and Epidemiligal Research. Lyon: Int. Agency for the Research on Cancer, 1991.

70. von Uexküll T: Psychosomatische Medizin. Munich, Germany: Urban and Schwarzenberg; 1990.

71. Vogel W, Boner DB: Stress immunity and cancer in stress and immunity. London: CRC Press; 1981.

72. Weismann AD: Vulnerability and the psychological disturbances in cancer patients. Psychosomatics. 1989; 30:80–85.

73. Wirsching M: Psychosomatische Medizin. Munich, Germany: C.H. Beck; 1996.

74. Wirsching M, Shirlin H, Weber G, Hoffmann F, Wirsching B: Brustkrebs im Kontext: Ergebnisse einer Vorhersagestudie und Konsequenzen für die Therapie. Z Psychosom Med. 1981; 27:239–252.

11 Biological Basis for Using High Dose Multiple Antioxidants as an Adjunct to Radiotherapy, Chemotherapy, and Experimental Cancer Therapies

Kedar N. Prasad[1], William C. Cole[1], Bipin Kumar[1], and K. Che Prasad[2]

Introduction

Radiation therapy and chemotherapy are major treatment modalities in the management of human cancer. Hyperthermia is also considered one of the important experimental cancer therapy modalities for some tumors. While impressive progress in radiation therapy (like more accurate dosimetry and more precise methods of radiation targeting to tumor tissue), and in chemotherapy (such as development of novel drugs with diverse mechanisms of action on cell death and growth inhibition) has been made, the value of these modalities in tumor control may have reached a plateau. At present, two opposing hypotheses regarding the use of antioxidants during radiation therapy or chemotherapy have been proposed. One hypothesis states that supplementation with high doses of multiple micronutrients including dietary antioxidants (vitamin C, vitamin E, and carotenoids) may improve the efficacy of these treatment modalities by increasing tumor response and decreasing some of their toxicity on normal cells. The other hypothesis suggests that antioxidants should not be used during treatment with standard cancer therapeutic agents because they would protect cancer cells against damage. Each of these hypotheses is based on different conceptual frameworks that are derived from results obtained from specific experimental designs, and thus, each may be correct within its parameters. This chapter analyses published data that are used in support of each hypothesis, and reveals how the current controversies can be resolved, if the results obtained from one experimental design are not extrapolated to the other. Here we also discuss the scientific rationale for a micronutrient protocol that includes high doses of dietary antioxidants (vitamin C, vitamin E succinate, and natural β-carotene) that may improve the efficacy of radiation therapy and chemotherapy or experimental therapy, if used adjunctively.

Currently in the United States, the incidence of new cancer is approximately 1.2 million individuals per year with about 600 000 deaths due to cancer each year. The incidence of a second primary malignancy among cancer survivors is about 10–12 % annually.

Standard cancer therapy, which includes radiation therapy, chemotherapy, and surgery (whenever feasible and needed), has been useful in producing increased cure rates in certain tumors including Hodgkin disease, childhood leukemia, and teratocarcinoma. However, the risk of a second malignancy and nonneoplastic diseases such as aplastic anemia, retardation of growth in some children, and delayed necrosis in some organs such as brain, liver, bone, and muscle exists. In addition, acute damage to normal tissues occurs during radiation therapy and chemotherapy, and in some instances, such damage becomes the limiting factor for the continuation of therapy. At this time, the efficacy of standard cancer therapy has reached a plateau for most solid tumors in spite of impressive progress in radiation therapy, such as dosimetry and more efficient methods of delivery of radiation doses to tumors, and in chemotherapy, like development of novel drugs with diverse mechanisms of action on cell death and growth inhibition. Since very few of the standard cancer therapeutic agents have selective effects on cancer cells, modifying agents that can selectively either enhance the effect of radiation and chemotherapeutic drugs on cancer cells without producing similar effects on normal cells, or protect normal cells without protecting cancer cells, may improve the efficacy of treatment with these therapeutic agents. In spite of extensive research and clinical evaluation of potentially useful chemical modifying agents, most have been ineffective in the management of human cancer, because none were selective for tumor or normal cells and because most were found to be toxic in humans (1, 2). Although amifostine (WR-2731), an analogue of cysteamine, protected normal cells without protecting most cancer cells (3–5) except glioma cells (4) against radiation damage, at protective doses, it can cause nausea, vomiting, hypotension, and marrow hypoxia in humans (6, 7).

Certain nontoxic antioxidants may selectively enhance the effect of therapeutic agents on cancer cells while protecting normal cells against some of their toxicities. However, the results on the effects of antioxidants in modifying damage produced by radiation and chemotherapeutic agents on normal and cancer cells, using different experimental conditions, have led to opposing hypotheses. Our hypothesis states that supplementation with multiple micronutrients including high doses of dietary antioxidants (vitamin C, vitamin E, and β-carotene) may improve the efficacy of radiation therapy and chemotherapy by increasing tumor response and decreasing some of their toxicity on normal cells (8–10). The other hypothesis suggests that antioxidants (dietary or endogenously made) should not be used during radiation therapy or chemotherapy because they would protect cancer cells against damage produced by these modalities (11, 12). At present, most oncologists believe the second hypothesis and do not recommend antioxidants to their patients during standard cancer therapy, believing that they may protect both normal and cancer cells against damage. Some of them may recommend a multiple vitamin preparation that contains low doses of antioxidants after completion of standard cancer therapy. In spite of this reservation of oncologists, over 70 % of their patients are taking nutritional supplements including antioxidants, with or without their knowledge. These practices by patients and their oncologists may be harmful for two reasons; first, because certain antioxidants, such as low doses of endogenously made antioxidants (SH compounds) (1, 2) or dietary antioxidants (13, 14) that do not affect the growth of cancer cells, may protect these cells against damage; and second, because low doses of individual antioxidants taken alone such as vitamin C (15, 16) and polar carotenoids (17) may stimulate the growth of some cancer cells. Therefore, supplementation with low doses of dietary or endogenously made antioxidants may be counterproductive during and after standard cancer therapy.

Each of the proposed hypotheses is based on a different conceptual framework that is derived from specific experimental designs, and thus, each may be correct within its parameters. This review has discussed the biological basis of current controversies, and has revealed that the failure to recognize differences between two distinct conceptual frameworks, each of which is based on specific experimental designs, is responsible for the current debate regarding the use of antioxidants during standard cancer therapy. This review has also discussed the scientific rationale for a micronutrient protocol that includes high doses of dietary antioxidants which can be used as an adjunct to standard cancer therapy in a clinical trial.

▬ Antioxidants

Definition of Types of Antioxidants and Their Doses

It is important to distinguish between dietary (such as vitamin A, vitamin C, vitamin E, and carotenoids) and endogenous antioxidants (such as SH compounds, like glutathione and antioxidant enzymes), because they modify the effects of irradiation or chemotherapeutic agents on normal and cancer cells differently. It is equally important to define doses of these antioxidants, because their effects differ depending upon the dose.

Antioxidant doses are often referred to as low, high, and toxic without specific reference to any biological criteria.

- For this review, **low doses** are referred to those that do not affect the growth of normal or cancer cells. In humans, antioxidant micronutrient supplements at about RDA doses can be defined as low dose. In tissue culture, vitamin C doses of up to 50 µg/mL, vitamin E (α-tocopherol) doses of up to 5 µg/mL, D-α-tocopherol succinate (α-TS) doses of up to 2 µg/mL, retinoid doses of up to 5 µg/mL, and β-carotene doses of up to 1 µg/mL can be defined as low dose.

- **High doses** are referred to those that inhibit the growth of cancer cells without affecting the growth of normal cells. Based on human studies, oral supplementation with vitamin C up to 10 g/day, vitamin E up to 1000 IU/day, vitamin A doses of up to 10 000 IU/day, and natural β-carotene doses of up to 60 mg/day can be defined as high dose. In tissue culture, vitamin C doses of up to 200 µg/mL, vitamin E doses of up to 20 µg/mL, retinoid doses of up to 25 µg/mL, and carotenoid doses of up to 15 µg/mL can be considered high dose.

- **Toxic doses** are referred to those that can inhibit the growth of both normal and cancer cells; and therefore, they are not used in any experimental systems. Although oral retinoic acid doses of 300 000 IU/day, vitamin E doses of 2000 mg/day, β-carotene doses of 150 mg/day, and vitamin C doses of 20 g or more per day have been used in cancer patients, their toxicities are limited to organs, such as liver and skin toxicity with retinoids, defect in blood clotting with vitamin E, diarrhea with vitamin C, and bronzing of skin with β-carotene.

Conceptual Framework of Hypotheses

Conceptual Framework of Our Hypothesis
This hypothesis is based on the following concepts:
- Dietary antioxidants such as vitamin A, vitamin C, vitamin E, and β-carotene, at high doses, can produce some biological effects on cancer cells by mechanisms that are not related to their antioxidant action.
- Dietary antioxidants at high doses inhibit the growth of cancer cells in culture, in animal and human tumor models without affecting the growth of normal cells.
- Dietary antioxidants at high doses enhance the effect of roentgen ray irradiation and chemotherapeutic agents on cancer cells, but protect normal cells against some of their damage.
- Prolonged treatment time before and after irradiation or chemotherapeutic agents is necessary for selectively enhancing the effect of these agents on tumor cells.

Conceptual Framework of Other Hypothesis
This hypothesis is based on the following concepts:
- The only function of antioxidants is to destroy free radicals.
- Antioxidants do not affect the growth of cancer cells.
- Antioxidants protect cancer cells and normal cells against damage produced by radiation or chemotherapeutic agents, since one of their mechanisms of damage is mediated via free radicals.
- No considerations are given to doses and types of antioxidants, and treatment period with antioxidants.

Thus, there are major differences in the conceptual frameworks of the two proposed hypotheses. These differences appear to be primarily due to differences in experimental designs that have utilized different doses and types of antioxidants, and treatment period before and after standard cancer therapeutic agents.

Experimental Designs of Our Hypothesis
This hypothesis is based on the results obtained on the following experimental conditions:
- Dietary antioxidants are given several hours to days before and after roentgen ray irradiation in more than one dose for the entire experimental period.
- High doses of dietary antioxidants are generally used in combination with radiation or chemotherapeutic agents.
- One or more dietary antioxidants are used in combination with standard cancer therapeutic agents.

Experimental Designs of Other Hypothesis
This hypothesis is based on the results obtained on the following experimental conditions:
- Antioxidants (dietary or endogenously made) are given shortly before roentgen ray irradiation or chemotherapeutic agents one time in a single dose, and generally removed immediately after treatment with therapeutic agents.
- Low doses of antioxidants are used in combination with radiation or chemotherapeutic agents.
- Only one antioxidant is used in combination with cancer therapeutic agents.

Types of Antioxidants
Our hypothesis is based on the effect of dietary antioxidants in modifying damage due to irradiation or chemotherapeutic agents on normal and cancer cells. The other hypothesis does not distinguish between dietary and endogenously made antioxidants in modifying injuries produced by cancer therapeutic agents.

Thus, if the conceptual framework and its respective experimental designs of one hypothesis are not extrapolated to the other, the current debates regarding the use of antioxidants during radiation therapy or chemotherapy can easily be reconciled without questioning the validity of the conceptual framework of each hypothesis.

In order to understand better the biological basis of our proposed hypothesis, it is essential that the effects of individual dietary and endogenously made antioxidants and their mechanisms of action are briefly described. All studies described below have been performed with high doses of dietary antioxidants and under experimental conditions in which the agents are present before and after the treatment with cancer therapeutic agents for the entire experimental period.

Effect in Experimental Analysis

Effect of High Doses of Individual Dietary Antioxidants

Several studies have now established that high doses of individual antioxidant micronutrients such as vitamin A (including retinoids) (16–19), vitamin C (16, 17, 20), vitamin E (21–26), and carotenoids including β-carotene (27–30) inhibit growth and cause differentiation and apoptosis in cancer cells in culture. They also reduce the growth of tumors in animal models (27, 31–34) and certain human tumors (35–41) without affecting the growth of normal cells. More recently, we have shown that D-α-tocopheryl succinate (α-TS) inhibits the growth and reduces the levels of mitotic accumulation in human cervical cancer cells and human ovarian carcinoma cells, but it has no such effect on three lines of human normal fibroblasts (42). α-Tocopheryl succinate also increases the level of chromosomal damage in cancer cells without producing such effects on normal cells (43). The growth-inhibitory doses of these antioxidant micronutrients vary from one species to another for the same tumor type. They also vary from one tumor type to another within the same species.

The extent and type of effect on tumor cells depends upon the type and form of micronutrients. For example, α-TS induces cell differentiation (Fig. 11.**1**), growth inhibition, and apoptosis in murine melanoma cells in culture, but α-tocopherol, α-tocopheryl acetate (α-TA), and α-tocopheryl nicotinate at similar concentrations were ineffective (21). α-Tocopheryl succinate induces only growth inhibition in human melanoma cells (17). Certain cancer cells such as rat glioma cells (C6) are more sensitive to natural (DL)-α-TS than to synthetic (DL)-α-TS on the criterium of growth inhibition whereas other tumors are equally sensitive to both natural and synthetic forms of α-TS (10).

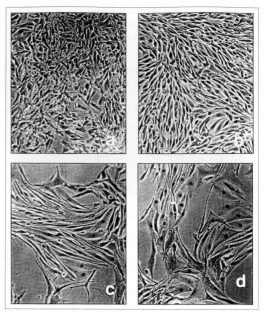

Fig. 11.1 Melanoma cells (10⁵) were plated in tissue culture dishes (60 mm), and D-α-tocopheryl succinate (α-TS) and sodium succinate plus ethanol were added to separate cultures 24 hours after plating. Drugs and medium were changed at two and three days after treatment. Photomicrographs were taken four days after treatment. Control cultures showed fibroblastic cells as well as round cells in clumps **a**; cultures treated with ethanol (1%) and sodium succinate (5–6 g/mL) also exhibited fibroblastic morphology with fewer round cells **b**; α-TS-treated cultures 5 g/mL **c**, and 6 μg/mL **d**, showed a dramatic change in morphology. Magnification × 300 (21).

Mechanisms of Action of High Doses of Dietary Antioxidants on Tumor Cells

To study the mechanisms of differential effects of antioxidant nutrients in cancer cells, it is important to establish whether the greater sensitivity of cancer cells to dietary antioxidant micronutrients (vitamin A, vitamin C, vitamin E, and carotenoids) is due to increased accumulation of antioxidants in these cells in comparison to that found in normal cells or whether cancer cells and normal cells accumulate the same levels of these antioxidant micronutrients, with cancer cells being more sensitive to these micronutrients than normal cells.

Accumulation of Dietary Antioxidants in Normal and Cancer Cells

Some studies have shown that tumor cells accumulate more vitamin C than normal tissue following

Table 11.1 Accumulation of D-α-tocopheryl succinate (α-TS) in human cervical cancer cells (HeLa) and normal human fibroblasts after 24 hours of treatment with α-TS

Concentrations of α-TS	Accumulation of α-TS (µg/mg protein)	
	Fibroblasts	HeLa cells
20 µg/mL (37.6 µM)		
Experiment 1	1.07	1.23
Experiment 2	0.89	1.02
10 µg/mL (18.8 µM)		
Experiment 1	1.38	1.87
Experiment 2	1.04	0.93

α-TS was extracted in hexane and α-tocopheryl acetate was used as an internal standard to determine the efficiency of extraction procedure. The α-TS levels for 24 hours were similar in both HeLa cells and normal fibroblasts. Each measurement was repeated twice and they were reproducible within the same experiment (43).

the administration of radioactively labeled vitamin C into animals carrying transplanted tumor (44). A similar observation was made earlier in patients with leukemia (37). Thus, increased accumulation of vitamin C by tumor cells following high-dose supplementation may be responsible for its anticancer activity. Our results show that human cervical cancer cells (HeLa cells) and normal human fibroblasts in culture accumulate similar levels of α-TS within 24 hours of treatment (Table 11.1). This suggests that tumor cells acquired increased sensitivity to α-TS for growth-inhibition, differentiation, and/or apoptosis during transformation. The relative uptake of other antioxidant micronutrients such as retinoids and carotenoids by normal and cancer cells in culture has not been studied.

The analysis of the basal levels of antioxidant micronutrients in human tumors and their adjacent normal tissues shows that the levels of individual antioxidant micronutrients in tumor tissue may be higher, lower, or the same in comparison to those found in the adjacent normal tissues (45–48). The exact reasons for these variations are not known. Several factors may account for the above results. They include differences in the dietary intake, vascularity, and uptake and subsequent intracellular metabolism of antioxidant micronutrients between normal and cancer cells.

Dietary Antioxidant-Induced Alterations in Gene Expression in Cancer Cells

Since high-dose vitamin A, vitamin C, vitamin E and carotenoids inhibit the growth of cancer cells but not of normal cells (16–20, 22–24, 26–43, 49), studies on the expression of genes that are involved in differentiation, growth regulation, trans-

Table 11.2 Effects of retinoids, β-carotene, and vitamin E on gene expression in tumor cells in culture

Reduced gene expression and/or activity	Increased gene expression and/or activity
p53 mutant	p53 wild-type
c-myc	p21
H-ras	c-fos
Bcl₂	c-jun
c-neu	HSP70
c-erB₂	HSP90
VEGF	connexin
Phosphotyrosine kinase	TGF-β
Protein kinase C	MAP kinase
Caspase	Cyclin A, cyclin D, and their kinases
Tumor necrosis factor	
Transcription factor E2F	
Fas	

Summarized from reviews (8, 10). Effects of retinoids, β-carotene, and α-tocopheryl succinate on gene expression and enzyme activity in various tumor cells in culture were studied. Alterations in gene expressions and enzyme activity were observed.

formation, and apoptosis have been carried out only in cancer cells. These studies reveal that retinoids, vitamin E, and β-carotene attenuate the levels of those cell-signaling systems and gene expressions that can lead to decreased cell proliferation rate, increased differentiation, and/or apoptosis. They include expression of c-*myc*, H-*ras* (50, 51), N-*myc* (51), mutated p53 (27), protein kinase C (52, 53), caspase (54), tumor necrosis factor (55), transcriptional factor E2F (25), and Fas (24). Retinoids, vitamin E, and β-carotene enhance the levels of those cell signaling pathways and gene expression that can lead to reduced growth rate, increased differentiation, and/or apoptosis, and they include the expression of wild-type p53 (27) and p21 (32), transforming growth factor β (TGF-β) (22), and the *connexin* gene (28). The above changes (Table 11.2) in gene expression may be one of the major factors that account for the growth-inhibitory effects of these dietary antioxidant micronutrients on cancer cells. It should be pointed out that most of the effects of dietary antioxidant micronutrients such as vitamin A, vitamin C, vitamin E, and carotenoids on gene expression in cancer cells may not be due to their classical antioxidant action.

In addition to changes in gene expression, a novel mechanism of action of α-TS has been reported in an animal tumor model. α-TS inhibits the growth of tumor cells in vivo without affecting normal cells (33). It also reduces the expression of vascular endothelial growth factor (VEGF), and thus acts as an antiangiogenesis factor at a concentration that is not toxic to normal cells. It is unknown whether retinoids, vitamin C, and β-carotene, which also inhibit the growth of cancer cells, can cause similar effects on angiogenesis in vivo.

Effect of Low Doses of Individual Dietary Antioxidants

In contrast to the effect of high doses of dietary antioxidant micronutrients, low doses of these micronutrients can have no effect on the growth of cancer cells and normal cells, or they can stimulate the growth of some cancer cells without affecting the growth of normal cells. For example, vitamin C at a low dose stimulated the growth of human parotid carcinoma cells in culture (16) and human leukemic cells in culture (15), but had no effect on the growth of human melanoma cells in culture (16) or murine neuroblastoma cells (20). Polar carotenoids at low doses can stimulate the growth of human melanoma cells in culture (17). In addition, certain amounts of antioxidants are needed for the growth of normal and cancer cells. Therefore, we do not recommend low doses of individual or multiple antioxidants during radiation therapy.

Effect of Multiple Dietary Antioxidants

A mixture of dietary antioxidants is more effective in reducing the growth of cancer cells than the individual antioxidants. A mixture of retinoic acid, α-TS, vitamin C, and polar carotenoids produced approximately 50% growth inhibition in human melanoma cells in culture at doses which produced no significant effect on growth when used individually (Table 11.3). Doubling the dose of vitamin C in the mixture caused a dramatic enhancement of growth inhibition. Similar observations were made on human parotid carcinoma cells in culture (16). A reduction of 50% in the dose of each micronutrient in a mixture did not affect the growth of human melanoma cells in culture. Each of the dietary antioxidants has different modes of

Table 11.3 Effect of a mixture of four antioxidant micronutrients on growth of human melanoma cells in culture

Treatments	Cell number (% of controls)
Vitamin C (50 µg/mL)	102 ± 5[a]
PC (10 µg/mL)	96 ± 2
α-TS (10 µg/mL)	102 ± 3
RA (7.5 µg/mL)	103 ± 3
Vitamin C (50 µg/mL) + PC (10 µg/mL) + α-TS (10 µg/mL) + RA (7.5 µg/mL)	56 ± 3
Vitamin C (100 µg/mL)	64 ± 3
Vitamin C (100 µg/mL) + PC (10 µg/mL) + α-TS (10 µg/mL) + RA (7.5 µg/mL)	13 ± 1

Data were summarized from a previous publication (17). a, standard error of the mean; α-TS, α-tocopheryl succinate; PC, polar carotenoids, originally referred to as β-carotene (30); RA, 13-*cis*-retinoic acid; vitamin C, sodium ascorbate.

action and therefore, it is essential that multiple dietary antioxidants are used in combination with radiation therapy.

Effect of Individual Endogenously Made Antioxidants

The effect of endogenously made antioxidants on cancer cells appears to be dose dependent. For example, the overexpression of manganese superoxide dismutase (Mn–SOD) reduces the growth and suppresses the malignant phenotype of glioma (56) and melanoma cells (57) in culture. Glutathione-elevating agents such as N-acetylcysteine (NAC) at high doses inhibit the growth of cancer cells in vitro and in vivo (58).

▬ Experimental Basis of Our Hypothesis

This section is divided in four parts. The first part will discuss the results obtained with antioxidants and radiation, the second part with antioxidants and chemotherapeutic agents, and the third part with antioxidants and experimental therapeutic agents.

High Doses of Dietary Antioxidants Enhance the Effect of Irradiation on Cancer Cells

Dietary antioxidants enhance the effect of irradiation selectively on cancer cells while protecting normal cells against some of the injuries. To observe this effect, antioxidants must be given before and after irradiation at high doses, and they must be present throughout the experimental period. The extent of enhancement of radiation damage by dietary antioxidant micronutrients depends upon the dose of radiation, dose and types of antioxidants, treatment period, and type of tumor cells.

Vitamin A, vitamin C, vitamin E, and carotenoids under the above experimental conditions may protect normal cells against radiation damage, but may enhance the effect of irradiation on cancer cells. For example, retinoic acid enhances the effect of irradiation on tumor cells by inhibiting the repair of potential lethal damage in cancer cells more effectively than that produced in normal fibroblasts (59). Retinoic acid with interferon-α2a (IFN-α2a) enhances radiation-induced toxicity in neck and head squamous cell carcinoma cells in culture (60). We have reported that the dose of vi-

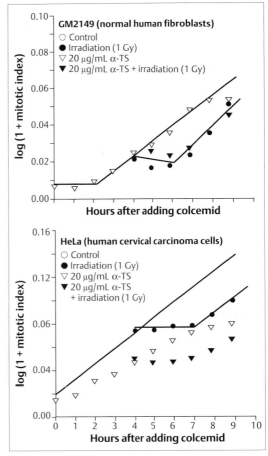

Fig. 11.2 Effect of α-TS on mitotic accumulation in human cancer cell lines and normal human fibroblasts. Decreased mitotic accumulation is seen in cancer cells, but not in normal fibroblasts. Each point represents an average of six samples. Significant difference at $P = 0.05$ was observed in all tumor cell lines at 20 mg/mL of α-TS at all points in comparison to controls (42).

tamin E (α-TS) which inhibited the growth of human cervical cancer cells in culture, but not of normal human fibroblasts in culture, when given in a single high dose before irradiation, enhanced the levels of radiation-induced decrease in mitotic accumulation (Fig. 11.**2**) and chromosomal damage (Fig. 11.**3**) in cancer cells. This form of vitamin E was present in the growth medium before and after irradiation for the entire observation period. On the other hand, the same dose of α-TS did not modify the effect of irradiation on mitotic accumulation in normal cells (42), but it protected normal cells

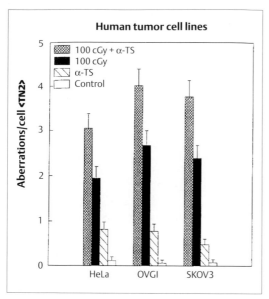

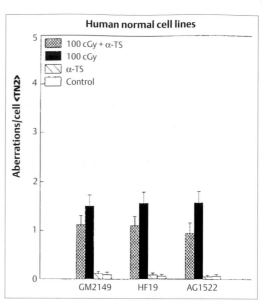

Fig. 11.3 Effect of D-α-tocopheryl succinate (α-TS) on the level of radiation-induced chromosomal damage in human cervical cancer cells (HeLa), ovarian carcinoma cell lines (OVG1 and SKOV3), and in human normal skin fibroblasts (GM2149, HF19 and AG1522). D-α-tocopheryl succinate treatment alone increased chromosomal damage in all three cancer cell lines, but not in any normal cell lines. D-α-tocopheryl succinate treatment also enhanced the levels of radiation-induced chromosomal damage in cancer cells but it protected normal cells against such damage. The bar is standard error of the mean; and the difference between control and experimental groups, and between irradiation alone and irradiation plus α-TS is significant at $P = 0.05$ (43).

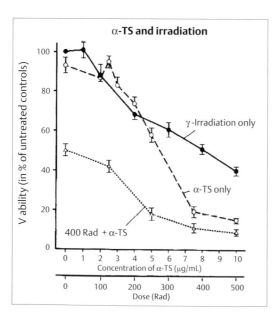

Fig. 11.4 Neuroblastoma cells (NBP2) were plated in tissue culture dishes (60 mm), and the cells were γ-irradiated 24 hours after plating. α-tocopheryl (α-TS) succinate or the solvent (ethanol 0.25 % and sodium succinate 5 μg/mL) was added immediately before irradiation. The drugs and medium were changed after two days of treatment. The number of cells per dish was determined after three days of treatment. Each experiment was repeated at least twice involving three samples per treatment. The average value ($172 \pm 7 \times 10^4$) of untreated control NB cells was considered 100 %, and the growth in treated cultures was expressed as a % of untreated controls. The bar at each point is standard error of the mean (61).

against chromosomal damage (43). In another study, we have reported that an aqueous form of α-tocopheryl and α-TS enhanced the level of radiation-induced growth inhibition in neuroblastoma (NB) cells (Fig. 11.**4**) (43, 61). Vitamin C enhanced the effect of irradiation on neuroblastoma (NB) cells, but not on glioma cells in culture (20). Dehydroascorbic acid (DHA), the major metabolite of ascorbic acid, acts as a radiosensitizer for hypoxic tumor cells (62). These studies show that certain antioxidant micronutrients in a single high dose, when given before irradiation, can protect normal cells against some of the effects of radiation damage, as well as enhance the effect of irradiation on cancer cells in culture provided they are present throughout the experimental period. A similar observation has been made in an animal model. For example, vitamin A (retinyl palmitate) or β-carotene at high doses given daily through dietary supplement before x-ay irradiation and throughout the experimental period enhanced the levels of radiation damage on transplanted breast adenocarcinoma in mice, and protected normal tissue against some of the toxicity of local irradiation (Table 11.**4**) (34). The administration of vitamin C through drinking water before and after roentgen ray irradiation decreased the survival of ascites tumor cells in mice without causing a similar effect on normal cells (63). The administration of multiple antioxidant micronutrients (vitamin A, vitamin C, and vitamin E) protected normal cells against damage produced by radioimmunotherapy in mice without protecting cancer cells (64). The doses of these multiple antioxidants may have been low; and therefore, the radiosensitizing effect of these micronutrients could not be observed. A few human studies have confirmed the differential modification of radiation injuries on normal and

cancer cells by these antioxidants. For example, retinoic acid and IFN-α2a enhanced the efficacy of radiation therapy of locally advanced cervical cancer (36).

High Doses of Dietary Antioxidants Enhance the Effect of Chemotherapeutic Agents on Cancer Cells

The direct interaction between antioxidants and cancer therapeutic agents can initially best be tested on cancer cells in culture. Several cell culture studies have revealed that vitamin C, α-TS, α-TA, vitamin A (retinoids), and polar carotenoids including β-carotene enhance the growth inhibitory effect of most of the chemotherapeutic agents on some cancer cells in culture (8–10). Chemotherapeutic agents used in these studies include 5-fluorouracil (5-FU), vincristine, adriamycin, bleomycin, dacarbazine, cisplatin, tamoxifen, cyclophosphamide, mutamycin, chlorozotocin, and carmustine. The extent of this enhancement depends on the dose and form of the antioxidants, the dose and type of chemotherapeutic agent, and the type of tumor cell. Some examples of antioxidant-induced enhancement of the effect of chemotherapeutic agents are described below. An aqueous form of vitamin E (α-TA) enhances the effect of vincristine on neuroblastoma cells in culture (10) (Fig. 11.**5**). Vitamin C enhances the effect of 5-FU on neuroblastoma cells in culture (20) (Fig. 11.**6**). α-Tocopheryl succinate enhances the effect of adriamycin on human prostate carcinoma cells in culture (65). Recently, we have found that α-TS increases the effect of adriamycin on human cervical cancer cells (HeLa) without modifying the effect of adriamycin on normal human fibroblasts in culture (unpub-

Table 11.4 Effect of vitamin A, β-carotene, and local roentgen radiation on the survival of mice with transplanted breast adenocarcinoma

Treatments	No. of mice	One year survival (no. of mice)
3000 rads, single dose (control)	24	0
Vitamin A	24	0
β-Carotene	24	0
Vitamin A plus roentgen rays	24	22
β-Carotene plus roentgen rays	24	22

Data were summarized from Seifter et al (34). Diets were supplemented with vitamin A (3000 IU/mouse) and β-carotene (270 µg/mouse), and these doses were about 10 times greater the RDA for mice.

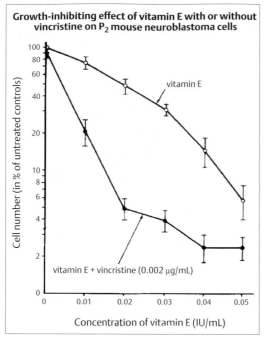

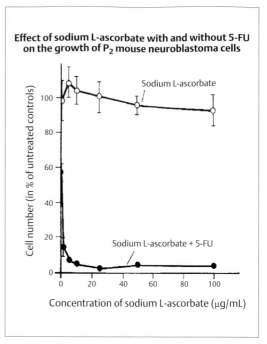

Fig. 11.5 Neuroblastoma cells (NBP2) (50 000 per dish) were plated in tissue culture dishes (60 mm), and vincristine and an aqueous preparation of vitamin E (D-α-tocopheryl acetate) were added 24 hours later. Drugs and medium were changed two days after treatment. The cell number and the number of trypan blue-stained cells were determined three days after treatment. The number of stained cells was subtracted from the total number of cells to obtain viable cells per dish. The average of control cultures was considered 100 %. Each value represents an average of at least six samples. The bar of each point is standard deviation (10).

Fig. 11.6 Neuroblastoma cells (50 000 per dish) were plated in tissue culture dishes (60 mm), and 5-fluorouracil (5-FU) (0.08 µg/mL) plus sodium ascorbate, or sodium ascorbate alone, was added 24 hours after plating. The drug and medium were changed every day, and the number of cells per dish was determined three days after treatment. Each value represents the mean of six to nine samples. The bar of each point is standard deviation. The bars not shown in figure were equal to sizes of symbol (20).

lished observation (Table 11.5). α-Tocopheryl succinate also enhances the effect of carmustine on rat glioma cells in culture (unpublished observation). A few in-vivo studies support the concept that antioxidants selectively enhance the effect of chemotherapeutic agents on tumor cells by increasing tumor response. For example, vitamin A (retinyl palmitate) or synthetic β-carotene at doses which are 10-fold higher than the RDA for these nutrients, in combination with cyclophosphamide, increased the cure rate from 0 % to over 90 % in mice with transplanted adenocarcinoma of the breast (34). A recent study using a thiol-containing antioxidant, pyrrolidine dithiocarbamate (PDTC), and a water-soluble vitamin E analogue (6-hydroxy-2,5,7,8-tetramethylchroman-2-carboxylic

acid), showed that antioxidant treatment enhanced the antitumor effects of 5-FU and doxorubicin in vitro against several cancer cell lines, as well as the effect of 5-FU in vivo against two colorectal cancer cell lines (32). The synthetic retinoid, fenretinide, is effective against a human ovarian carcinoma xenograft and potentiates cisplatin activity (31). The effect of individual antioxidant vitamins in combination with roentgen ray irradiation or chemotherapeutic agents has not been tested in human tumors in vivo in a systematic manner; however, some studies reveal that certain antioxidants in combination with irradiation and chemotherapeutic agents may be beneficial in the management of human tumors. Eighteen nonrandomized patients with small cell lung cancer received multiple antioxidant treatment with chemotherapy and/or radiation. The median sur-

Table 11.5 Modification of adriamycin effect on human cervical cancer cells (HeLa) and human normal skin fibroblasts in culture by D-α-tocopheryl succinate

Treatments	HeLa cells	Fibroblasts
Solvent control	99 ± 2.6*	104 ± 3.4
Adriamycin (0.1 µg/mL)	57 ± 6.2	77 ± 2.4
α-TS (10 µg/mL)	99 ± 1.6	101 ± 3.7
Adramycin (0.1 µg/mL) plus α-TS	20 ± 7.9	77 ± 1.7
Adriamycin (0.25 µg/mL)	14 ± 2.9	68 ± 1.0
Adriamycin (0.25 µg/mL) plus α-TS	5 ± 0.8	62 ± 1.8

Cells (20 000 per well) were plated in a 24-well chamber, and adriamycin and α-tocopheryl succinate (α-TS) were added at the same time. Drug, α-TS, and fresh growth medium were changed at two days after treatment and the viability of cells was determined by MTT assay. Growth in experimental groups was expressed as the % of the untreated control. Each experiment was repeated at least twice, and each value represents an average of six to nine samples ± SEM. (Kumar et al unpublished observation)

Table 11.6 Preliminary results of a randomized clinical trial using high-dose multiple antioxidants as an adjunct to chemotherapy

Treatments	Arm chemotherapy (no. of patients = 29)	Arm chemotherapy ± antioxidant (no. of patients = 28)
Median number of completed chemotherapy cycles	3	6
Number of patients completing 6 cycles	11	16
Complete response	0	1
Partial response	9	16
Stable disease	5	4
Progressive disease	15	8
Overall survival at 1 year	7 months	14 months

Ascorbic acid, 6100 mg/day; D-α-tocopherol, 1050 mg/day; β-carotene, 60 mg/day; copper sulfate, 6 mg/day; manganese sulfate, 9 mg/day; zinc sulfate, 45 mg/day, and selenium, 900 µg/day. Antioxidant treatment was started 48 hours before chemotherapy and continued for one month after completion of therapy, and then reduced to half dose as a maintenance regimen. (Pathak et al, unpublished observation)

vival time was markedly enhanced and patients tolerated chemotherapy and irradiation well (39). Similar observations were made in several private practice settings (40). A randomized trial with non-small cell lung carcinoma patients revealed that the tumor response in groups receiving chemotherapy plus multiple antioxidants was better than that observed in groups receiving chemotherapy alone (Table 11.**6**). β-Carotene supplementation reduced radiation therapy and chemotherapy-induced oral mucositis without interfering with their efficacy on tumor cells (66).

Effect of a mixture of dietary antioxidants in combination with certain chemotherapeutic agents on cancer cells. A mixture of antioxidants containing retinoic acid, vitamin C, α-TS, and polar carotenoids in combination with 5-(3,3-dimethyl-1-triazeno)-imidazole-4-carboxamide (DTIC), tamoxifen, cisplatin, or IFN-α2a inhibited the growth of human melanoma cells in culture more than that produced by the individual agents (17) (Table 11.**7**). This suggests that multiple antioxidants are also effective in enhancing the effect of certain chemotherapeutic agents on cancer cells. No such studies have been performed on normal cells.

Efficacy of Individual Antioxidants in Combination with Hyperthermia

Hyperthermia alone, or in combination with radiation, is primarily used in the management of local tumors where all other standard modalities have failed. Variable improvements in transient tumor

Table 11.7   Enhancement of the effect of certain chemotherapeutic agents by a mixture of four antioxidants on human melanoma cells in culture

Treatments	Cell number (% of controls)
Solvent	101 ± 4[a]
Cisplatin (1 µg/mL)	67 ± 4
Antioxidant mixture	56 ± 3
Cisplatin + antioxidant mixture	38 ± 2
Tamoxifen (2 µg/mL)	81 ± 3
Tamoxifen + antioxidant mixture	30 ± 2
DTIC (100 µg/mL)	71 ± 2
DTIC + antioxidant mixture	38 ± 2
Interferon-α2b	82 ± 5
Interferon-α2b + antioxidant mixture	29 ± 1

The antioxidant mixture consisted of vitamin C, 50 µg/mL; polar carotenoids, 10 µg/mL; α-tocopheryl succinate, 10 µg/mL, and 13-*cis*-retinoic acid, 7.5 µg/mL, added at the time of plating. Data were summarized from a previous publication (20). a, standard error of the mean; polar carotenoids were originally referred to as β-carotene (40).

Table 11.8   Effect of α-tocopheryl succinate (α-TS) on hyperthermia-induced growth inhibition in neuroblastoma cells in culture

Treatments	Cell number (% of controls)
Solvent (ethanol 0.25%) + sodium succinate (5 µg/mL)	102 ± 3[a]
α-TS (5 µg/mL)	50 ± 3
43 °C (20 min)	43 ± 1
α-TS + 43 °C	9 ± 1
41 °C (45 min)	56 ± 3
α-TS + 41 °C	21 ± 2
40 °C (8 h)	55 ± 2
α-TS + 40 °C	30 ± 2

Data were summarized from previous publications (10). a, standard error of the mean.

control have been observed. The temperatures used range from 43–45 °C. Hyperthermia, for the most part, has not proved to be of any significant value in improving the cure rate or survival time of any type of human cancer, but has proved to be of some value in improving quality of life for a variable period of time. Therefore, the current treatment approaches must be altered from local hyperthermia at higher temperatures to whole-body hyperthermia at lower temperatures that was tolerated without side effects. We have reported (10) that α-TS markedly increased the effect of low temperature (41 °C) and high temperature (43 °C) hyperthermia on neuroblastoma cells in culture (Table 11.**8**). We propose that multiple antioxidants in combination with hyperthermia (local or whole body) may further im-

prove the efficacy of hyperthermia in the treatment of human cancer.

Effect of Individual Antioxidant Vitamins in Combination with Certain Biological Response Modifiers

We have reported (10) that α-TS and polar carotenoids markedly enhanced the levels of cAMP-induced terminal differentiation in neuroblastoma cells (Fig. 11.**7**) and melanoma cells (Fig. 11.**8**) in culture. In addition, α-TS (Fig. 11.**9**) and vitamin C also enhance the growth-inhibitory effect of sodium butyrate (10) and IFN-α2b (17) on neuroblastoma and human melanoma cells. The observation on butyrate is of particular importance, because phenyl butyrate is in phase I trial for the treatment of human glioma that has been difficult to treat with chemotherapeutic agents. Retinoic acid in combination with IFN-α2a is highly active in the treatment of squamous cell carcinoma of the cervix in human (67), suggesting that it can enhance the growth-inhibitory effect of some biological response modifiers.

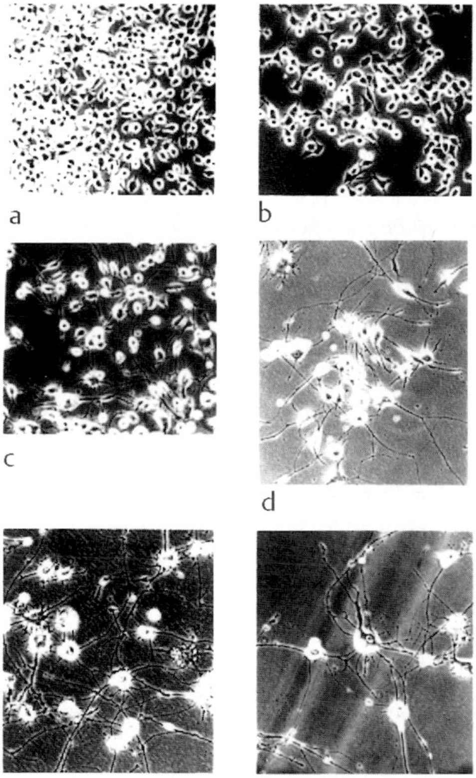

Antioxidants Selectively Protect Normal Cells against Damage Produced by Radiation and Chemotherapeutic Agents

Several studies have established the radioprotective value of vitamin A, vitamin C, vitamin E, and carotenoids in protecting normal cells (2, 63, 64, 68–70) but not cancer cells (43, 64):

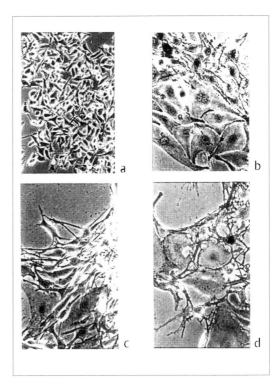

Fig. 11.7 Photomicrographs of neuroblastoma cells (NBP2) in culture after treatment with R020–1724 and β-carotene. X 200.
a Control cells at four days after plating (50 000 cells/ 60 mm dish), showing mostly round cells.
b Cells treated with β-carotene (20 μg/mL), showing no significant change in morphology after four days of treatment.
c Cells treated with R020–1724 (200 μg/mL), revealing increasing numbers of cells with neurites after four days of treatment.
d Cells treated with R020–1724 plus β-carotene, showing more differentiated cells after four days of treatment than cells treated with R020–1724 alone.
e Cells after eight days of treatment with R020–1724 plus β-carotene.
f Cells after 11 days of treatment with R020–1724 plus β-carotene (10).

Fig. 11.8 Photomicrographs of murine melanoma cells in culture after treatment with R020–1724 and α-TS for four days. X 450.
a Control cells varied in morphology.
b Cells treated with α-TS were elongated, had long cytoplasmic processes, and showed a net-like arrangement.
c Cells treated with R020–1724 (200 μg/mL) were large and elongated, had some long processes, and showed a net-like arrangement.
d Cells treated with R020–1724 plus α-TS showed a higher level of morphological differentiation than cells treated with each of the individual agents (10).

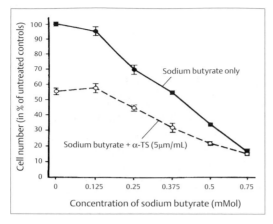

Fig. 11.9 Effect of D-α-tocopheryl succinate (α-TS) in combination with sodium butyrate on the growth of neuroblastoma cells in culture. Cells (50 000 cells/60 mm dish) were plated in tissue culture dishes, and α-TS and sodium butyrate were added one after another 24 hours later. Fresh growth medium and agents were changed at two days after treatment and growth was determined at three days after treatment. Each value represents an average of six samples. The bar at each point is standard deviation (73).

- Treatment with antioxidant micronutrients reduced the effect of irradiation on normal tissues in patients with small cell lung carcinoma (39, 40).
- β-Carotene reduced radiation-induced mucositis without interfering with the efficacy of radiation therapy in patients with cancer of the head and neck (66).
- Administration of vitamin E in a single dose to normal adult rodents before roentgen ray irradiation increased the survival of irradiated animals (1, 20, 70).
- The addition of vitamin C and vitamin E in a single dose before irradiation reduced the level of DNA damage to normal cells (171).
- Vitamin E in combination with pentoxifylline decreased the level of radiation-induced fibrosis (72). Vitamin E reduced bleomycin-induced lung fibrosis (73), adriamycin-induced cardiac toxicity (74, 75) and adriamycin-induced skin necrosis (76).
- Vitamin E also reduced adriamycin-induced toxicity in liver, kidney, and intestinal mucosa (77).

- Another study has reported that β-carotene and vitamin A (retinyl palmitate) reduced the adverse effects of cyclophosphamide in rats (34).
- Vitamin C and vitamin E have been shown to reduce the adverse effects of some chemotherapeutic agents on normal cells (78). Vitamin E and vitamin C supplements reduced the tamoxifen-induced hyperlipidemia in patients with breast cancer (79).

Thus, most of the studies clearly demonstrate that high-dose dietary antioxidant micronutrients (vitamin A, vitamin C, vitamin E, and carotenoids) selectively enhance the growth-inhibitory effect of irradiation and chemotherapeutic agents on cancer cells, and in some cases they protect normal cells against such damage. There are no published studies that show that high doses of these micronutrients under our experimental conditions have ever protected cancer cells against damage produced by irradiation or chemotherapeutic agents.

Mechanisms of Action of Dietary Antioxidant-Induced Enhancement of Radiotherapy and Chemotherapy

The exact reasons for the dietary antioxidant micronutrient-induced enhancement of damage produced by standard therapeutic agents on cancer cells are unknown. We propose the following:

- The treatment of tumor cells with high doses of these micronutrients before irradiation or radiotherapy or chemotherapy may initiate changes in the expression of genes that cause differentiation, growth inhibition, and/or apoptosis (22, 24, 26–28, 33, 49–56). The resulting damage will continue to progress during the entire therapeutic period.
- Free radicals produced by cancer treatment become irrelevant to antioxidant-affected cancer cells; however, other mechanisms of damage continue to exert their influence. Micronutrients such as retinoic acid inhibit the repair of radiation damage in cancer cells more than in normal cells (60). In contrast to cancer cells, normal cells are not harmed by these dietary antioxidants. When treated with radiation or chemotherapeutic agents, antioxidants protect them at least from damage by free radicals.

Modification of Radiation Damage by Endogenous Antioxidants

Extensive studies have been published to show that endogenous antioxidants such as SH compounds and their derivatives (cysteamine, glutathione, and others) protecte normal and cancer cells in vitro and in vivo when given before roentgen ray irradiation at doses which do not cause toxicity (1, 2). In fact, differential radiosensitivity, which is commonly observed during various phases of the cell cycle, is related to different levels of SH compounds. It has been shown that mitotic cells, which are most radiosensitive, have the lowest levels of SH compounds, and that S-phase cells, which are most radioresistant, have the highest levels of these compounds (80).

Antioxidant enzymes such as catalase, superoxide dismutase, and glutathione peroxidase play an important role in protecting normal cells against damage produced by reactive oxygen species. Therefore, one would predict that they play a similar role in cancer cells. Indeed, overexpression of antioxidant enzymes increased the radioresistance of tumor cells (81–84). Some studies have revealed that overexpression of mitochondrial manganese superoxide dismutase (Mn-SOD) suppressed the growth of some tumor cells and enhanced the radioresistance of a hepatocellular carcinoma cell line and other tumor cells, while it did not modify radiation damage to hypoxic cancer cells. For these reasons, we do not recommend raising the level of endogenous antioxidants by means of glutathione-elevating agents (N-acetyl cysteine and α-lipoic acid) or selenium, a cofactor for glutathione peroxidase, over the RDA amount during radiotherapy or chemotherapy.

Experimental Basis of the Other Hypothesis

Dietary antioxidants such as vitamin E (α-tocopherol) when given in a single low dose shortly before irradiation reduced the effectiveness of roentgen ray irradiation in an animal tumor model (14). Similarly, when vitamin C, vitamin E, or N-acetyl cysteine, a glutathione-elevating agent, were added to tumor cell culture in a single low dose that does not affect the growth of cancer cells, shortly before irradiation, they protected cancer cells

against radiation damage (11, 13, 14). These data have been used to suggest that antioxidants should not be used during radiation therapy or chemotherapy.

Comments on Current Controversies

The data presented in support of each the proposed hypotheses suggest that the current debates regarding the use of antioxidants during radiotherapy or chemotherapy primarily rest on an extrapolation of one conceptual framework based on specific experimental designs as compared to another one based on experimental conditions that are entirely different with respect to dose, treatment time, and type of antioxidants. Data show that high doses of dietary antioxidants that inhibit the growth of cancer cells but not of normal cells, when given before and after irradiation or chemotherapeutic agents for the entire observation period, may improve the efficacy of the therapy. However, results also show that low doses of dietary or endogenous antioxidants, when given in a single low dose that does not affect the growth of cancer cells shortly before irradiation, may protect cancer cells against radiation or chemotherapy damage.

Some oncologists recommend a multiple vitamin preparation containing low doses of antioxidants after completion of cancer therapy. This practice may be counterproductive, because like normal cells, tumor cells need certain amounts of antioxidants for growth and survival, and because low doses of antioxidants may stimulate the growth of residual tumor cells. Thus, it is essential that these factors should be taken into account while designing a clinical trial to test the efficacy of antioxidants in combination with radiation therapy and/or chemotherapy. In addition, data on antioxidants that are obtained on cancer prevention studies must not be used in designing cancer treatment investigations, because they were harmful. For example, low doses of N-acetyl cysteine or high levels of antioxidant enzymes may be very useful in cancer prevention, but they may be harmful when used in combination with radiation therapy, because they would protect cancer cells against radiation damage.

Clinical Studies with Multiple Dietary Antioxidant Micronutrients in Combination with Standard Therapy

A randomized placebo-controlled trial on the use of antioxidants during radiation therapy has not been performed as yet. Dr. Jae Ho Kim of the Henry Ford Hospital in Detroit, Michigan, has completed a randomized pilot trial with high-dose multiple micronutrients including dietary antioxidants (vitamin C and vitamin E, and natural β-carotene) in cancer patients receiving chemotherapy and radiation therapy. Results showed that all patients tolerated high-dose micronutrients well and that quality of life was improved during radiation therapy with no adverse effect on the efficacy of standard therapy (personal communication). A few oncologists have used high dose multiple antioxidants in combination with standard cancer therapy, and improved outcomes have been reported (39, 40). A preliminary randomized trial with high dose antioxidants in combination with chemotherapeutic agents (cisplatin and paclitaxel combination) in patients with advanced non-small cell lung carcinoma reported beneficial effects on tumor response and tolerance to chemotherapeutic agents for a follow-up period of one year (Table 11.**6**).

▬ Proposed Doses of Micronutrients To Be Used as an Adjunct to Radiation Therapy and/or Chemotherapy

The scientific rationale for the proposed micronutrient protocol has been discussed in detail in recent publications (8, 10). The micronutrient supplement protocol is divided into two categories: active treatment phase and maintenance phase.

- During the **active treatment phase**, daily micronutrients are given orally at least 48 hours before radiation therapy or chemotherapy, and continued for the entire treatment period. After the completion of treatment, doses of supplementary antioxidant micronutrients are reduced to half over a four-week period, which is maintained during the **maintenance phase** (lifetime). The rational for giving micronutrients at least 48 hours before standard cancer therapy is that antioxidant-induced damage is initiated in cancer cells but not in normal cells prior to initiation of cancer treatment with standard therapeutic agents.

- The rational for continuing micronutrient supplement throughout the treatment period is that these micronutrients continue to cause additional damage in cancer cells as well as inhibit the repair of damage.

The micronutrient protocol contains supplements described below. A baseline supplement contains multiple micronutrients:
- vitamin A, vitamin C, and vitamin E
- natural β-carotene
- vitamin D
- B vitamins
- appropriate minerals but not iron, copper, and manganese, because these three trace minerals interact with vitamin C to produce free radicals.

A brand name, Sevak (Premier Micronutrient Corporation, Nashville, Tennessee), which contains the above ingredients, is being sold commercially and is in a clinical trial. A preparation of multiple micronutrients is suggested because some of them may be depleted during radiation therapy or chemotherapy due to extensive cellular death, loss of appetite, and other side effects.

- An additional 8 g of vitamin C in the form of calcium ascorbate is recommended. Doses of vitamin C at 10 g or more have been used in human cancer treatment without toxicity (38, 85).
- This form of vitamin C was selected because ascorbic acid at high doses can cause an upset stomach in some patients (85).
- Calcium ascorbate rather than sodium ascorbate was selected because sodium ascorbate at high doses can increase the acidity of urine in the bladder and increase the risk of chemically induced bladder cancer in animals due to chronic irritation (86).
- An additional 800 IU of natural vitamin E in the form of α-TS is recommended. This form of vitamin E is the most potent form of vitamin E both in vitro and in vivo (8, 10). The natural form of vitamin E is used because animal studies have demonstrated that various organs selectively pick up the natural form of vitamin E over the synthetic form (87).
- An additional 60 mg/day of natural β-carotene is recommended. The natural form of β-carotene was selected because it is more effective than the synthetic form. For example, natural β-carotene protects against radiation-induced

transformation in vitro, whereas synthetic β-carotene is ineffective (88).

All micronutrient supplements described above should be taken orally and in two divided doses, one-half dose in the morning and one-half dose in the evening. The rationale for taking micronutrients twice a day is that the biological half-life of most micronutrients is about six to 12 hours. Micronutrient supplements can be started at least 48 hours prior to standard therapy and should be continued for one month after completion of standard therapy. Thereafter, the maintenance phase begins in which supplementery doses of vitamin C, vitamin E, and β-carotene can gradually (over a four-week period) be reduced to half the levels of the active treatment phase. Such maintenance doses of micronutrients may reduce the risk of recurrence of tumors as well as the risk of a second malignancy among cancer survivors.

References

1. Prasad KN. *Handbook of Radiobiology*. Boca Raton, FL: CRC Press, 1995.
2. Thomson J. *Radiation Protection in Mammals*. New York: Reinhold, 1962.
3. Capizzi RL, Oster W. Chemoprotective and radioprotective effects of amifostine: an update of clinical trials. *Int J Hematol* 2000; 72: 425–435.
4. Murray D, Rosenberg E, Allalunis-Turner MJ. Protection of human tumor cells of differing radiosensitivity by WR-1065. *Rad Res* 2000; 154: 159–162.
5. Orditura M, De Vita F, Roscigno A et al. Amifostine: a selective cytoprotective agent of normal tissues from chemo-radiotherapy induced toxicity (review). *Oncol Reports* 1999; 6: 1357–1362.
6. Hospers GA, Eisenhauer EA, De Vries EG. The Sulfhydryl containing compounds WR-2721 and glutathione as radio- and chemoprotective agents. A review, indications for use and prospects. *Br J Cancer* 1999; 80: 629–638.
7. Allalunis-Turner MJ, Walden TL Jr, Sawich C. Induction of marrow hypoxia by radioprotective agents. *Rad Res* 1989; 118: 581–586.
8. Prasad, KN, Kumar A, Kochupillai MD, Cole WC. High doses of multiple antioxidant vitamins: essential ingredients in improving the efficacy of standard cancer therapy. *J Am Coll Nutr* 1999; 18: 13–25.
9. Cole WC, Prasad KN. Contrasting effects of vitamins as modulators of apoptosis in cancer cells and normal cells: a review. *Nutr Cancer* 1997; 29: 97–103.
10. Prasad K, Cole W, Prasad K. Scientific rationale for using highdose multiple micronutrients as an adjunct to standard and experimental therapies. *J Am Coll Nutr* 2001; 20: 450S–463S.
11. Salganik R. The benefits and hazards of antioxidants: controlling apoptosis and other protective mechanisms in cancer patients and the human population. *J Am Coll Nutr* 2001; 20: 464S–472S.
12. Labriola D, Livingston R. Possible interactions between dietary antioxidants and chemotherapy. *Oncology*. 1999; 13: 1003–1008.
13. Witenberg B, Kletter Y, Kalir HH et al. Ascorbic acid inhibits apoptosis induced by x-irradiation in HL60 myeloid leukemia cells. *Rad Res* 1999; 152: 468–78.
14. Sakamoto K, Sakka M. Reduced effect of irradiation on normal and malignant cells irradiated in vivo in mice pretreated with Vitamin E. *Br J Rad* 1973; 46: 538–40.
15. Park CH. Vitamin C in leukemia and preleukemia cell growth. *Prog Clin Biol Res* 1988; 259: 321–330.
16. Prasad KN, Kumar R. Effect of individual antioxidant vitamins alone and in combination on growth and differentiation of human non-tumorigenic and tumorigenic parotid acinar cells in culture. *Nutr Cancer* 1996; 26: 11–19.
17. Prasad KN, Hernandez C, Edwards-Prasad J et al. Modification of the effect of tamoxifen, CIS-platin, dtic and Interferon-A2B on human melanoma cells in culture by a mixture of vitamins. *Nutr Cancer* 1994; 22: 233–245.
18. Amatruda TTD, Sidell N, Ranyard J, Koeffler HP. Retinoic acid treatment of human neuroblastoma cells is associated with decreased N-myc expression. *Biochem Biophys Res Commun* 1985; 126: 1189–1195.
19. Sporn MB, Roberts AB. Role of retinoids in differentiation and carcinogenesis. *Cancer Res* 1983; 43: 3034–3040.
20. Prasad KN, Sinha PK, Ramanujarn M, Sakamoto A. Sodium ascorbate potentiates the growth inhibitory effect of certain agents on neuroblastoma cells in culture. *Proc Natl Acad Sci USA* 1979; 76: 829–832.
21. Prasad KN, Edwards-Prasad J. Effect of tocopherol (vitamin E) acid succinate on morphological alterations and growth inhibition in melanoma cells in culture. *Cancer Res* 1982; 42: 550–555.
22. Kline K, Yu W, Zhao B. Vitamin E succinate: mechanisms of action as tumor cell growth inhibitor. *In:* K. Prasad, L. Santamaria, R. Williams (eds.), *Nutrients in Cancer Prevention and Treatment*, pp. 39–55. New Jersey: Humana Press, 1995.
23. Yu W, Israel K, Liao QY et al. Vitamin E succinate (ves) induces fas sensitivity in human breast cancer cells: role for MR 43,000 fas in ves-triggered apoptosis. *Cancer Res* 1999; 59: 953–961.
24. Turley JM, Fu T, Ruscetti FW, Mikovits JA et al. Vitamin E succinate induces fas-mediated apoptosis in

estrogen receptor-negative human breast cancer cells. *Cancer Res* 1997; 57: 881–890.

25. Turley J, Ruscetti F, Kim S-J et al. Vitamin E succinate inhibits proliferation of BT-20 human breast cancer cells: increased binding of cyclic amp negatively regulates E_2F transactivation activity. *Cancer Res* 1977; 57: 2668–2675.

26. Israel K, Yu W, Sanders BG et al. Vitamin E succinate induces apoptosis in human prostate cancer cells: role for fas in vitamin E succinate-triggered apoptosis. *Nutr Cancer* 2000; 36: 90–100.

27. Schwartz JL. Molecular and biochemical control of tumor growth following treatment with carotenoids or tocopherols. *In*: Prasad KN. Santamaria L, Williams RM (eds). *Nutrients in Cancer Prevention and Treat*, pp. 287–316. New Jersey: Humana Press, 1995.

28. Zhang LX, Cooney RV, Bertram JS. Carotenoids up-regulate connexin-43 gene expression independent of their provitamin A or antioxidant properties. *Cancer Res* 1992; 52: 5707–5712.

29. Krinsky N. Antioxidant functions of carotenoids. *Free Rad Biol Med* 1989; **7**: 617–635.

30. Hazuka MB, Edwards-Prasad J, Newman F et al. Betacrotene induces morphological differentiation and decreases adenylate cyclase activity in melanoma cells in culture. *J Am Coll Nutr* 1990; 9: 143–149.

31. Formelli F, Cleris L. Synthetic retinoid fenretinide is effective against a human ovarian carcinoma xenograft and potentiates cisplatin activity. *Cancer Res* 1993; 53: 5374–5376.

32. Chinery R, Brockman JA, Peeler MO et al. Antioxidants enhance the cytotoxicity of chemotherapeutic agents in colorectal cancer: a P53-independent induction of $P^{21Wafi/cipi}$ via C/E^{BPB}. *Nature Med* 1997; 3: 1233–1241.

33. Malafa MP, Neitzel LT. Vitamin E Succinate promotes breast cancer dormancy. *J Surg Res* 2000; 93: 163–170.

34. Seifter E, Rettura A, Padawar J et al. Vitamin A and B-carotene as adjunctive therapy to tumor excision, radiation therapy and chemotherapy. *In*: Prasad, KN (ed.), *Vitamins, Nutrition and Cancer*, pp. 1–19. Basel: Karger, 1984.

35. Meyskens FL Jr. Role of vitamin A and its derivatives in the treatment of human cancer. *In*: Prasad KN, Santamaria L, Williams RM (eds.). *Nutrients in Cancer Prevention and Treatment*, pp. 349–362. Totowa, New Jersey: Humana Press, 1995.

36. Lippman SM, Parkinson DR, Itri LM et al. 13-CIS retinoic acid plus interferon A-2_A: highly active systemic therapy for squamous cell carcinoma of the cervix. *J Natl Cancer Inst* 1995; 84: 241–245.

37. Hanck AB. Vitamin C and Cancer. *Prog Clin Biol Res* 1988; 259: 307–320.

38. Cameron E, Pauling L, Leibowitz B. Ascorbic acid and cancer. A review. *Cancer Res* 1979; 39: 663–681.

39. Jaakkola K, Lahteenmaki P, Laakso J et al. Treatment with antioxidant and other nutrients in combination with chemotherapy and irradiation in patients with small-cell lung cancer. *Anticancer Res* 1992; 12: 599–606.

40. Lamson DW, Brignall MS. Antioxidants in cancer therapy; their actions and interactions with oncologic therapies. *Alternative Med Rev* 1999; 4: 304–329.

41. Garewal H. Beta-carotene and antioxidant nutrients in oral cancer prevention. *In*: Prasad KN. Santamaria L, Williams RM (eds). *Nutrients in Cancer Prevention and Treatment*, pp. 235–247. NJ. Human Press, 1995.

42. Jha MN, Bedford JS, Cole WC et al. Vitamin E (D-A tocopheryl succinate) decreases mitotic accumulation in λ-irradiated human tumor, but not in normal cells. *Nutr Cancer* 1999; 35: 189–194.

43. Kumar B, Jha MN, Cole WC et al. D-alpha tocopheryl succinate (vitamin E) enhances radiation-induced chromosomal damage levels in human cancer cells, but reduces it in normal cells. *J Am Coll Nutr* 2002; 21: 339–343.

44. Agus DB, Vera JC, Golde DW. Stromal cell oxidation: a mechanism by which tumors obtain vitamin C. *Cancer Res* 1999; 59: 4555–4558.

45. Piyathilake CJ, Bell WC, Johanning GL et al. The accumulation of ascorbic acid by squamous cell carcinomas of the lung and larynx is associated with global methylation of DNA. *Cancer* 2000; 89: 171–176.

46. Liede KE, Alfthan G, Hietanen JH et al. Beta-carotene concentration in buccal mucosal cells with and without dysplastic oral leukoplakia after long-term beta-carotene supplementation in male smokers. *Eur J Clin Nutr* 1998; 52: 872–876.

47. Picardo M, Grammatico P, Roccella F et al. Imbalance in the antioxidant pool in melanoma cells and normal melanocytes from patients with melanoma. *J Invest Dermatol* 1996; 107: 322–326.

48. Langemann H, Torhorst J, Kabiersch A et al. Quantitative determination of water- and lipid-soluble antioxidants in neoplastic and non-neoplastic human breast tissue. *Int J Cancer* 1989; 43: 1169–1173.

49. Prasad KN, Cohrs RJ, Sharma OK. Decreased expressions of C-myc and H-ras oncogenes in vitamin E succinate induced morphologically differentiated murine B-16 melanoma cells in culture. *Biochem Cell Biology* 1990; 68: 1250–1255.

50. Cohrs RJ, Torelli S, Prasad KN et al. Effect of vitamin E succinate and a camp-stimulating agent on the expression of C-myc and N-myc and H-ras in mu-

rine neuroblastoma cells. *Int J Dev Neurosci* 1991; 9: 187–194.

51. Thiele CJ, Reynolds CP, Israel MA. Decreased expression of N-myc precedes retinoic acid-induced morphological differentiation of human neuroblastoma. *Nature (London)* 1985; 313: 404–406.

52. Gopalakrishna R, Gundimeda U, Chen Z. Vitamin E succinate inhibits protein kinase C: correlation with its unique inhibitory effects on cell growth and transformation. *In*: Prasad K, Santamaria L, Williams R. (eds). *Nutrients in Cancer Prevention and Treatment*, pp. 21–37. Totowa, New Jersey: Human Press, 1995.

53. Mahoney C, Azzi A. Vitamine E inhibits protein kinase C activity. *Biochem Biophys Res Commun* 1988; 154: 694–697.

54. Neuzil J, Svensson I, Weber T et al. Alpha-tocopheryl succinate-induced apoptosis in jurkat T cells involves caspase-3 activation, and both lysosomal and mitochondrial destabilisation. *Febs Lett* 1999; 445: 295–300.

55. Nakamura T, Goto M, Matsumoto A, Tanaka I. Inhibition of NF-kappa B transcriptional activity by alpha-tocopheryl succinate. *Biofactors* 1998; 7: 21–30.

56. Zhong W, Oberley LW, Oberley TD et al. Suppression of the malignant phenotype of human glioma cells by over expression of manganese superoxide dismutase. *Oncogene* 1997; 14: 481–490.

57. Church SL, Grant JW, Ridnour LA et al. Increased manganese superoxide dismutase expression suppresses the malignant phenotype of human melanoma cells. *Proc Natl Acad USA* 1993; 90: 3113–3117.

58. De Flora S, D'Agostini F, Masiello L et al. Synergism between N-acetylcysteine and doxorubicin in the prevention of tumorigenicity and metastasis in murine models. *Int J Cancer* 1996; 67: 842–848.

59. Rutz H, Little J. Modification of radiosensitivity and recovery from X-ray damage *in vitro*, by retinoic acid. *Int J Rad Oncol, Biol, Phys* 1981; 16: 1285–1288.

60. Delaney TF, Afridi N, Taghian AG et al. 13-CIS-retinoic acid with alpha-2A-interferon enhances radiation cytotoxicity in head and neck squamous cell carcinoma in vitro. *Cancer Res* 1996; 56: 2277–2280.

61. Sarria A, Prasad KN. DL-alpha tocopheryl succinate enhances the effect of gamma-irradiation on neuroblastoma cells in culture. *Proc Soc Exp Biol Med* 1984; 175: 88–92.

62. Koch CJ, Biaglow JE. Toxicity, Radiation sensitivity modification, and metabolic effects of dehydroascorbate and ascorbate in mammalian cells. *J Cellular Physiology* 1978; 94: 299–306.

63. Tewfik FA, Tewfik HH, Riley EF. The influence of ascorbic acid on the growth of solid tumors in mice and on tumor control by x-irradiation. *Int J Vit Nutr Res – Supplement* 1982; 23: 257–263.

64. Blumenthal RD, Lew W, Reising A et al. Anti-oxidant vitamins reduce normal tissue toxicity Induced by radio-immunotherapy. *Int J Cancer* 2000; 86: 276–280.

65. Ripoli E, Rawa B, Webber M. Vitamin E enhances the chemotherapeutic effects of adriamycin on human prostate carcinoma cells in vitro. *J Urol* 1986; 136: 529–531.

66. Mills EE. The modifying effect of beta-carotene on radiation and chemotherapy induced oral mucositis. *Br J Cancer* 1988; 57: 416–417.

67. Lippman SM, Kavanagh JJ, Paredes-Espinoza M et al. 13-cis-Retinoic acid plus interferon-α2a in locally advanced squamous cell carcinoma of the cervix. *J Natl Cancer Inst* 1993; 85: 241–245.

68. Srinavasan V, Jacobs AL, Simpson SA et al. Radioprotection by vitamin E. Effect on hepatic enzymes, delayed type hypersensitivity and post-irradiation survival in mice. *In*: Meyskens, FLJ and Prasad, KN (eds). *Modulations Mediations of Cancer Cells by Vitamins*, pp. 119–131. Basel: Karger, 1983.

69. Malick MA, Roy RM, Sternberg J. Effect of vitamin E on post-irradiation death in mice. *Experientia* 1978; 34: 1216–1217.

70. Londer HM, Myers CE. Radioprotective effects of vitamin E. *Am J Clin Nutr* 1978; 31: 705A.

71. Konopacka M, Widel M, Rzeszowska-Wolny J. Modifying effect of vitamins C, E and beta-carotene against gamma-ray-induced DNA damage in mouse cells. *Mutation Res* 1998; 417: 85–94.

72. Delanian S. Striking regression of radiation-induced fibrosis by a combination of pentoxifylline and tocopherol. *Br J Rad* 1998; 71: 892–894.

73. Yamanaka N, Fukishima M, Koizumi K et al. Enhancement of DNA chain breakage by bleomycin and biological free radical producing systems. *In*: DeDuve C, Hayashi T (eds). *Tocopherol, Oxygen and Biomembranes*. New York: North Holland, 1978; 59–69.

74. Van Vleet JF, Greenwood L, Ferands VJ, Rebar AH. Effect of selenium-vitamin E on adriamycin-induced cardiomyopathy in rabbits. *Am J Vitamin Res* 1978; 39: 997–1000.

75. Wang YM, Madanat FF, Kimball JC et al. Effect of vitamin E against adriamycin-induced toxicity in rabbits. *Cancer Res* 1980; 40: 1022–1027.

76. Svingen BA, Powis A, Abbel PL, Scott M. Protection against adriamycin-induced skin necrosis in the rat by dimethylsulfoxide and alpha-tocopherol. *Cancer Res* 1981; 41: 3395–3399.

77. Geetha A, Sankar R, Marar T, Devi CSS. Alpha-tocopherol reduces doxorubicin-induced toxicity in rats hiatological and biochemical evidences. *Indian I Physiol Pharmacol* 1990; 34: 94–98.

78. Trizna Z, Schantz SP, Lee JJ et al. In vitro protective effect of chemopreventive agents against bleomycin-induced genotoxicity in lymphoblastoid cell lines and peripheral lymphocytes of head and neck cancer patients. *Cancer Detect Prev* 1993; 17: 575–583.

79. Babu JR, Sundravel S, Arumugam G et al. Salubrious effects of vitamin C and vitamin E on tamoxifen-treated women in breast cancer with reference to plasma lipid and lipoprotein levels. *Cancer Lett* 2000; 151: 1–5.

80. Sinclair WK. Cysteamine: differential X-ray protective effect on Chinese hamster cells during the cell cycle. *Science* 1968; 159: 442–444.

81. Hirose K, Longo DL, Oppenheim JJ et al. Overexpression of mitochondrial manganese superoxide dismutase promotes the survival of tumor cells exposed to interleukin-1, tumor necrosis factor, selected anticancer drugs, and ionizing radiation. *FASEB Journal* 1993; 7: 361–368.

82. Sun J, Chen Y, Li M et al. Role of antioxidant enzymes on ionizing radiation resistance. *Free Rad Biol Med* 1998; 24: 586–593.

83. Motoori S, Mazima H, Ebara M, et al. Overexpression of mitochondrial manganese superoxide dismutase protects against radiation-induced cell death in the human hepatocellular carcinoma cell line HLE. *Cancer Res* 2001; 61: 5382–5388.

84. Urano M, Kuroda M, Reynolds R et al. Expression of manganese superoxide dismutase reduces tumor control radiation dose: gene-radiotherapy. *Cancer Res* 1995; 55: 2490–2493.

85. Creagan ET, Moertel CG, O'Fallon JR. Failure of high-dose vitamin C (ascorbic acid) therapy to benefit patients with advanced cancer. *New Engl J Med* 1979; 301: 687–690.

86. Fukushima S, Imaida K, Shibata M-K et al. L-ascorbic acid amplification of second-stage bladder carcinogenesis promotion by NAHCO$_3$. *Cancer Res* 1988; 48: 6317–6320.

87. Ingold KU, Burton GW, Foster DO et al. Biokinetics of and discrimination between dietary RRR- and SRR-alpha-tocopherols in the male rat. *Lipids* 1987; 22: 163–172.

88. Kennedy AR, Krinsky NI. Effects of retinoids, B-carotene and canthaxanthene on U.V. and x-ray-induced transformation of C3H10T 1/2 cells in vitro. *Nutr Cancer* 1994; 22: 219–232.

▃ 12 Selenium in Oncology

G. N. Schrauzer

▃ Introduction

Selenium is an essential trace element recognized as a cancer-protective agent and is increasingly employed as an adjuvant in cancer therapy. Whereas for cancer prevention organic nutritional forms of selenium (Se) are used, sodium selenite is the preferred form of selenium for therapeutic applications. Sodium selenite is administered primarily to reduce side effects of chemotherapy and radiation therapy. Patients are typically receiving 300–1000 µg Se/day as sodium selenite orally or by infusion for one to five days prior to and during chemotherapy or radiation, and subsequently oral doses of 100–300 µg Se/day for maintenance. Sodium selenite is also used in conjunction with biological therapies and in the management of secondary or postoperative lymphedema.

▃ Selenium in Cancer Prevention

Epidemiological and Case–Control Studies

Evidence for cancer protective properties of selenium was first obtained through comparisons of U.S. cancer mortalities in low and high selenium regions and by correlating cancer mortalities in different countries with dietary selenium intake parameters (1–5). The cancer-protective properties of selenium were subsequently demonstrated in animal studies, as well as in vitro with various tumor cell lines. Further supporting evidence for cancer-protecting effects of selenium was obtained through case–control studies (6–11) which, for the most part, demonstrated that low serum or plasma selenium levels, or, in later studies, levels of selenoprotein P (12, 13), were indicative of increased cancer risk. Other workers using toenail selenium levels as indices of selenium status reached similar conclusions for cancers of lung (14), stomach (15), and invasive prostate cancer (16).

Effects of Selenium-Antagonistic Elements

The cancer-protecting effects of selenium are counteracted by selenium-antagonistic elements that may be found in foods, the drinking water, or the environment (17–23). Some of these elements, arsenic (As), lead, mercury, and cadmium, for example, are known to inhibit selenium-dependent enzymes, impede selenium uptake, or to form unreactive selenides accumulating in organs and tissues, while others counteract the cancer-protective effects of selenium indirectly by stimulating oxygen radical production. Accordingly, the selenium requirement increases in the presence of such elements. These findings are relevant to occupational medicine: A Swedish study (24) revealed that lung tissues from foundry workers who had died from lung and other types of cancer exhibit much higher arsenic/selenium ratios than those from foundry workers who had died from heart disease or accidents. Higher arsenic/selenium ratios were observed in the scalp hair of miners of a tin mine in China who developed lung cancer than those who did not (25). This prompted studies to reduce the cancer risk of exposed workers by means of selenium. In one such study (26), supplemental selenium at 300 µg Se/day increased blood and hair selenium as well as plasma glutathione peroxidase (GSH-Px) activity and reduced the concentration of lipid hydroperoxides compared with placebo. In addition, measurements of unscheduled DNA synthesis revealed the DNA of lymphocytes of the selenium-supplemented miners to be less damaged than that of miners receiving placebo, a result consistent with a reduction of cancer risk in the supplemented group. For accurate assessments of cancer risk multielement analyses are necessary and are producing promising results (for additional discussion see refs. 27–29). Zinc, while itself essential for normal cellular functions, also abolishes the cancer-protecting effects of selenium if supplied in excessive amounts (29). Zinc in addition is specifically required by the tumor for growth and progression and accumulates in its actively growing surface layer (30), and there is evidence for its direct interaction with selenium in vivo (31, 32).

Cancer Prevention Trials with Selenium

From the 1980s onward, several cancer prevention trials with selenium have been conducted. The first trial which showed a protective effect of selenium A was performed from 1985–1989 in Qidong, a region north of Shanghai with a high incidence of primary liver cancer (PLC) and hepatitis B (HB) (33–35). Subjects in one commune in the center of the endemic area receiving table salt fortified with sodium selenite experienced a drop of PLC and HB incidence to approximately one-half of the incidences observed in control populations maintained on ordinary salt. Another intervention trial was conducted from 1984 to 1991 in Linxian, Henan Province, China, a region with high incidence of esophageal cancer (36). In this trial the cancer protective effects of several vitamins and minerals including selenium were tested against a placebo. While supplemental retinol, zinc, riboflavin, niacin, molybdenum, and vitamin C were ineffective, supplemental selenium combined with β-carotene and vitamin E lowered the total mortality by 9 % and the cancer mortality by 13 %. However, best known is the trial directed from 1983–1996 by L.C. Clark et al. (37), which involved 1332 conservatively treated, mostly male, former nonmelanoma skin cancer patients. The consecutively enrolled subjects either received selenium (200 μg/day) in the form of selenomethionine incorporated in yeast or a placebo for up to seven years. In the selenium-supplemented group, lung cancer mortality was reduced by 53 %, the incidence of cancer of prostate by 63 %, of colon and rectum by 58 %. Selenium supplementation had no effect on skin cancer recurrence, which, however, is not unexpected as selenium at the dosage chosen does not act on premalignant or transformed cell populations that the study subjects may have harbored. In view of the significant protective effects observed, a new trial designated "SELECT" was started in May 2001. In this largest cancer prevention trial ever to be conducted, 32 000 men will be enrolled in 400 centers in the United States, Canada, and Puerto Rico. Study subjects will receive 200 μg of selenium as L-selenomethionine (in this case not in yeast), with or without vitamin E, or a placebo (38). Its primary aim is to show if a supplement of sele-nium in the form of selenomethionine will lower the incidence of prostate cancer, and whether the protective effect of selenium can be further increased by vitamin E. Secondary end points, i. e., cancers developing at other sites, will also be monitored, the study is scheduled to be completed in 2012.

Mechanisms of Anticarcinogenic Action

The mechanisms by which selenium protects against the development of cancer are complex. They depend on the dosage and chemical form of selenium and the nature of the initiating agent and hence are probably multifactorial. In the following only some of the many mechanisms will be delineated.

Effects of Selenium Deficiency on Gene Expression

Cells grown or maintained in selenium deficient media do not become spontaneously malignant, they still require a carcinogenic stimulus, which may be chemical, physical, viral or genetic. However, an insufficient supply of selenium evidently results in adaptive changes facilitating the malignant transformation of cells. The extent of these changes has recently been elucidated through a study (39) with cells from the intestine of mice. When these cells were grown under conditions of selenium deficiency, as many as 44 of their genes were up-regulated, among them genes associated with DNA repair and the protection against oxidative stress and genes controlling cell cycle. In addition, at least 24 genes were down-regulated, those involved with selenoprotein synthesis, the synthesis of enzymes involved in detoxification (cytochrome P450, GSH S-transferase, epoxide hydrolase) as well as the synthesis of enzymes regulating lipid transport, angiogenesis, cell adhesion, cell cycle, and cell growth. All these changes point to diminished resistance to carcinogenic stress factors. The loss of cell cycle control alone, for example, may increase the error rate during DNA replication and prevent DNA repair. The down-regulation of the detoxifying enzymes may prevent carcinogens to be metabolized.

Antimutagenic and Antiviral Effects

The down-regulation of selenoprotein synthesis will result in low activities of key selenoenzymes protecting cellular DNA against free radical-induced mutations. The glutathione peroxidases, as is well known, prevent the accumulation of H_2O_2 and of lipid hydroperoxides in cells and tissues. Cells deficient in GSH-Px thus will more likely suffer mutations that will push them further toward becoming malignant. The protective action extends to the genomes of viruses that might be present in a dormant state but which may be activated and become pathogenic through an oxygen radical-induced mutation, as was demonstrated with a nonpathogenic coxsackie B3 virus strain (40). It has been suggested (41, 22), by analogy, that selenium could prevent mutations of other viruses, preventing them from becoming oncogenic.

The Putative Role of the Thioredoxin Reductases

In addition to GSH-Px, thioredoxin reductases (TRxRs) (42) deserve particular attention, whose primary function is to catalyze the reduction of the oxidized forms of thioredoxins back into their reduced forms. Thioredoxins are ubiquitous low molecular weight proteins containing two Cys–SH groups in their active reduced forms and a disulfide (Cys–S–S–Cys)-linkage in their oxidized forms. Thioredoxins serve as electron donors in a multitude of biologically important reactions, such as DNA synthesis, DNA repair, gene transcription, cell growth, apoptosis, detoxification reactions, including those involving carcinogens, and they in addition help to maintain the functioning of the immune system. The TRxRs have surprisingly low substrate specificity. In addition to the thioredoxins they also reduce protein disulfide isomerase, selenite, selenodiglutathione, nitrosoglutathione, glutathione peroxidase, H_2O_2, and lipid hydroperoxide reductase, alloxan, and vitamin K, NK lysine disulfide, lipoic acid, dehydroascorbic acid, and the ascorbyl free radical (43). In the physiological hierarchy of the selenoenzymes, the TRxRs fall behind the GSH-Px. Thus, for optimal TRxR activity, higher amounts of selenium are required than for the saturation of GSH-Px activity. The cancer-protective effects of selenium undoubtedly also involves other selenoproteins, of which 25 are encoded in the human genome (44) and whose functions have not been elucidated.

Effect on DNA Methylation

However, some protective functions of selenium are not associated with any selenoenzyme. The interaction of selenium with toxic or carcinogenic metals as discussed above belongs to this category; the methylation of selenium is another. Selenium is methylated under physiological conditions. As an acceptor of biogenic methyl groups selenium was shown to prevent the hypermethylation of DNA (45), an early activating step in benzo(α) pyrene carcinogenesis (46).

Oncogene Inactivation

Among the effects on the genomic level of tumor cells, selenium has been shown to inactivate the oncogene c-*myc* and to activate c-*fos*, causing the partial retransformation of human hepatoma cells (47). Related to these effects of selenium is the inactivation of MAZ, the c-*myc* activating zinc finger protein, which regulates the activation of c-*myc* (48). These effects of selenium are counteracted by zinc, providing a deeper insight into the mechanism of the zinc–selenium antagonism mentioned above. Selenium has also been shown to inhibit the activation of the nuclear transcription factor NFκB, to activate p53, and to induce apoptosis (49). Selenium may be viewed, in these processes, to act as a catalyst of cellular respiration; the interdependence of its anticarcinogenic effects on oxygen availability has been stressed (50).

▬ Selenium in Cancer Chemotherapy

Reduction of Side Effects of Chemotherapeutic Agents

Cancer patients as a rule present with subnormal blood selenium levels and signs of increased lipid peroxidation (51). They thus are in a state of weakened resistance to oxidative stress to begin with and will suffer more damage during therapy as oxygen radical production is increased by many cytotoxic agents as well as during radiation therapy. The administration of selenium thus is indicated as a general supportive measure, as well as a means of diminishing additional oxygen radical damage occurring during chemotherapy and radiation. For example, the nephrotoxicity of cisplatin, believed to be caused by the stimulation of oxygen radical production in the kidney, was prevented by selenium in rats if administered one hour prior to the cytostatic agent (52–54). In humans, selenium protected even when given after cisplatin: In patients with ovarian cancer treated with cisplatin, sodium selenate and vitamin E prevented the rise of Creatine Kinase serum values, an indicator of kidney damage (55). In addition, the selenium treatment prevented the drop of the leukocyte counts in these patients so that blood transfusions were not required. In other studies sodium selenite was shown to reduce the cardiotoxicity of adriamycin (56, 57) caused by oxidative damage of the cardiac muscle. The reduction of toxic side effects by sodium selenite also extends to cytotoxic agents not necessarily caused by oxidative damage, such as the highly cytotoxic polyamine synthase inhibitors MGBG, EHNA, ARA-A, and DFMO, administered to rats with transplanted human prostate cancer cells (58). The question whether selenium interferes with the therapeutic efficacy of cytotoxic agents has since also been addressed in in-vitro studies with different human cancer cell lines (59). The therapeutic efficacy of doxorubicin, docetaxel, 5-FU, MTX, and mafosfamide against MDA-MB-231 breast cancer cells in vitro was not affected by increasing amounts of sodium selenite in the culture medium. In addition, the antiproliferative activities of cisplatin, etoposide, gemcitabine, or mitomycin C against human A549 lung cancer cells remained unaltered, while the inhibitory activity of docetaxel against these cells was actually increased. An enhancement of the antiproliferative or inhibitory activities of 5-FU, oxaliplatin, and irinotecan by selenite was also observed with HCT116 and SW620 colon cancer cells.

Current Therapeutic Selenite Dosage Recommendations

Patients receiving chemotherapy are given, orally or by infusion, 1000 µg of selenium as sodium selenite per day for 1–5 days prior to and during chemotherapy. The dosage is subsequently lowered to 500, 300, 200, and 100 µg selenium/day.

Sodium selenite administered according to this scheme is generally well tolerated as even at the maximum of 1000 µg selenium/day, which is given only for a few days, it is still below the "individual toxic level" of 1600 µg/day for long-term selenium intake (60). Additional sodium selenite dosage schemes for specific applications are also given in Chapter 21 (p. 247), as well as in a recently published monograph (61).

Anti-Inflammatory Effects

Inflammatory reactions are known to occur after treatment with certain chemotherapeutic agents. Vinorelbine is one such agent. Given by infusion, this agent causes phlebitis of the arm in sensitive patients, which often forces the interruption or cessation of the treatment. A pretreatment of such patients with sodium selenite prior to Vinorelbine infusion was found to significantly reduce or prevent this adverse reaction (62).

Diminution of Drug Resistance

The enhanced production of oxygen radicals and *increased* lipid peroxidation during cytotoxic drug therapy activates antioxidative defense mechanisms of tumor cells (63) resulting in an increase of their intracellular glutathione (GSH) concentrations and ultimately the development of drug resistance (64–66). Selenite reacts with GSH to yield *selenodiglutathione*, GSSeSG, and related species, which in the presence of oxygen catalyze the oxidation of GSH to GSSG. Depletion of the tumor cells of GSH resensibilizes them against the cytostatic agent and may simultaneously induce p53 activity and apoptosis resulting in cell destruction (67).

Radioprotective Effects

Following the first demonstration of the radioprotective effects of organic selenium compounds by Breccia in 1969 (68), additional studies were conducted which confirmed that sodium selenite or seleno amino acids increased the survival of rats exposed to whole-body irradiation (69). Selenium compounds in combination with common radioprotective drugs such as glucan and amifostine (WR-2721) produced synergistic and even super-additive effects as evidenced by longer survival and measurement of bone marrow cell counts at similar radiation dose (70). In addition, selenite reduced the toxicity of amifostine without affecting its radiotherapeutic efficiency. The radioprotective effects of sodium selenite (selenase) were also investigated with normal human fibroblasts and tumor cells under standardized in-vitro cell culture conditions (71). Whereas selenite in the medium increased the survival rate of the fibroblasts, it had no detectable protecting effect on the tumor cells. In fact, the selenite-treated tumor cells exhibited greater radiosensitivity and increased apoptosis. Another study with normal human endothelial cells and several different tumor cell lines produced similar results, i. e., normal cells pretreated with sodium selenite (selenase) exhibited concentration-dependent protective effects, no such effect was apparent with the tumor cells. Finally, sodium selenite at certain concentrations as well as WR-1065 (a metabolite of WR-2721) protected cells against radiation-induced mutations. On combined administration the protective effects were additive, although the two agents appear to protect by different mechanisms (72).

▬ Immunoprotective Effects

Supplemental sodium selenite enhances the functions of natural killer cells and lymphokine-activated killer cells, supporting its use for the maintenance of patients after conventional therapy (73). In an observational study performed from 1977–1986, selenium at individualized dosages in the form of selenium yeast was administered daily for several months to 70 conservatively treated, hospitalized cancer patients that were receiving low-dose chemotherapy (CMF) and BCG for immunostimulation (74). The recurrence rate in this group of patients was significantly lower than in historical controls receiving the same therapy without selenium. Other clinical studies demonstrate the immunoprotective properties of sodium selenite: In patients with solid tumors treated with chemotherapy, radiation therapy, and selenite the decline of immune cell counts was diminished by one third compared with control patients receiving the same therapy without sodium selenite (75). The selenite-treated patients did not require cell growth-stimulating agents that normally have to be administered after the second

and third therapy cycle. In addition, these patients only seldom required antiemetic drugs. On the whole, sodium selenite treatment had a positive effect on the general condition and the quality of life of these patients. Sodium selenite also reduced side effects of radiation in patients with cancer of the cervix or corpus uteri, preventing or alleviating tenesmus and irritation of the bladder, two conditions which often force interruption or early termination of the treatment (76). Last but not least the results of a preliminary study should be mentioned in which 22 patients with precancerous oral cavity lesions were receiving 300 μg of selenium/day as sodium selenite in solution (eight individuals) or in organic form in capsules (14 individuals), in three four-week cycles. At the end of the therapy there were two complete responses, five partial responses, six minor responses, and five stable diseases with an objective response of 38.8 % (77). Progression after suspension of therapy occurred in seven of 18 patients. The authors stress the need for a longer treatment period and, in view of the encouraging results of their preliminary work, the need for controlled studies.

▬ Sodium Selenite in the Management of Secondary Lymphedema

Lymphedema of the Arm

Secondary lymphedema develop in cancer patients after surgical interventions and radiation therapy. Due to removal of lymph nodes and diminished functioning of the lymphatic passages excess lymph accumulates in the affected extremity. The diminished oxygen supply may trigger the invasion of polymorphous neutrophilic leukocytes and the production of reactive oxygen radical species, resulting in inflammatory reactions and ultimately progressive degenerative changes in the affected extremity. The administration of sodium selenite (selenase), in some cases even after single oral dose of 800 μg selenium, causes spontaneous volume reductions of the affected extremity and has anti-inflammatory effects; selenite supplementation in addition diminished the serum levels of 2-hydroxynonenal and malondialdehyde, two parameters of lipid peroxidation (78–80). Selenite in addition increased the contractility of the lymphatic vessels, improved the effect of manual decongestion therapies by about 15 % compared with patients treated by manual decongestion therapy only. Patients are typically receiving 1000 µg selenium/day during the first week of manual decongestive therapy, and 300 µg selenium/day thereafter. Patients receiving this treatment for five months remained free of erysipelas infections and required no antibiotics. In contrast, during the same period erysipelas infections occurred in 50 % of patients treated conventionally without selenite (81). Treated patients maintained on sodium selenite also showed improved condition of the skin, which otherwise, under heavy tension, tends to roughen and thicken due to hyperkeratotic changes. Additionally, 30 % of the selenite-treated patients reported an improvement of nycturia and incontinence; also noticed was a significant improvement of vision, and all reported a generally improved quality of life (81, 82).

Lymphedema in the Head–Neck Area

Interstitial lymphedema develop in most patients with head–neck tumors after surgery, chemotherapy, and radiation therapy. Patients developing endolaryngeal edema under these conditions require effective therapy if tracheostomy is to be avoided. The treatment of such patients with sodium selenite (selenase) was found to be helpful, as evidenced by the results of a recent clinical study (83). Of 30 such patients 20 developed endolaryngeal edema on average four weeks after radiotherapy, accompanied by breathing difficulties and whistling noises during respiration. In 16 of the 20 patients with endolaryngeal edema sodium selenite (orally, 3×200 µg Se/day) effected a significant reduction of the edema over a period of eight weeks. Of the 30 patients, 12 were also treated with proteolytic enzymes, but this treatment proved effective in only two individuals. In 13 of 20 patients, tracheostomy was not necessary; of the seven tracheostomies that had to be performed in the remaining patients, five were temporary and only two were permanent.

In another study with 20 patients with cancer of the floor of the mouth and tongue at stages T3 and T4, 10 received sodium selenite (selenase) for 21 days, prior to, during, and after neck dissection at 1000 µg Se/day. Already during the first week, a clear reduction of the lymphedema was apparent, compared with the patients receiving placebo, which persisted during the remaining two weeks of treatment (84). This result is important since the secondary lymphedema developing after neck dissection causes significant hydrostatic, metabolic, and immunological disturbances. In addition, in the affected regions sclerotic connective tissue replaces subcutaneous adipose layers, and secondary inflammatory processes result in further tissue damage.

Sodium Selenite in the Maintenance of Brain Tumor Patients

In an observational study sodium selenite at dosages of 1000 µg Se/day along with oxygen and other supportive measures was found to be beneficial in the maintenance of conservatively treated brain tumor patients exhibiting the typical symptoms of increased intracranial pressure (85). In 76 % of the treated patients a definite improvement and in 24 % a slight improvement of the general condition and a decrease of symptoms such as nausea, emesis, headache, vertigo, unsteady gait, speech disorders, and a decrease of Jacksonian seizures were observed.

Answers to Some Frequently Asked Questions

Germany's Selenium Status and the Recommended Daily Selenium Intake

The German Nutritional Society is presently recommending for adults a daily selenium intake of 30–70 µg/day, the current American recommendation is 55 µg/day. These intake recommendations were derived primarily from the amount of selenium required to achieve maximum GSH-Px activity in serum. A recent study revealed the selenium intakes of German adults are presently in the order of 30 µg/day for women and 42 µg/day in men (86). Of the women and men examined approximately 20 % took only 20 or 25 µg per day, respectively, resulting in a negative selenium balance. This result reaffirms the conclusions of a previous study that concluded that a significant percentage of the German population is in a state of compensated selenium deficiency (87).

Optimal Selenium Intakes for Cancer Prevention

Blood selenium concentrations in different countries vary widely, but each country tends to regard its average or median value as "normal." From epidemiological studies blood selenium levels of 0.25–0.30 µg/mL were estimated as adequate for cancer protection. An adult of 75 kg body weight desirous of reaching this level must maintain an average dietary selenium intake of 250–300 µg/day, which requires an additional 200 µg of selenium to be taken in the form of supplements. This recommended intake for cancer prevention is below the reference dose (RfD) for selenium, the amount generally recognized as safe for adults for indefinite periods (88). It corresponds to 5 µg Se/kg per body weight and equals five times the recommended dietary allowance (RDA). Blood selenium levels of 0.25–0.30 µg/mL are presently attained by the populations of selenium-rich parts of Venezuela as well as by people in Japan, Thailand, and Malaysia subsisting on the traditional Asian diets. However, the increasing Westernization of the diets in the latter countries results in a diminution of the selenium intakes so much so that concern has been voiced about the likely negative public health effects, namely, the increase of the cancer incidence rates (89).

Therapeutic and Nutritional Forms of Selenium

Sodium selenite in appropriate galenic preparations and different dosages for oral intake or infusions are approved in Germany, Austria, and in several other EU countries for the treatment of selenium deficiency, as occurring in cases of cancer, rheumatoid arthritis, or in patients in intensive care. Nutritional selenium supplements are available containing selenium in the form of L-selenomethionine, mainly in yeast, some with additional vitamins and minerals.

Sodium selenite is the preferred form of selenium in the therapy and maintenance of patients suffering from diseases such as cancer, chronic or acute inflammatory conditions, lymphedema, heart disease etc. as well as of patients in intensive care. Selenomethionine is suitable for nutritional supplementation and used whenever a slow, lasting improvement of selenium status is desired. Selenomethionine, a naturally occurring toxic amino acid, is also the major nutritional form of selenium and is normally found in trace amounts in cereals, grains, soy, rice, and other foods of plant origin. As is true for methionine, selenomethionine cannot be synthesized efficiently in the human organism. Since from selenomethionine all biologically important forms of selenium can be formed (90) it fulfills the criteria as an essential amino acid. Selenocysteine, in contrast, can be synthesized in the human organism but is not a major nutritional form of selenium. Selenomethionine is actively absorbed to the extent of 96% but is as such not immediately bioavailable. Some of it is incorporated into body proteins in place of methionine, more at deficient methionine intakes, or metabolized predominantly to selenide via selenocystathione and selenocysteine. At the selenide stage selenium becomes available for selenoprotein synthesis. Excess selenide is methylated and excreted. During normal protein turnover a fraction of the protein-incorporated selenomethionine is released along with methionine. At constant dietary intakes of selenomethionine and methionine, a steady state is established. The blood and tissue selenium contents thus are essentially proportional to the dietary selenomethionine intakes. Selenite, in contrast to selenomethionine, is passively absorbed and is not significantly stored in body proteins. Absorbed or infused selenite is transferred from the plasma into the erythrocytes, reduced and re-released into the plasma. It remains in the so-called selenite exchangeable selenium pool and is available for selenoprotein biosynthesis and metal detoxification. Prior to excretion it is methylated; the major excretory form is the trimethylselenonium ion. At high levels of intake some of the selenium is also exhaled in form of dimethyl selenide or dimethyl diselenide, giving the breath a characteristic garliclike odor.

Incompatibility of Vitamin C with Sodium Selenite

Sodium selenite contains selenium in a reducible form and reacts with vitamin C rapidly to form elemental selenium, which has low bioavailability. If vitamin C is to be administered it should never be given shortly before, with, or shortly after selenite. It is recommended to take sodium selenite in the morning on an empty stomach and to wait at least one hour before vitamin C is taken. When vitamin C is to be given by intravenous infusion, the recommended time interval after selenite is two hours. Selenomethionine, in contrast to selenite, is compatible with vitamin C, and both can be taken jointly.

Upper Safe, Permissible, and Toxic Dosages

Selenium intakes of up to 350 µg/day by adults of normal weight are recognized as safe for indefinite periods. The reference dose (RfD) for selenium of 350 µg/day is equal to 5 µg Se/kg per body weight and equals five times the recommended dietary allowance (RDA) (89). Apart from the RfD several other selenium dosage limits have been defined by different regulatory agencies. For example, the British Committee on Medical Aspects of Food Policy of the Department of Health in 1991 defined 450 µg Se/day as the "maximal safe intake" for indefinite periods (91). Another reference value is the "Tolerable Upper Intake Level" (UL) of 400 µg/day, representing the highest level of daily selenium intake that is likely to pose no risk of adverse health effects to almost all individuals in the general population (89). The UL for selenium is equal to one half of the "No observed adverse effect level" (NOAL) of selenium of 800 µg/day. From observations in high selenium regions of China an "individual toxic level" of 1595 or 1600 µg Se/day was deduced (92). This level was defined as "capable of causing the development of chronic overt toxic selenosis after long-term intake." Previously, observations in high selenium regions of the USA suggested that mild, reversible signs of toxic selenosis occur after intakes of 2400–3000 µg Se/day for many months (93). This apparent discrepancy may be due to the fact that selenium toxicity is lower if protein intake is high. Therapeutically, sodium selenite at dosages of 1000–2000 µg of selenium is administered before and during therapy only for several days. Higher dosages are not recommended, although, according to one report (94), 10 mg and even 20 mg of selenium as sodium selenite can be given by intravenous infusion for five consecutive days to patients without apparent side effects. However, the same author reports that 50 mg selenium (as sodium selenite) produced nausea and vomiting and could only be given once. The acute toxicity of sodium selenite was deter-

mined in various animal species to range from 1–5 mg/kg body weight, corresponding to 70–350 mg (as elemental selenium) in a 70 kg adult. The minimum lethal dose of sodium selenite on intravenous administration in mice is 3.0 mg/kg body weight and corresponds to 60% of the LD_{50} of 5.0 ± 0.62 mg/kg. The LD_{50} of selenomethionine on intravenous administration was determined to be 22.0 ± 3.43 mg/kg body weight, the minimum lethal dose, 10 mg/kg body weight (95).

References

1. Shamberger RJ, Frost DV: Possible inhibitory effect of selenium on human cancer. Can. Med. Ass. J. 1969; 100: 682.
2. Schrauzer GN, Rhead WJ: Interpretation of the methylene blue reduction test of human plasma and the possible cancer protecting effect of selenium. Experientia 1971; 27: 1069–1071.
3. Shamberger RJ, Willis CE: Selenium distribution and human cancer mortality. CRC Critical Reviews in Clinical Laboratory Sciences 1971; 211–221.
4. Schrauzer GN, Rhead WJ, Evans GA.: Selenium and cancer: chemical interpretation of a plasma "cancer test." Bioinorg. Chem. 1973; 2: 329–370.
5. Schrauzer GN, White DA, Schneider CJ: Cancer mortality correlation studies. III. Associations with dietary selenium intakes. Bioinorg. Chem. 1977; 7: 23–34.
6. Willett WC, Morris JS, Pressel S, et al.: Prediagnostic serum selenium and risk of cancer. The Lancet 1983; 2 (8342U): 130–134.
7. Salonen JT, Alfthan G., Huttunen JK, Puska P: Association between serum selenium and the risk of cancer, Am. J. of Epid. 1984; 120: 342–339.
8. Fex G., Petterson B, Akesson B: Low plasma selenium as a risk factor for cancer in middle aged men. Nutr. Cancer 1987; 10: 221–229.
9. Itoh Y, Kikuchi H: Serum selenium contents and the risk of cancer. Biomed Res. Trace El. 1997; 8: 75–76.
10. Aaseth J., Glattre E., Frey H., Norheim G. Ringstad J., Thomassen, Y: Selenium in the human thyroid gland. In: Proc. 6th Int. Trace El. Symp. 1989, Vol 3, Anke M, Baumann W, Bräunlich H, Brückner C, Groppel B, Grün M.(eds), VEB Krongress- u. Werbedruck, Jena, 1989; pp. 911–914
11. Glattre .M, Thomassen Y, Thorensen SQ, et al.: Prediagnostic serum selenium in a case-control study of thyroid cancer. Int. J. Epid. 1989; 18: 45–49.
12. Persson-Moschos M, Alfthan G, Åkesson B: Plasma selenoprotein P levels of healthy males in different selenium status after oral supplementation with

different forms of selenium. Eur. J. Clin. Nutr. 1998; 52: 363–367.

13. Persson-Moschos M, Stavenow L, Åkesson B, Lindgärde F: Selenoprotein P in plasma in relation to cancer morbidity in middle-aged Swedish men. Nutr. Cancer 2000; 34: 19–26.

14. van den Brandt PA., Goldbohm A, van't Veer P, et al.: A prospective cohort study on selenium status and the risk of lung cancer. Cancer Res.1993; 53: 4860–4865.

15. van den Brandt PA, Goldbohm RA, van't Veer P, et al.: A prospective study on toenail selenium levels and risk of gastrointestinal cancer. J. Natl. Cancer Inst. 1993; 85: 224–229.

16. Yoshizawa K, Willett WC, Morris SJ, et al.: Study of prediagnostic selenium level in toenails and the risk of advanced prostate cancer. J. Natl. Cancer Inst.1998; 90: 1219–1124.

17. Schrauzer GN, White DA, Schneider CJ: Inhibition of the genesis of spontaneous mammary tumors in C3H mice: Effects of selenium and of selenium-antagonistic elements and their possible role in human breast cancer. Bioinorg. Chem. 1976; 6: 265–270.

18. Schrauzer GN: Trace elements in carcinogenesis. In: Draper, H.H. (ed.), Advances in Nutrition Research. Plenum Press, New York, N.Y., 1979; 2: 219–244

19. Schrauzer GN, Kuehn K, Hamm D: Effects of dietary selenium and lead on the genesis of spontaneous mammary tumors in mice. Biol. Trace El. Res. 1981; 3: 185–196.

20. Schrauzer GN, White DA, McGinness JE, Schneider CJ, Bell LJ: Arsenic and cancer. Effects of the joint administration of selenium and arsenic on the genesis of spontaneous mammary tumors in mice. Bioinorg. Chem. 1978; 9: 245–253.

21. Schrauzer GN: Effects of selenium antagonists on cancer susceptibility: new aspects of chronic heavy metal toxicity. In: Brown SS, Kodama, T (eds): Toxicology of Metals. Ellis Horwood, Chichester 1987, pp. 91–98.

22. Schrauzer GN, White DA, Schneider CJ: Inhibition of the genesis of spontaneous mammary tumors in C3H mice: Effects of selenium and of selenium-antagonistic elements and their possible role in human breast cancer. Bioinorg. Chem. 1976; 6: 265–270.

23. Schrauzer GN: Anticarcinogenic effects of selenium. CMLS (Cellular and Molecular Life Sciences) 2000; 57: 1864–1873.

24. Wester PO, Brune D, Norberg GL: Arsenic and selenium in lung, liver, and kidney tissue from dead smelter workers. Brit. J. Industr. Med. 1981; 38: 179–184.

25. Wang,W, Xu H, Xiang S, Guo L: A study of the relation of the Se/As ratio in the hair of workers to lung cancer at the Yunnan Tin Mine. In: Proc. Internatl. Symp. on Environmental Life Elements and Health, Beijing, P.R.C., p. 216 (1988).

26. Yu S-Y, Mao BL, Xiao P, et al.: Intervention trial with selenium for the prevention of lung cancer among tin miners in Yunnan, China. Biol. Trace El. Res. 1990; 24: 105–108.

27. Singh V, Garg AN: Trace element correlations in the blood of Indian women with breast cancer. Biol. Trace El. Res. 1998; 64: 237–245.

28. Sky-Peck HE: Distribution of trace elements in normal and neoplastic human tissues by energy dispersive x-ray fluorescence. In: Moro R, Cesareo R (eds), XRF and PIXE Applications in Life Sciences, World Scientific, Teaneck, N.J. 1989, pp. 31–47.

29. Schrauzer GN: Inorganic element levels in neoplasia. In: Handbook of Metal Ligand Interactions, Berthon G. (ed), Marcel Dekker, Inc., New York, Basel, Hong Kong, 1995; pp. 1060–1067.

30. Ujiie S., Itoh, Y, Kikuchi H, Wakui A: Zinc distribution in malignant tumors. Biomed. Res. Trace Elements 1994; 5: 81–82.

31. Eybl V, Sykora J, Mertl F: In vivo interaction of selenium with zinc. Acta Pharmacol. Toxicol. Suppl. 1986; 59: 547–8.

32. Chmielnicka J, Zareba, G., Witasik, M., and Brzesncka E: Zinc–selenium interaction in the rat. Biol. Trace El. Res. 1988; 15: 267–276.

33. Yu Sh-Y, Zhu Y-J, Li W-G: Protective role of selenium against hepatitis B virus and primary liver cancer in Qidong. Biol. Trace El. Res. 1997; 56: 117–124.

34. Yu Sh-Y, Zhu Y-J, Li W-G, et al.: A preliminary report of the intervention trials of primary liver cancer in high risk populations with nutritional supplementation of selenium in China. Biol. Trace El. Res. 1991; 29: 289–294.

35. Yu Sh.-Y, Li W-G, Zhu Y-J, Yu W-P, Hou C: Chemoprevention trial of human hepatitis with selenium supplementation in China. Biol. Trace El. Res. 1989; 20: 15–22.

36. Blot WJ, Li JY, Taylor PR, et al.: Nutrition intervention trials in Linxian, China: Supplementation with specific vitamin/mineral combinations, and disease-specific mortality in the general population. J. Natl. Cancer Inst. 1993; 85: 1483–1492.

37. Clark LC, Combs GF, Turnbull BW, et al.: Effects of selenium supplementation for cancer prevention in patients with carcinoma of the skin. J. Am. Med. Assoc. 1996; 276: 1957–1963.

38. Klein EA, Thompson IM, Lippman SM, et al.: SELECT The next prostate cancer prevention trial. Vitamin E and Selenium Cancer Prevention Trial. J. Urol. 2001; 166: 1311–1315.

39. Rao L, Puschner B, Prolla TA.: Gene expression profiling of low selenium status in the mouse intestine. J. Nutr. 2001; 131: 3175–3181.

40. Beck MA.: Selenium as an antiviral agent. In: Hatfield DL (ed.), Selenium. Its Molecular Biology and Role in Human Health. Kluwer Academic Publications, Boston, Dordrecht, London 2001; pp.235–245.

41. Taylor EW, Nadimpalli RG, Ramanathan CS: Genomic structure of viral agents in relation to the synthesis of selenoproteins. Biol. Trace El. Res. 1997; 56: 63–91.

42. Gallegos A., Berggren M, Gasdaska JR, Powis G: Mechanism of the regulation of thioredoxin reductase activity in cancer cells by the chemopreventive agent selenium. Cancer Res. 1997; 57: 4965–4970.

43. Homgren A : Selenoproteins of the thioredoxin system. In: Hatfield DL (ed.), Selenium. Its Molecular Biology and Role in Human Health. Kluwer Academic Publications, Boston, Dordrecht, London 2001; pp.179–188.

44. Kryukov, G.V, Castellano S, Novoselov SV, et al.: Characterization of mammalian selenoproteomes. Science 2003; 300: 1439–1443.

45. Cox R: Selenite: a good inhibitor of rat liver DNA methylase. Biochem. Int. 1985; 10: 63–69.

46. Flesher JW, Myers SR, Stansbury KH: The site of substitution of the methyl group in the bioalkylation of benzo-α-pyrene. Carcinogenesis 1990; 11: 493–496.

47. Yu S-Y, Lu XP, Liao SD: The regulatory effect of selenium on the expression of oncogenes associated with the proliferation and differentiation on tumor cells. In: Collery P, Poirier LA, Manfait M, Etienne JC, (eds): Metal ions in Biology and Medicine. John Libbey Eurotext, Paris 1990, pp. 487–489.

48. Nelson KK, Bacon B, Christensen MJ: Selenite supplementation decreases the expression of MAZ in HT29 human colon adenocarcinoma cells. Nutrition and Cancer 1995; 26: 73–81.

49. Otsuka G, Nagaya K, Mizuno M, Yoshida J, Sao H: Inhibition of nuclear factor κ B activation confers sensitivity to tumor necrosis factor-α by impairment of cell cycle progression in human glioma cells. Cancer Res. 1999; 59: 4446–4452.

50. Schrauzer GN: Sauerstoff und Selen in der Onkologie. Z. Onkol./J. Oncol. 2000; 32: 17–22.

51. Look M, Crissafidou A: Vollblutselenspiegel und Lipidperoxide bei Tumorpatienten unter Chemotherapie: "DNA-Effekte" von Sauerstoffradikalen am Beispiel des Transkriptionsfaktors NFkB und des p53-Tumorsuppressorgens. Med Klin 1995; 90: Suppl. 1: 18–22.

52. Ohkawa K, Tsukada Y, Dohzono H, Koike K, Terashima Y: The effects of co-administration of selenium and cis-platin (CDDP) on CDDP-induced toxicity and antitumor activity. Br J Cancer 1988; 58: 38–41.

53. Vermeulen NP, Baldew GS, Los G, McVie JG, De Goeij JJ: Reduction of cisplatin nephrotoxicity by sodium selenite. Lack of interaction at the pharmacokinetic level of both compounds. Drug Metab Dispos. 1993; 21: 30–36.

54. Baldew G.S, van den Hamer CJA, Los G, Vermeulen NPB, de Goeij JJM, McVi. JG: Selenium-induced protection against cis-diamminedichloroplatinum(II) nephrotoxicity in mice and rats. Cancer Res. 1989; 49: 3020–3023.

55. Dimitrov NV, Hay MB, Hudler DA, Charamella LJ, Ullrey DE: Abrogation of adriamycin-induced cardiotoxicity by selenium in rabbits. Am J Pathol. 1987; 126: 376–383.

56. Boucher F, Coudray C, Tirard V, et al.: Oral selenium supplementation in rats reduces cardiac toxicity of adriamycin during ischemia and reperfusion. Nutr 11: 708–711, 1995.

57. Myers CE, McGuire WP, Liss RH, Ifrim I, Grotzinger, Young RC: Adriamycin: the role of lipid peroxidation in cardiac toxicity and tumour response. Science 1977; 8: 165.

58. Kuehn K, Dunzendorfer U, Whitmore WF, Schrauzer GN: Chemotherapy and trace element levels in blood and tissue of rats implanted with prostate tumor cells. Biol. Trace El. Res: 1985; 8: 237–250.

59. Schroeder, CP, Goeldner, EM, Schulze-Forster, K, Eickhoff, CA, Holtermann, P, Heidecke H.: Effect of selenite combined with chemotherapeutic agents on the proliferation of human carcinoma cell lines. Biol. Trace El. Res. 2004; 99: 17–25.

60. Yang G, Xia Y: Studies on human dietary requirements and safe range of dietary intakes of selenium in China and their application in the prevention of related endemic diseases. Biomed. Environ. Sci. 1995; 8: 187–201.

61. Schumacher K: Therapie maligner Tumoren. Integration konventioneller und komplementärer Therapie. Manual f. Klink und Praxis. Schatauer Verlag Stuttgart, New York 2000.

62. Holzhauer P: Kann durch die prophylaktische Gabe von Natriumselenit die Inzidenz und der Schweregrad der durch Vinorelbin induzierten lokalen Phlebitis beeinflusst werden? Dtsch Z Onkol 2002; 34: 14–16.

63. Hercberg A, Brok-Simoni F, Hltzman F, Bar-Am J, Leith JT, Brenner HJ: Erythrocyte glutathione and tumour response chemotherapy. The Lancet 1992; 339: 1074.

64. Caffrey PB, Frenkel GD: Selenite cytotoxicity in drug resistant and nonresistant human ovarian tumor cells. Cancer-Res 1992; 52: 4812–4816.

65. Gouyette A: Resistance associated with the glutathione system. Bull Cancer (Paris) 1994; 81: 69S–73S.

66. Caffrey PB, Frenkel GD: Selenite and drug resistance in cancer chemotherapy. The sixth international Symposium on Selenium in Biology and Medicine, Peking 1996.

66.b Shallom J, Juvekar A, Chitnis M: Selenium (Se) cytotoxicity in drug senslitive and drug resistant murine tumour. Cancer Biother. 1995; 10: 243–248.

67. Lanfear J, Fleming J, Wu L, Webster G, Harrison PR: The selenium metabolite selenodiglutathione induces p53 and apoptosis: relevance to the chemopreventive effects of selenium? Carcinogenesis 1994;15: 1387–1392.

68. Breccia A, Badiello R, Trenta A, Mattii M: On the chemical radioprotection by organic selenium compounds in vivo. Radiation Res. 1969; 38: 483–492.

69. Weiss, JF, Srinivasan V, Kumar KS, Landauer, MR. Patchen ML: Radioprotection by selenium and other metals. Abstract, 4th International Congress on Trace Elements in Medicine and Biology, Trace Elements and Free Radicals in Oxidative Diseases, Chamonix, France, April 5th–9th 1993.

70. Patchen ML, MacVittie TJ, Weiss JF: Combined modality radioprotection: The use of glucan and selenium with WR-2721. Int J Radiat Oncol Biol Phys 1990; 18: 1069–1075.

71. Schleicher UM, Cotarelo CL, Andreopoulos D, Ammon J, Mittermayer CH: In-vitro-Strahlensibilität verschiedener Zellen nach Natriumselenit-Inkubation. DEGRO-Congress November 7–10, 1998, Nuremberg, Germany.

72. Diamond A.M, Dale P, Murray JL, Grdina DJ: The inhibition of radiation-induced mutagenesis by the combined effects of selenium and the aminothiol WR-1065. Mut Res 1996; 356: 147–154.

73. Kiremidjian-Schumacher L, Roy M, Wishe HI, Cohen MW, Stotzky G: Supplementation with selenium augments the functions of natural killer and lymphokine-activated killer cells. Biol. Trace El. Res. 1996; 52: 227–239.

74. Donaldson R, VA Hospital St. Louis, see: Schrauzer GN, Selen, Neue Entwicklungen aus Biologie, Biochemie und Medizin, 3rd ed., 1998, Johann Ambrosius Barth Verl.Heidelberg, Leipzig, Germany, pp. 189–192.

75. Tittel R: Lecture at Symposium "Chancen nutzen in der Onkologie – komplementär-medizinische adjuvante Strategien", 2nd BIOMEDICINA on May 1 1998, Dresden, Germany.

76. Hehr T, Rodemann HP: In-vitro-Untersuchungen zur radioprotektiven Wirkung von Natriumselenit. Abstract, 23rd German Cancer Congress: Satellitensymposium Selen in der Onkologie. Ein essentielles Spurenelement auf dem Prüfstand. Berlin, Germany, June 8.–12, 1998.

77. Toma S, Micheletti A, Giachero A, et al.: Selenium therapy in patients with precancerous and malignant oral cavity lesions: Preliminary results. Cancer Detec Prev 1991; 15 (6): 491–494.

78. Schrauzer GN: Selen in der Therapie des chronischen Lymphödems – mechanistische Perspektiven

und praktische Anwendungen. Z Lymphol 1997; 21: 16–19.

79. Brenke R, Siems, W. Grune T: Therapieoptimierungsmaßbahmen beim chronischen Lymphödem. Z Lymphol 1997; 21: 20–22.

80. Siems WG., Brenke R, Beier A., et al.: Therapieoptimierung beim chronischen Lymphödem chirurgisch behandelter Tumorpatienten durch Natriumselenit. Dtsch Z Onkol 1994; 26: 128–132.

81. Kasseroller R: Therapieoptimierung des chronischen Lymphödems mit Natriumselenit. Z Lymphol 1997; 21: 23–25.

82. Kasseroller R, Schrauzer, GN: Treatment of secondary lymphedema of the arm with physical decongestion therapy and sodium selenite. Am. J. Therapeutics 2000; 7: 273–279.

83. Büntzel J, Weinaug R, Glatzel M, Fröhlich D, Micke O, Schuller P, Küttner K: Sodium selenite in the treatment of interstitial post-irradiation edema of the neck and head area. Trace Elements and Electrolytes 2002; 19: 33–37.

84. Zimmermann T, Leonhardt H, Kersting S, Albrecht S, Range U, Eckelt U: Sodium selenite reduces the postoperative lymphedema after oral tumor surgery. Biol. Trace El. Res. In press.

85. Pakdaman A: Symptomatic treatment of brain tumor patients with sodium selenite, oxygen and other supportive measures. Biol. Trace El. Res. 1998; 62: 1–6.

86. Anke M, Dröbner C, Röhrig B, Schäfer U, Müller R: Der Selenbestand der Fauna und der Selengehalt pflanzlicher und tierischer Lebensmittel Deutschlands. Ernährungsforsch. 2002; 47: 67–79.

87. Oster O: Zum Selenstatus in der Bundesrepublik Deutschland. Universituatsverlag Jena GmbH, Jena, Germany, 1992.

88. Patterson B, Levander OA: Naturally occurring selenium compounds in cancer chemoprevention trials: A workshop summary. Cancer Epidemiol. Biomarkers and Prevention 1997; 6: 63–69.

89. Ujiie S, Kikuchi H: The relation between serum selenium value and cancer in Miyagi, Japan: 5-year follow-up study. Tohoku J. Exp. Med. 2000; 196: 99–109

90. Schrauzer GN: The nutritional significance, metabolism and toxicology of selenomethionine. Adv. Food Nutr. Res. 2003; 47:73–112.

91. Department of Health, UK. Dietary reference values for food energy and nutrients for the United Kingdom, Report on Health and Social Subjects, No. 41, 1991. London, Her Majesty's Stationery Office.

92. Yang G, Xia Y: Studies on human dietary requirements and safe range of dietary intakes of selenium in China and their application in the prevention of related endemic diseases. Biomed. Environ. Sci. 1995; 8, 187–201.

93. NRC (National Research Council). Selenium. Medical and Biologic Effects of Environmental pollutants. National Academy of Sciences, Washington D.C. 1976, p.28.

94. Röhrer H: Verträglichkeit hochdosierter Selengaben in der Onkologie, Erfahrungsheilk. 1989; 38: 761.

95. Ammar EM, Couri D: Acute toxicity of sodium selenite and selenomethionine in mice after ICV and IV administration. Neurotoxicology 1981 2: 383–386.

— 13 Proteolytic Enzymes

Joseph Beuth

— Introduction

The oral administration of proteolytic enzymes (systemic enzyme therapy) has its origins in experience-based medicine and can be traced back, depending on the culture, to 1000-year-old records.

The enzyme-deficiency theory of cancer was articulated by the Scottish embryologist John Beard around the turn of the last century. His collected articles on the topic were published in book form in 1911 (1). This work was gradually forgotten. About 40 years ago, Max Wolf developed the concept of **systemic enzyme therapy** for oncology. The observation that tumor patients' sera had reduced cytotoxic activity against tumor cells, which was restored after the addition of proteolytic enzymes, formed the basis of the therapy. In addition, it was noted that malignant tumors were more common in old age with a concurrent reduction in the production of pancreatic enzymes as well as hydrolytic activity in the serum.

This led to the attempts to restore the oncolytic activity of the serum through the administration of oral proteolytic enzyme mixtures. Proteolytic enzymes are large molecules that can be absorbed. They then disperse into different compartments in the body in various concentrations (Table 13.1).

Initial animal experiments showed that the growth of experimental tumors was reduced and that the hydrolytic activity of the serum was normalized (8).

During this time, the role of proteolytic enzymes in clotting and fibrinolysis was also discovered. Metastases and their organotropic tendencies were explained at the time by "fibrino-lytic stickiness," through which tumor cells docked onto other organs and evaded immune surveillance. Research in immunology in the following years increasingly brought to light explanations for the mechanisms of action of systemic enzyme therapy.

Pharmacological Examinations

- It was observed that tumor cells emitted factors that blocked the immune system (**blocking factors**). In this manner, tumor cells protect themselves by shedding surface structures (soluble antigens) from being recognized by antibodies and from the attack by cells of the immune system. Through soluble antigens, antibodies are caught, creating immune complexes that inhibit unspecified immune cells such as monocytes/macrophages and natural killer (NK) cells. The prevailing hypothesis at the time was that these blocking factors could be reduced through systemic enzyme therapy (9).

- Infiltrates of leucocytes during the rejection process provided indications of the interaction between macrophages and NK cells in the defense against foreign tissue and tumor cells. Aggregations of leucocytes are formed by means of **adhesion molecules** on tissues and immune cells.

For example, the adhesion molecule ICAM-1 on endothelial cells indicates an area of inflammation where leucocytes dock via the adhesion molecule LFA-1. Tumor cells can also carry adhesion molecules. The adhesion molecule CD44 plays a prominent role in metastasizing cells,

Table 13.1 Distribution of proteolytic enzymes, four to six hours after oral administration			
	Rabbit—4 h after application (% of applied dose)	Guinea pig—4 h after application (% of applied dose)	Sprague-Dawley rats—6 h after application (% of applied dose)
Plasma	2.29	8.49	24.60
Liver	1.35	3.51	0.30
Kidneys	0.45	0.58	1.58
Muscles	17.01	18.90	18.39

because through them tumor cells are able to adhere to lymph nodes or organ tissues.

Various adhesion molecules belong to the so-called "superfamily" of immunoglobulins, such as antibodies, for example. Since the immune complex level was reduced after enzyme therapy, it was examined to what extent enzymes were able to alter comparable adhesion molecules. It was thereby demonstrated that not only was CD44 reduced, but the amount of adhesion molecules of the immune globulin super family on the surface was also reduced on target cells.

A contribution to the reduction of **metastatic risk** could therefore be seen in a reduction in the amount of CD44 on tumor cells. The increase in immune response against tumor cells plays a part in this (Table 13.**2**).

The blocking of cytotoxic activity of macrophages and NK cells through immune complexes has been examined in vitro. Through treatment of macrophages and NK cells with enzymes this blockage was reversed and cytotoxicity increased. This effect depends on the basic initial activity of the cells. Activated cells can only be stimulated to a small degree, or not at all. In tumor patients the immune system often shows a reduced activity because of tumor destructive therapy, but also because some tumor cells emit immune suppressive mediator substances (cytokines) such as transforming growth factor-beta (TGF-β) interleukin-4 (IL-4).

Changes of the in-vitro cytokine profile of NK cells and macrophages following administration of proteolytic enzymes were examined in isolated lymphocytes of plasmacytoma patients. **Tumor necrosis factor-alpha (TNF-α)** plays a critical role in the defense against tumor cells and is often inactive in tumor patients. In blood samples treated with proteolytic enzymes, the inactive TNF-α became tumoricidal again. When the isolated leucocytes were simultaneously incubated with proteolytic enzymes and proinflammatory cytokine interferon-γ, IL-6 was secreted.

Interleukin-6 (IL-6) belongs to the inflammatory cytokines, which indicates that enzymes regulate the interplay of inflammatory cytokines.

In the last few years the Th1/Th2 scheme of immune response has moved to the center of research. The Th1 and Th2 immune reactions (T helper lymphocytes) are determined by different cytokine patterns, each representing another path of the immune response (3).

In studies looking at the pathogenesis of multiple sclerosis it was shown that proteolytic enzymes regulate the **balance of Th1/Th2 cytokines.** The cytokine TGF-β proved to be a key molecule. It regulates the repair of tissues, is an anti-inflammatory cytokine, and inhibits autoimmune diseases. In combination with an elevated level of TGF-β, one finds fibroses, scleroses (arterioscleroses), tumor growth, and metastases. Apparently the tumor growth and metastases through the immune suppressive effect of TGF-β is promoted. In a study on TGF-β-induced nephritic fibrosis in diabetes mellitus it was shown, that orally administered proteolytic enzymes inhibit fibrosis and simultaneously reduce TGF-β.

The reason for this is offered by a fundamental realization of systemic enzyme therapy: When proteolytic enzymes gain entrance into the blood circulation, they bind enzyme inhibitors, especially to α_2-macroglobulin. During the

Table 13.2 Effects of individual enzymes and a standardized enzyme mixture on different components of the immune system				
	Papain	**Chymotrypsin**	**Trypsin**	**sE**
Immune complex splitting	+++	++	–	+++
Inhibition of IC splitting	–	+	++	++
Complement activation	–	–	+++	+++
NK cells	+	+	++	+++
Macrophage induction	+	+	++	+++
Receptor modulation	++	++	++	+++

+/–, effects of the enzymes on receptors or adhesion molecules; IC, immune complex; sE, standardized enzyme mixture made up of papain, chymotrypsin, trypsin.

binding of hydrolases/proteases to the α_2-macroglobulin the molecule changes its form and characteristics. This α_2-macroglobulin-hydrolase/protease complex can bind a variety of cytokines. If the complex is removed from the circulation, elevated cytokine levels can be reduced in this way (4).

▬ Experimental Studies

- In experience-based medicine proteolytic enzymes are orally administered for a **reduction of side effects** of chemotherapy and radiation therapy. In animal studies this empirical finding has been verified.
  - The cytostatic agent **bleomycin** induced the production of TGF-β, which causes fibrosis of the lungs. With concomitant administration of proteolytic enzymes the pulmonary cytotoxicity of bleomycin was significantly reduced.
  - The cytostatic agent **cisplatin**, used in the therapy of ovarian cancer as well as head and neck tumors, causes damage of the spleen. With the concomitant administration of proteolytic enzymes these damaging effects can be clearly reduced depending on the dosage in rats.
- Influence of tumor growth and metastasis: the efficacy of systematic enzyme therapy can be proved for two types of tumors in mice (B16 melanoma and Lewis lung cancer). The survival time of animals with melanoma was significantly prolonged and was associated with histologically smaller metastases. In the Lewis cancer the positive effect of proteolytic enzymes was even more pronounced. Animals that had received proteolytic enzymes 24 hours before tumor transplantation showed a significantly increased survival rate compared with the control group during the period of observation (7).

▬ Clinical Studies

For defined, standardized mixtures of proteolytic enzymes (as well as for the enzyme bromelain alone) the following effects were verified:
- immune modulation
- immune stimulation
- antitumor activities
- antimetastatic activities
- anti-infectious activities.

In addition, several well-documented application observations exist that demonstrate an influence on the defense readiness and quality of life in plasmacytoma, breast, and colorectal cancer patients (reduced side effects of tumor-destructive measures). These application observations were ultimately verified in Good Epidemiological Practices (GEP)-compliant (2, 5, 6) cohort studies, which have been accepted by the European Union as proof of efficacy. Therefore, the Food and Drug Administration recognized a first cohort study for the indication of plasmacytoma (enzyme therapy as a complementary measure to the standard therapy regimen) giving it "orphan drug" status. Enzyme therapy has therefore successfully made the leap into "evidence-based medicine."

Plasmacytoma

Since 1987, Sakalová in Bratislava has treated a proportion of her plasmacytoma patients with oral proteolytic enzymes complementary with standard therapy. In 1997, the data of all patients treated and documented for plasmacytoma in the context of an optimized retrospective cohort study in parallel groups was gathered. The proper conditions for such a study were adhered to.

Out of 333 identified patients, 265 fulfilled the inclusion and exclusion criteria. Patients with stages I–III plasmacytoma according to Durie and Salmon, who had received optimized chemotherapy, were allocated to the therapy group if they had received a minimum of six months of proteolytic enzyme therapy. The patients of the control group had not received enzyme therapy. The initial decision by the examiner, whether the patient should receive therapy was completely at random and not determined by any prognostic considerations. The dose-standardized enzyme therapy started together with chemotherapy and continued with a reduced dosage after the second year.

As a basic therapy patients received an optimized chemotherapy (Methyl prednisolone, Vincristine, Cyclophosphamide, CCNU, Melphalan [MOCCA] or Vincristine, Melphalan, Cyclophosphamide, Prednisone [VMCP]) in four-week to six-week intervals until occurrence of a remission and following that in four-month to eight-month intervals. From stage IIA onwards patients with bone lesions either received bisphosphonates and/or vitamin D.

The data were collected according to the current standard and subjected to an independent audit. The evaluation was carried out with various statistical testing procedures, where the primary efficacy criterion was the survival of the patients examined with Kaplan–Meier analysis and Cox regression analysis.

Secondary efficacy criteria were the first positive response to therapy, the duration of the first remission, and the tolerability of systemic enzyme therapy.

For patients with stage III the median survival time of 47 months in the control group was prolonged to 83 months through oral enzymes ($P_{logrank}$ = 0.0014). A significant prolongation of survival was also verified for the overall group of patients with all stages I–III (adjusted sample $P_{logrank}$ = 0.0003). Due to the insufficient time of observation, no median survival time was given. The significant prolongation of survival was still valid, when in an "intention-to-treat" analysis all patients who had received proteolytic enzymes at least once were allocated to the therapeutic group.

Sensitivity analyses resulted in no indications as to relevant differences between the patient groups. The covariates age, sex, and known risk factors proved to be without influence (secretory myeloma type, paraprotein in the serum, osteolysis, recurrent infections). The disease stage was of relevance, where the risk increased with the advancement of the stage, and the therapy with proteolytic enzymes reduced the estimated mortality risk by 50–60%. Through systematic enzyme therapy the response rate was higher and the duration of remission was longer. An early and long-lasting first remission was an important prognostic factor for patient survival.

Proteolytic enzymes were tolerated without problems by the patients: only 3.6% of patients showed low to moderate gastrointestinal complaints. In the context of this study, the mixture of proteolytic enzymes was therefore recognized with an "orphan drug" status.

Breast Cancer

The influence of disease symptoms and the influence of side effects through other therapeutic measures were chosen as primary efficacy criteria.

Overall, data from 2339 patients who suffered from primary nonmetastasizing breast cancer and received all standard therapies (surgical operation with adjuvant tumor-destructive chemotherapy, radiotherapy, and hormone therapy) were collected. Further complementary medicine measures were also possible. In the therapeutic group, 1283 patients were complementarily treated with proteolytic enzymes over a median duration of about 10 months. The control group consisted of 1056 patients who had not received complementary enzymes.

Since the data of a sufficiently large number of patients without complementary therapy (n = 410) were available, a relevant subgroup was formed for analysis of the results: systemic enzyme therapy *without* further complementary medical measures (n = 239).

The **tolerability of enzymatic therapy** was studied in the overall sample of all 1283 patients. In over 2.3% of all patients side effects were reported that were attributed to enzyme therapy. These were mainly low to moderately pronounced gastrointestinal complaints, which were controlled, if necessary, through a reduction in dose. By nature, one must assume that in such a retrospective retrieval of data the incidences of side effects would be lower than in prospective studies. Nonetheless, similar studies in which the control group received a standard therapy, showed that serious side effects were most definitely recorded by the therapist in patient charts. In conclusion it can therefore be said that proteolytic enzymes as a complementary therapy of breast cancer basically do not cause any additional problems with respect to tolerability.

For the proof of efficacy, 239 enzyme-treated patients were compared with 410 patients in the control groups for the initial monotherapy groups. The outcome showed a significant and clinically relevant superiority of the enzyme group. Enzymes stabilized and improved the condition of the patients, partially due to a significant reduction in the number and severity of side effects induced by radiation and chemotherapy.

In the control group 45% of patients showed side effects, whereas the incidence was only 25%

in the enzyme-treated group. Enzymes had an especially beneficial effect on the therapy or disease-specific symptoms of nausea, loss of appetite, gastrointestinal complaints, headache, fatigue/exhaustion, disturbances in memory and concentration, fatigue, and restlessness. The total symptom score was significantly influenced to a clinically relevant degree.

In the monotherapy groups, an explorative analysis was conducted for the time until appearance of events such as tumor remission, metastasis, and death for the various UICC stages. The patient numbers and period of observation were sufficient for the UICC stages IIA/IIB in order to obtain a significant outcome trend: the time until emergence of an event (tumor remission, metastasis, and death) was significantly longer in the enzyme group (2).

Colorectal Cancer

The study design and conductance complied for the most part with the approach described for breast cancer. Overall, data were collected from 1242 patients with a primary tumor of variable size and dissemination. The 616 patients in the enzyme-treated group received defined amounts of the standardized enzyme preparation over a median period of about nine months.

In the control group without enzyme therapy, 626 patients were retrieved that had received a basic tumor-destructive therapy, as had the patients in the enzyme group. Both groups were divided into subgroups that had either received additional complementary therapies (combination therapy group) or not (monotherapy group).

The groups were comparable in regard to their basic data, risk factors, prognostic criteria, and conventional therapies. The tolerability of enzyme therapy was practically identical with the observa-

tions made in the group of breast cancer patients (see above).

The influence on symptoms of disease and the influence on side effects of toxic therapeutic measures were considered as primary efficacy parameters. Besides the multivariate analysis of disease symptoms and side effects of chemotherapy or radiation therapy (Mann–Whitney test)—a method utilized solely, at first, in breast cancer—the data were evaluated in an independent propensity-matched pairs analysis, which revealed the significant and clinically relevant superiority of complementary, systematic enzyme therapy. A matched pairs analysis confirmed the results.

Proteolytic enzymes administered as a complementary treatment improved the therapy-specific and disease-specific symptoms of nausea, vomiting, loss of appetite, diarrhea, headaches, fatigue, depression, disturbances in concentration and memory, restlessness, and sleep disturbances. A notable reduction in the number and severity of chemotherapy and radiation therapy-induced side effects was seen in the enzyme-treated group. In the control group 24.1 % of patients reported side effects, whereas the incidence in the enzyme-treated group was merely 9.5 %.

For the overall sample size of all 1242 patients, the survival time for the various Dukes stages an explorative analysis was performed with the propensity-matched pairs technique. For patients with stage Dukes D, a prolongation in survival was documented in the enzyme group (5).

The analysis of survival time was not a primary objective of the study in both breast cancer and colorectal cancer. The periods of observation were insufficient for a comprehensive and complete Kaplan–Meier analysis. These data can therefore only be first hints of a possible life-prolonging effect of complementarily administered enzymes. It is planned to obtain the missing observation times through a follow-up evaluation of survival times of

Table 13.3 Proteolytic enzymes as complementary treatment								
Study	Tumor	Agent	QoL	AE	Remission/ metastases	Survival time	References
Retrospective	Breast cancer	sE	↑ *	↓ *	↓ *	↑	2
Retrospective	Colorectal cancer	sE	↑ *	↓ *	↓ *	↑	5
Retrospective	Plasmacytoma	sE	↑ *	↓ *	↓ *	↑ *	6

*A statistically significant study is required; QoL: quality of life; retrospective: GEP-compliant cohort study (EBM-level 2); sE: standardized enzyme mixture (papain, trypsin, chymotrypsin); AE: adverse effects.

the patients from these retrospective studies (Table 13.**3**).

Summary

Systematic enzyme therapy has stood the test as a complementary measure to the established tumor-destructive standard therapies in oncology. Valid study outcomes prove that side effects of tumor-destructive therapies can be reduced. This has a direct, positive influence on the quality of life of the patient on the one hand, and also enables the optimal administration of chemotherapy and radiation therapy cycles, which can be decisive from an overall therapeutic viewpoint. Patients whose tumor diseases are diagnosed and treated at an early stage, profit from the therapy with proteolytic enzymes, partially due to immunomodulatory, antiedematous effects that cause reduction in swelling of tissues and promote wound healing, while the improvement in quality of life is therapeutically relevant in the palliative area.

References

1. Beard J: The Enzyme Therapy of Cancer. London, UK: Chatto and Windus Publ.; 1911.
2. Beuth J, Ost B, Pakdaman A, et al.: Impact of complementary oral enzyme application on the postoperative treatment results of breast cancer patients. Results of an epidemiological multicentre retrospective cohort study. Cancer Chemother. Pharmacol. 2001; 47:45–54.
3. Desser L, Holomanova D, Zavadova E, Pavelka K, Mohr T, Herbacek I: Oral therapy with proteolytic enzymes decreases TGF-β levels in human blood. Cancer Chemother. Pharmacol. 2001; 47:10–15.
4. Lauer D, Müller R, Otto A, Naumann M, Birkenmeier G: Modulation of growth factor binding properties of α-2 macroglobulin by enzyme therapy. Cancer Chemother. Pharmacol. 2001; 47:4–9.
5. Popiela T, Kulig J, Hanisch J, Bock PR: Influence of a complementary treatment with oral enzymes on patients with colorectal cancers. An epidemiological retrospective cohort study. Cancer Chemother. Pharmacol. 2001; 47:55–63.
6. Sakalova A, Bock PR, Dedik L, et al.: Retrospective cohort study of an additive therapy with an oral enzyme preparation in patients with multiple myeloma. Cancer Chemother. Pharmacol. 2001; 47:38–44.
7. Wald M, Olejar T, Seokova V, Zadinova M, Boubelik M, Ponchkova P: Mixture of trypsin, chymotrypsin and papain reduces formation of metastases and extends survival time of C57Bl6 mice syngeneic melanoma B-16. Cancer Chemother. Pharmacol. 2001; 47:16–22.
8. Wolf M, Ransberger K: Enzymtherapie. Vienna, Austria: Mandrich Verlag; 1970.
9. Wrba H: Kombinierte Tumortherapie. Grundlagen, Möglichkeiten und Grenzen der adjuvanten Methoden; Stuttgart, Germany: Hippokrates Verlag; 1995.

14 Lectin-Standardized Mistletoe Extracts

Josef Beuth

Origin of the Mistletoe Extract Therapy

Mistletoe (*Viscum album* L.) has been prescribed as a natural remedy by Hippocrates, by the Druids, and by Arabian physicians long before Rudolf Steiner in the 1920s promoted aqueous extracts from mistletoe for treating tumors according to so-called anthroposophical considerations.

Aqueous mistletoe extracts have a complex composition. Since the early 1950s, various mistletoe constituents have been isolated, e. g., low molecular weight substances (phenolic vegetable acids, flavonoids) and high molecular weight compounds (viscotoxins, polysaccharides, glycoproteins/lectins).

It was only through further development of analytical test procedures at the beginning of the 1980s that it became possible to isolate active plant substances in larger quantities, characterize them, and evaluate at least some of their pharmacological activity.

In the context of these studies, it became clear that the immunological effect of mistletoe extracts partly depended on their lectin content. Qualitatively, mistletoe lectins are divided into two groups according to their sugar specificity: galactoside-specific (Gal) lectin and *N*-acetylgalactosamine-specific (GalNAc) lectin.

The Gal lectin (mistletoe lectin 1, ML-1) predominates in mistletoes from deciduous trees, while the GalNAc lectin is found primarily in mistletoes of coniferous trees.

At present, several mistletoe preparations are available on the German market that are manufactured according to different processes. Mistletoes from different host trees are harvested and processed at different times of the year. Defined anthroposophical manufacturing procedures subject the mistletoe extract to fermentation by *Lactobacillus* species, a process that partly degrades the ML-1 lectin.

So far, aqueous mistletoe extracts have been classified by evidence-based medicine as falling into the group of therapeutics that have a supposed, but not yet sufficiently proved, clinical efficacy. In order to allow for their responsible application according to scientific criteria, mistletoe preparations were tested for their biological activity. It is primarily due to the identification of an immunoactive component (ML-1) and the evaluation of its properties that the clinical administration of mistletoe extracts was standardized and thus became relevant for scientifically oriented medicine (1).

Mechanism of Action and the Application of Mistletoe Extracts in Medicine

The following mechanisms of action are currently postulated for mistletoe extracts:
- cytotoxicity
- modulation of the immune response
- stimulation of the immune response
- induction of apoptosis
- stabilization of DNA.

The cytotoxic effect of mistletoe extracts is dose dependent and can be demonstrated in vitro. Apart from mistletoe lectins, there are obviously other components responsible for the cytotoxic effect, but their detailed analysis is still pending.

It has been demonstrated for ML-1, as well as other mistletoe lectins, that their in-vitro cytotoxicity is nonspecific. Depending on the mode of application (intratumoral, intravenous, intracavitary), this property could possibly be used for treatment in oncology.

The immunomodulator activity of mistletoe extracts seems promising, for example, in the treatment of rheumatoid diseases, which are usually characterized by immunological dysregulation of T lymphocyte subpopulations (helper/inducer T cells, CD4; suppressor/cytotoxic T cells, CD8). The CD4/CD8 cell ratio is characteristically altered in rheumatoid diseases and manifests itself especially through an increase in CD4 cells, resulting finally in an increased ratio. The starting point for immunomodulation in rheumatoid diseases seems to be the regulation of both CD4/CD8 ratio and Th1/Th2 ratio, and this is usually followed by the suspension of symptoms. It is currently not completely established which of the components of mistletoe extracts are in the end responsible for immunomodulation. Although ML-1 is a potent immunomodulating component, it is the efficacy of homeopathic and ML-1-deficient mistletoe extracts that seems to indicate that other components must be involved in the immunomodulating activity (9).

Mistletoe extracts contain several immunostimulating principles, e. g., polysaccharides, vesicular structures, and mistletoe lectins. While polysaccharides and vesicles have not yet been sufficiently evaluated with respect to their immunological activities, it is especially the immunological reactivity of mistletoe lectins that has been demonstrated in recent years.

There are diverse application schemes for inducing optimal effects by mistletoe extracts. For immunomodulation, mistletoe extracts are taken orally and by inhalation or are administered by intracutaneous, subcutaneous, intravenous, and sometimes intracavitary injections. When using mistletoe extracts as an immunomodulating substance, it should be noted that ML-1 especially must be administered in the optimal dose, because otherwise the immunomodulation achieved might be less than optimal. This measure is valid for all forms of application.

If the cytotoxicity of mistletoe lectins is to be used therapeutically, higher dosages are usually required than in the case of immunoactivation or immunomodulation. Such **high-dose therapies** can be administered by intravenous, intratumoral, or intracavitary injection, but they have not been evaluated scientifically. The mistletoe extracts would be assessed in this case like cytostatic agents, no matter which of its components is responsible for the effect.

Considering the multiple mechanisms of action and forms of application of mistletoe extracts, with special reference to the introduction of mistletoe preparations by R. Steiner to anthroposophical cancer therapy, it is no wonder that in various medical fields (such as anthroposophy, naturopathy, homeopathy) mistletoe therapy has been practiced for a long time in oncology patients, while evidence-based medicine has so far rejected this type of treatment because of insufficient evaluation.

From the scientific point of view, anthroposophical as well as homeopathic preparations of mistletoe extract are prepared according to their respective doctrines. Manufacturers declare procedures for the standardization of manufacturing (such as procedure standardization, biological standardization, dilution according to the regulations of the German Homeopathic Pharmacopeia, HAB 1). The scientific relevance of these standardization procedures remains in dispute (4).

▬ Experimental Studies

Under the impression that the lectin–carbohydrate interaction plays a role in immunoregulation and that obvious successes of mistletoe therapy can be traced back to the presence of defined components in the extract, various experimental studies focused on proving the efficacy of ML-1. Initial in-vitro studies (Table 14.**1**) confirmed the immunomodulating activity of ML-1:

- significantly increased expression of activation markers on human/murine mononuclear immunocytes following incubation with ML-1 [e. g., interleukin-2 (IL-2) receptors on T lymphocytes; HLA-DQ antigens on B lymphocytes]
- significantly increased cytokine secretion by human/murine mononuclear immunocytes [e. g., IL-1, IL-2, interferon-γ (IFN-γ), and TNF-α following incubation with ML-1]
- no increased proliferation of tumor cells by ML-1 incubation
- cytotoxic effect on tumor cells (with higher ML-1 doses)
- significantly increased phagocytic activity (chemiluminescence test) of human polymorphonuclear leukocytes (granulocytes) following incubation with ML-1 (1, 4, 8).

Initial designs of in-vivo experiments (Table 14.**1**) yielded results suggesting an involvement of cytokines in the ML-1-induced immunomodulation. In mouse and rabbit models, administration of the optimal ML-1 dose was followed by increased body temperature, increased activity of defined immunocytes, and also by a significant thymus-activating effect, suggesting that ML-1 strengthens the body's defense mechanism.

Experiments on the immunoactive effect of the GalNAc lectin in the corresponding murine model did not show comparable effects on the number and activity of immunocytes or on the proliferation, maturation, and emigration of thymocytes.

Other experimental studies in murine tumor models indicated a statistically significant reduction of lung metastases (L-1 sarcoma) and liver metastases (RAW 117-H10 lymphosarcoma) following administration of the optimal immunomodulating dose of ML-1. In connection with this experimental design, it also became clear that, in the BALB/c mouse model, regular injections of ML-1 significantly raised the number and activity of cells of the mononuclear phagocyte system (MPS, and other macrophages) as well as the weight of the thymus gland (as the correlate of the lymphatic system).

Because it was feared that ML-1 injections might cause an increase in connective tissue or shift of fluid into the thymus, both of which would imitate thymus-cell proliferation, the number of thymocytes per mg organ weight was determined. Quantitative analysis of the number of thymocytes confirmed the effect of ML-1 on thymocyte proliferation. Statistically, the number of thymocytes was significantly higher after administration of ML-1 than in control animals. This experimental design demonstrates that subcutaneous administration of the optimal immunoactive ML-1 dose obviously induces vigorous proliferation of thymocytes and acts as a stimulus for the maturation of lymphatic cells of both helper/inducer CD4+ phenotype and suppressor/cytotoxic CD8+ phenotype, as demonstrated by means of flow cytometry using monoclonal antibodies. It is interesting to note that the number of double-labeled (CD4+/CD8+) immature thymocytes was also significantly higher in the treatment group than in the control group. Obviously, the injection of ML-1 resulted in an increase in thymocyte proliferation as well as an accelerated maturation into the helper/inducer and suppressor/cytotoxic phenotypes (see above).

It is assumed that accelerated maturation of the lymphatic cells of the thymus is followed by increased emigration of such cells into the peripheral blood. The numbers of peripheral blood lymphocytes (PBL) were therefore analyzed in order to explain the effect of ML-1 on this parameter. It turned out that the absolute PBL number was clearly higher after treatment with ML-1. This increase was not statistically significant when compared with the untreated control group, but it clearly was higher than the biological or statistical range of scatter.

The state of PBL activity was analyzed by flow cytometry, and the analysis showed a statistically significant enhancement in the expression of activation markers (IL-2 receptors) on the PBL of ML-1-treated mice as compared with untreated control animals.

Administration of the optimal immunoactive ML-1 dose in BALB/c mice is followed by the maturation and emigration of T lymphocytes, and activated stages of these cells can be detected in the peripheral blood. Further studies are aimed at understanding the basic mechanisms of this seemingly selective process, which is reminiscent of the activity of thymic hormones or cytokines.

The effects of hydrocortisone as immunosuppressant and of ML-1 as immunoprotective substance (with respect to proliferation, maturation, and emigration of T lymphocytes) were studied in the BALB/c mouse model. The immunosuppressive character of hydrocortisone regarding the parameters investigated (number and maturation of thymocytes, number of lymphocytes and monocytes in the peripheral blood) was confirmed. The immunomodulating ML-1 (in the form of lectin-standardized extract) showed distinct immunoprotective properties when administered in the optimal dose. This was evident from wide-ranging normalization of values following administration of hydrocortisone 24 hours prior to the start or after the completion of ML-1 therapy (1).

Table 14.1 Experimental data on the in-vitro/in-vivo effects of ML-1 and ML-1-standardized mistletoe extract	
In vitro	**In vivo (murine model)**
↑ Activation of immunocytes	↑ Number of immunocytes (peripheral blood)
↑ Release of cytokines	↑ Activation of immunocytes
↑ Cytotoxicity	↑ Proliferation, maturation, emigration of thymocytes
↓ Proliferation of tumor cells	↑ Immunoprotection under cortisone
↑ Phagocytotic activity of granulocytes	↑ Antibacterial effect
	↑ Antimetastatic effect
	∅ Cellular toxicity following long-term application

▬ Clinical Studies

General Remarks

Within the scope of application-related observations and clinical studies, mistletoe extracts are being administered to cancer patients. Here, too, special emphasis is given to the question whether there are verifiable benefits for the patients. Verification of such benefits, in a scientifically understandable way, is only possible when administering standardized or normalized extracts in an optimal, individualized dose. For this reason, immunological data obtained with nonstandardized or nonnormalized mistletoe extracts must be put in perspective. On the one hand, reproducibility seems questionable; on the other hand, a final verdict would only be possible under statistically defined conditions. Therefore, almost all data obtained so far must be regarded as clues or trends, the adequate statistical evaluation of which is still pending. Another weak point of all existing data on the immunoactive effect of standardized or normalized mistletoe extracts is the small number of probands in the older studies. This always raises the question of how the patients were selected for treatment. Selection bias (overrating of positive results, neglecting negative results) should also be considered, and the data obtained so far should be put into perspective.

It is understood that all criticism and objections are also valid for research results obtained with ML-1 or ML-1-normalized mistletoe extracts. Nevertheless, it should be mentioned here that all protagonists try to record—descriptively and, in some cases, also quantitatively—as many immunological aspects of the respective therapy as possible, for example:

- statistically significant increase in number and activity of defined immunologically competent cells (immunocytes) in cancer patients
- statistically significant increase in acute phase proteins in the serum of cancer patients, induced by the secretion of inflammatory cytokines
- immunoactive effects during or after tumor-destructive measures
- statistically significant increase in plasma β-endorphins, correlating with an increase in the quality of life of cancer patients
- enhancement of ex-vivo or in-vitro release of cytokines (IL-2, IFN-γ, TNF-α) by mononuclear immunocytes of cancer patients following adequate stimulation (3).

All these data strongly suggest immunomodulation in cancer patients following the administration of ML-1-normalized mistletoe extract. Therapeutically, this seems to make sense in so far as the initial tumor-destructive measures are normally followed by (in some cases, long term) immunosuppression in the patient, thus encouraging recurrence and metastasis of tumors and also the development of opportunistic infections. Accordingly, any immunostimulation or immunoprotection induced by ML-1-normalized mistletoe extracts may be regarded as a benefit for the patients. However, the final proof is still pending.

Especially the release of cytokines through activation of mononuclear immunocytes seems important. On the one hand, very different types of tumors (e. g., renal cell carcinoma, colorectal carcinoma, malignant melanoma) are treated in conventional oncology—in part, successfully—by means of cytokine-induced immunotherapy, direct cytokine therapy, combined immunotherapy, and chemotherapy. On the other hand, cytokine induction by ML-1-normalized mistletoe extracts seems to exclude defined tumor types such as lymphoma and leukemia from treatment.

The induction of cytokine secretion by mistletoe extracts seems to be advantageous for **carcinoma** because it stimulates, and keeps going, the complete (anticarcinogenic, anti-infective) cascade of immune reactions. In addition to the optimal dose, the form of application and treatment intervals are important for inducing optimal immunomodulation or immunostimulation by mistletoe extracts.

Within the scope of the discussion on "mistletoe therapy as an experimental form of treatment with preclinically verified risk potential," experimental in-vitro data of tumor cell proliferation induced by mistletoe lectin or cytokines (especially IL-6) as well as experimental in-vivo data of a chemically-induced urinary bladder carcinoma model in the rat are cited, for example, as a basis for assessing the risk potential. The scientific relevance of repeatedly reproduced data in review articles appears to be more than questionable for the following reasons:

- Results of in-vitro or in-vivo studies based on animal experiments cannot be directly applied to the clinical situation.

- In in-vitro experiments, experts of international reputation could detect neither the proliferation of tumor cells nor the release of the cytokine IL-6.

So far, an increased tendency for growth or metastasis of syngeneic murine tumors in vivo could not be demonstrated by means of administering standardized or lectin-normalized mistletoe extracts. However, indisputable anticarcinogenic or antimetastatic effects of standardized or lectin-normalized mistletoe extracts were observed in experimental animal models (1, 4, 8). Seen from this angle, one should always question the topic-oriented expertise of study groups, because they tend to turn experimental in-vitro or in-vivo data into direct proof of a risk potential.

The **dosage of mistletoe extracts** is determined based on the immunoactive component ML-1; for anthroposophical preparations, this is done according to differently weighted application schemes and according to homeopathic criteria. Whereas local reactions are to be expected with intracutaneous application, subcutaneous administration of mistletoe extracts has proved to be an acceptable form of application with few side effects, and it is reliably followed by immunostimulation (e.g., increased number and activity of immunocytes, positive intracutaneous test).

The optimal dosage of mistletoe extracts (and also that of ML-1 and ML-1-normalized extracts) has not undergone sufficient scientific verification for other forms of application, such as intravenous, intracavitary, intratumoral, and oral applications (3, 4, 8).

Special Applications

The majority of clinical studies using standardized mistletoe extracts are flawed with respect to randomization, blinding, stratification, or patient numbers, thus making an adequate scientific evaluation impossible. The shortcomings include:
- unacceptable documentation of the disease (diagnosis, stage, and duration of disease; previous therapies; evaluation of prognostic factors)
- therapeutic intervention, result, and statistics are not understandable or verifiable by the observer
- comparison of data with historic control group
- lack of recording or identifying dropouts.

• This means that the existing data on therapeutic studies using standardized mistletoe extracts fail to meet the scientific criteria currently in force and, therefore, have not yet provided definitive evidence of the efficacy of this therapeutic approach. It should be emphasized here once again that there is always the suspicion of **selection bias**, namely, the tendency to publish positive results and to neglect negative ones. Even though this phenomenon may not apply wholesale to the studies at issue, one should nevertheless notice that almost all existing therapeutic studies have been published in journals without adequate scientific assessment (peer review).

This is the current state of studies on lectin-normalized mistletoe therapy from the scientific point of view. It underlines the need for action regarding further evaluation of studies dealing with this complementary therapeutic measure.

Scientific evaluation of the therapeutic principle of immunomodulation or immunostimulation through lectin-normalized mistletoe extracts has been initiated and partly completed (prospective randomized clinical study; scientifically acceptable documentation and cohort evaluation of application and therapeutic effect with respect to defined tumor types, both in practice and clinic). Table 14.**2** lists landmark studies on lectin-normalized mistletoe therapies.

• At present, there are only two studies available (in the form of peer reviewed publications) which more or less meet the current scientific demands for a prospective randomized, multicenter, controlled study design. In both of these studies, patients with squamous cell carcinoma of the head and neck received adjuvant/complementary treatment with a lectin-normalized mistletoe preparation; patients in the control group received only the consensus standard therapies. Within the scope of these studies, it could not be documented that patients benefit from adjuvant lectin-normalized mistletoe therapy. The measured parameters included quality of life, undesired drug reactions of the tumor-destructive standard therapy, time free of relapses and metastases, survival time, and immunological responses. Based on data existing so far, the authors concluded that head-and-neck squamous cell carcinoma—

Study	Tumor	Mistletoe preparation	IM	QoL	ST	Publication
Table 14.2 Studies on lectin-standardized mistletoe therapy						
1. Prospective, randomized, multicenter, placebo-controlled	Mammary carcinoma	Lektinol		+*		(12)
2. Prospective, randomized, multicenter	Head-and-neck (metastatic) SCC	Eurixor				(11)
3. Prospective, randomized, multicenter	Head-and-neck SCC	Eurixor				(11)
4. Prospective, randomized	Glioblastoma	Eurixor	+*	+	+[1]	(7)
5. Prospective, randomized	Mammary carcinoma	Eurixor	+*	+		(6)
6. Prospective, randomized	Colon carcinoma	Eurixor	+*	+		(5)
7. Cohort study	Mammary carcinoma	Eurixor		+*		(10)

[1] Grade IV; +, improved; * statistically significant; IM, immunomodulation; QoL, quality of life; SCC, squamous cell carcinoma; ST, survival time.

which is very difficult to treat and often resistant to treatment—does not belong to the indications of lectin-normalized mistletoe therapy (11).

Transferring the data from these studies to other tumor types or stages is scientifically not permissible; it is even wrong. This is especially so because the adjuvant therapeutic concepts (chemotherapy or radiation therapy in addition to surgery) are not yet very promising for patients with (advanced) head-and-neck squamous cell carcinoma, and also because defined risk factors (such as alcohol and nicotine consumption) jeopardize therapeutic interventions or patient compliance.

Especially the local, mucosa-specific immunosuppression that accompanies the chronic addictive constellation of many patients with squamous cell carcinoma of the head and neck (i.e., alcohol and nicotine abuse) were responsible for this patient cohort's failure to benefit from adjuvant lectin-normalized mistletoe therapy. According to the authors, more detailed studies are required in order to counteract a possible distortion of study results (bias), for example, by certain risk constellations especially in cases of head-and-neck squamous cell carcinoma.

Detailed analysis seems to be essential in order to arrive at a final verdict on adjuvant lectin-normalized mistletoe therapy in patients with head-and-neck squamous cell carcinoma. The most important parameters for such studies include:

- analysis according to stage and location of the tumor and according to the surgical method used
- consideration of risk factors and prognosis
- evaluation of patient compliance
- exploration of patient histories and possible biometric correction of other complementary measures (using the propensity score)
- identification of center-associated effects with respect to surgery or surgery plus radiation therapy.

• In a study that conformed to good clinical practices (GCP-compliant study), women patients with **mammary carcinoma** received a lectin-normalized mistletoe preparation to complement standard therapy. After surgery, at the start of CMF chemotherapy, the patients received the medication to be studied (lectin-normalized mistletoe preparation) or a placebo over a period of 15 weeks. The intention-to-treat analysis resulted in a significant advantage for the treatment group as compared with the placebo group with respect to the criterion of the main objective, namely, to influence undesired drug reactions of the standard therapy or the quality of life (10).

So far, this landmark study has not been published in a peer-reviewed journal, and the results must therefore be regarded as preliminary. The design of the study (including documentation and biometric analysis) meets all requirements of evidence-based medicine and, once published in adequate form, will require conventional medicine to redefine its position toward mistletoe therapy. Until recently, conventional oncology has assigned mistletoe therapy to natural philosophy, pseudomedicine, or even magic. The result of this study is confronting us with a new situation, because even "the skeptical conventional physician can no longer ignore certain forms of mistletoe preparation" (G. Nagel, Freiburg, Germany).

- Thirty-eight patients with **malignant glioma (WHO grades III/IV)** were enrolled in a controlled clinical trial (7). All patients were subjected to the internationally recommended standard oncological therapy (microsurgical tumor extirpation, radiation, basic clinical attendance according to consensus and indication) and randomized into treatment and control groups. The treatment group received complementary immunotherapy with lectin-normalized mistletoe extract, whereas the control group received no complementary treatment. The final analysis of this study showed:
  - a significant improvement of immunity and quality of life in the treatment group as compared with the control group
  - a tendency toward a prolonged relapse-free period for patients in the treatment group (17.4 ± 8.2 months) as compared with the control group (10.5 ± 3.9 months)
  - a statistically significant (Breslow $P = 0.035$) extension of total survival time for WHO Grade IV glioblastoma patients in the treatment group (20.5 ± 3.5 months) as compared with the control group (9.9 ± 2.1 months).

These promising findings should be confirmed in a GCP-compliant, prospective, randomized multicenter study. The final proof of the efficacy of the lectin-normalized mistletoe therapy in the case of glioblastoma has not yet been produced.

▬ Summary

In the studies carried out so far, the immunoactive effect of ML-1 was demonstrated unambiguously. So far, no adverse effects worth mentioning have occurred under therapeutic ML-1 administration. We might therefore consider an adequate immunotherapy for cancer patients to expand the therapeutic spectrum by controlled strengthening of the body's defense mechanisms. From a scientific, complementary medicine point of view, one should administer ML-1-normalized preparations because the immunoactive effect of aqueous mistletoe extracts is predominantly induced by ML-1. One possibility is the regular injection of an optimal immunostimulating ML-1 dose without having to worry about harmful overdosing or ineffective underdosing.

▬ Outlook

The documentation of improvements in the quality of life with lectin-normalized mistletoe preparations should be viewed as a start of the further scientific and clinical development of this classic phytotherapy. The purpose of subsequent controlled clinical studies should be to examine the anticancer effects of lectin-normalized mistletoe extracts, pure ML-1, and recombinant ML-1, all of which have been demonstrated in animal experiments. In addition, it should be checked whether improvement in the quality of life by lectin-normalized mistletoe therapy also increases compliance of cancer patients so that optimization of tumor-destructive therapeutic measures becomes possible.

▬ References

1. Beuth J, Köhler W, Pulverer G (eds): Specific Adherence Mechanisms in Microbiology and Immunology. D. Akademie der Naturforscher Leopoldina, 1997.
2. Beuth J, Stoffel B, Pulverer G: Mistletoe lectins. Clinically relevant immunomodulators. Nova Acta Leopoldina. 1997; 75:89–94.
3. Beuth J: Clinical relevance of immunoactive mistletoe lectin-1. Anticancer Drugs. 1997; 8:53–55.
4. Büssing A (ed.): Mistletoe. The Genus Viscum. Harwood Academic Publ., 2000.
5. Heiny BM, Albrecht V, Beuth J: Lebensqualitätsstabilisierung durch Mistellektin-1-normierten Extrakt beim fortgeschrittenen kolorektalen Karzinom. Onkologe. 1998; 1:35–39.
6. Heiny BM, Beuth J: Mistletoe extract standardized for the galactoside-specific lectin (ML-1) induces β-endorphin release and immunopotentiation in breast cancer patients. Anticancer Res. 1994; 14: 1339–1342.

7. Lenartz D, Dott U, Menzel J, Beuth J: Survival of glioma patients after complementary treatment with galactoside-specific lectin from mistletoe. Anticancer Res. 2000; 20:2073–2076.
8. Scheer R, Bauer R, Becker H, Berg PA, Fintelmann V (eds): Die Mistel in der Tumortherapie. Grundlagenforschung und Klinik. Essen, KVC Verlag, 2001.
9. Scheer R, Becker H, Berg PA (eds): Grundzüge der Misteltherapie. Stuttgart, Hippokrates Verlag 1996.
10. Schumacher K, Schneider B, Reich G, et al.: Influence of complementary treatment with lectin-standardized misteltoe extract on breast cancer patients. A controlled epidemiological multicentric retrolective cohort study. Anticancer Res. 2003; 23: 5081–5088
11. Steuer-Vogt M, Bonkovsky V, Ambrosch P, et al.: The effect of adjuvant mistletoe treatment programme in resected head and neck cancer patients. A randomized controlled clinical trial. Eur. J. Cancer. 2001; 37:23–31.
12. Semiglasov VF, Stepula VV, Dudov A, et al.: The standardized mistletoe extract PS76A2 improves QoL in patients with breast cancer receiving adjuvant CMF chemotherapy: a randomized, placebo-controlled, double-blind multicenter clinical trial. Anticancer Res. 2004; 24: 1293–1302.

15 Mistletoe Extracts from the Anthroposophical Point of View

Arndt Büssing

Introduction

Treatment of cancer patients with extracts from *Viscum album* L., the white-berried European mistletoe, is one of the most widely used forms of complementary cancer therapy in Europe. Many scientists have pointed out the obvious discrepancy between the popularity of mistletoe extracts in cancer treatment and its classification, by conventional medicine, as a treatment modality of unproved efficacy. Reservations about this form of adjuvant cancer therapy still exist.

Mistletoe extracts have been used in the treatment of cancer patients since the beginning of the twentieth century. Their introduction in cancer therapy by the philosopher Rudolf Steiner was not based on an empirical acquisition of knowledge through experiments, as is standard procedure today, but on ideas in the field of Humanities (13). The therapeutical principles of mistletoe uses in Anthroposophical Medicine are described in detail by Fintelmann (for a review, see ref. 13). Upon Steiner's suggestion, injectable mistletoe preparations were developed for the treatment of cancer patients, and these have been used exclusively by anthroposophical physicians. Meanwhile, mistletoe therapy has stepped out of the sphere of anthroposophy and has also been used by physicians who see themselves as belonging to a more conventionally oriented medicine. In Germany, the approval of mistletoe extracts for treating cancer patients is based on the monographs of Commission C (*Anthroposophic Medicine*) and Commission E (*Phytotherapy*) of the former Federal Health Department.

Mistletoe Extracts

Unlike manufacturers of phytotherapeutic mistletoe extracts, the pharmaceutical companies claiming to produce mistletoe extracts according to Steiner's suggestions use juices from mistletoe harvested in both summer and winter. These juices are then mixed by using a special whirling process. From the anthroposophical point of view, it is this special process that creates the effective medication.

The fresh leaves, short branches, and mistletoe berries—and sometimes the layer (rooting shoot)—are used for producing the extracts (Table 15.**1**). Depending on the manufacturer, the mistletoe plant is either subjected to fermentation, pressed, or extracted with cold water (8).

Pharmaceutical manufacturers with an anthroposophical orientation offer mistletoe preparations derived from different host trees. Mistletoe from apple trees is primarily used for treating women with mammary carcinoma, while mistletoe from oak or pine trees is used more frequently for tumors in men. This peculiarity also goes back to recommendations by Steiner, who assigned mistletoe plants derived from certain host trees to certain organ systems. There is still no definite evidence of a tumor-specific effect of mistletoe from certain host trees. One cannot suggest that the application of mistletoe extract from a defined host tree should be recommended for the treatment of a particular type of cancer. Nevertheless, when choosing a preparation for the patient, it may be of advantage to know that mistletoes derived from different host trees are believed to have different potencies.

In anthroposophical medicine, only the specially mixed mistletoe juice, rather than a single defined ingredient, is regarded as effective medication. Nevertheless, clinically relevant reactions can still be assigned to certain constituents (Fig. 15.**1**).

In the 1990s, the main interest of scientific research on mistletoe (to which anthroposophical medicine is not explicitly in opposition) was directed toward mistletoe lectins. These proteins have reproducible pharmacological activities even in nanogram concentrations, whereas other substances require distinctly higher concentrations.

Currently, the most important effects that have been confirmed experimentally are:

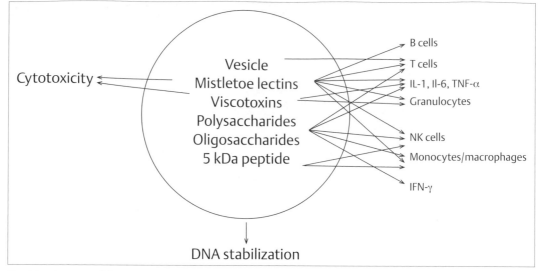

Fig. 15.1 Overview of the immunomodulating effects of defined *Viscum album* constituents.

– induction of programmed cell death (apoptosis)
– modulation of the immune response
– protection of DNA against chemotherapeutic agents (8, 9).

The cytotoxic effects of mistletoe extracts can be assigned to mistletoe lectins as well as viscotoxins, while the immunomodulating effects are not restricted to mistletoe lectins but are also induced by polysaccharides and oligosaccharides, and viscotoxins (Fig. 15.**1**).

▬ Experimental Studies

After administering mistletoe extract to cancer patients by injection, a circumscribed reddening of the skin may occur at the injection site, and this may be accompanied by a rise in body temperature. If one imagines the tumor as "condensed cold," this "cold" can then be "dispersed" by the "heat" of the mistletoe. The patient is thus motivated to tackle the tumor as well as his/her surroundings; the patient is stimulated to become more active again, to "warm" to his/her social milieu. According to Steiner, the tumor can only disperse if one succeeds in "wrapping the growth into a warm coat," i.e., if the mistletoe injection produces fever. The local reaction and febrile condi-

tion are immunological reactions to the injection of "foreign" material to which the body must respond. The "warm coat" can be compared with peritumoral (inflammatory) infiltration: the immunocompetent cells begin to attack the tumor cells.

To explain the therapeutic approach of using mistletoe extract, at least three hypotheses are being discussed that can be tested in scientific studies: cytotoxicity, immunomodulation, and enhancing the quality of the patient's life. They are discussed in detail in the following sections.

Cytotoxicity

Generally speaking, there is a higher tendency toward cell proliferation within the tumor than in the normal tissue; the tumor cells have become largely independent from the death signals that limit the growth of cells. Mistletoe extracts induce apoptotic cell death in tumor cells as well as nonmalignant cells (8, 9). The apoptosis-inducing potentials of mistletoe extracts derived from different host trees correlate closely with the contents of cytotoxic mistletoe lectins, while necrotic cell death is rather caused by viscotoxins—as becomes evident when using very high concentrations of viscotoxins.

Table 15.1 Affected lymphocyte populations (2)	
Mistletoe lectin I	• Eliminates primarily CD16$^+$/CD56$^+$ CD8-NK cells
Mistletoe lectin III	• Eliminates primarily CD8$^+$ lymphocytes (phenotype of suppressor/memory CD8$^+$ CD28$^+$ CD62L^{lo} T cells)
Less sensitive to mistletoe lectin III	• CD8$^+$ CD28$^+$ CD62L^{hi} naïve/cytotoxic T cells • CD4$^+$ T helper/inducer lymphocytes • CD19$^+$ B cells

Mistletoe Lectins

Mistletoe lectins are ribosome-inactivating proteins that differ from each other with regard to sugar specificity and molecular weight (50–63 kDa). Mistletoe lectin I binds to D-galactose, while mistletoe lectin II and mistletoe lectin III bind to N-acetylgalactosamine (8, 9).

Mistletoe lectins cause inhibition of protein biosynthesis in cell-free systems and apoptosis in cultured cells. A few minutes after incubating human lymphocytes with mistletoe lectins, there is an increase in intracellular Ca^{2+}, which is regarded as expression of a "receptor-mediated signal." A few hours later, membrane changes (blebbing) and chromatin condensation with the following aftereffects can be observed (2, 3, 5, 8, 9):
- production of mitochondrial oxygen intermediary products
- expression of mitochondrial Apo-2.7 molecules
- mitochondrial release of cytochrome c
- caspase activation with subsequent degradation of various proteins and kinases
- translocation of phosphatidylserine from the inner to the outer layer of the mitochondrial membrane
- fragmentation of DNA.

Conventional "death receptors" such as Apo-1/Fas (CD95) or TNF receptor type 1—which are of special importance for apoptotic signaling and caspase activation—do not seem to be directly stimulated by mistletoe lectins (8, 9).

In patients with metastasizing tumors (and also in HIV patients), suppressor/memory T cells predominate, while cytotoxic T lymphocytes are underrepresented. Hence, a possible therapeutic approach could be the elimination of these cells in favor of cytotoxic T lymphocytes by treatment with ML-III (Table 15.**2**). It should be investigated whether this selective effect can be utilized in clinical applications.

Incubation of human lymphocytes with mistletoe lectins caused a significant up-regulation of CD95L surface molecules in the surviving lymphocytes (6). This Fas ligand induces apoptosis in Fas$^+$ target cells; hence, the tumor cells should also be attacked by stimulated Fas ligand-positive lymphocytes, in addition to direct mistletoe lectin-induced cell death. It should be clarified how the subcutaneous injection of a mistletoe preparation can yield a "distant" effect by means of activated lymphocytes, although these do not seem to proliferate.

Viscotoxins

- Viscotoxins belong to the family of α-thionines and β-thionines, a group of alkaline cysteine-rich polypeptides with a molecular weight of 5 kDa. The toxicity of viscotoxins has been determined primarily in animal experiments. In cats, intravenous administration of viscotoxins at a final concentration of 0.1 mg/kg body weight resulted in the death of all animals, while the LD$_{50}$ in mice was 0.5 mg/kg body weight (27). Application of viscotoxins at low concentrations caused a drop in blood pressure, bradycardia, and negative inotropy of the heart.
- Incubation of human lymphocytes or Molt-4 leukemia cells with viscotoxins caused rapid permeabilization of the cell membrane, swelling of mitochondria associated with a loss of their cristae, and the formation of oxygen metabolites within a few minutes or hours (3–5). This indicated accidental (necrotic) cell death. Unlike in granulocytes, it seemed as if the formation of reactive oxygen metabolites in lymphocytes and tumor cells was no longer compensated by the cellular redox systems (such as glutathione) (4).
- Viscotoxins thus induce necrotic cell death, which leads to rupture of the cell membrane and release of cell organelles into the intercellular space and, therefore, causes inflammatory

tissue reactions. By contrast, mistletoe lectins cause apoptotic cell death, which causes condensation of the cell into apoptotic bodies that are phagocytosed by the neighboring cells without inducing inflammatory tissue reactions.

- According to the above-mentioned working model, viscotoxins cause a "dispersing reaction" (or "heat"), while mistletoe lectins cause a "condensing reaction" (or "cold")—which is the physiological state of the body.
- The direct cytotoxic effect of mistletoe extracts can be demonstrated in an impressive way in cell cultures and animal experiments (9, 18). In a clinical setting, however, subcutaneous and intravenous administration hardly yields such an effect. This might be due to the induction of anti-ML antibodies during mistletoe therapy (9, 18), but—even before the formation of antibodies—also to inhibition of mistletoe lectin activity by serum glycoproteins and lipids (25, 26).
- In animal experiments, a clear inhibition of growth and/or prolonged survival times can be achieved by injection of mistletoe extracts in case of the following tumors (9):
  - B16F10 melanoma
  - Dalton lymphoma
  - ascites sarcoma 180
  - Ehrlich carcinoma
  - MB49 bladder carcinoma
  - methylcholanthrene-induced fibrosarcoma.
- It has been shown that intraperitoneal application of a mistletoe extract over a period of 15 weeks can significantly inhibit the develop-

ment of methylcholanthrene-induced sarcoma in C57BL/6 mice (20).

Clinically relevant, mistletoe lectin-mediated cytotoxicity is most likely to be expected with intratumoral application of the extracts, and this has also been described in several individual cases (12, 22–24, 28, 38). When administered systemically, this phenomenon is only observed in exceptional cases and with very high doses.

Immunomodulation

When the immune system is not able to prevent or restrict tumor growth, mistletoe extracts are supposed to activate certain components of the immune system, thus leading to improved immunosurveillance and/or to improved anticancer responses. The nonspecific immune system reacts to the injection of mistletoe extract in multiple ways. It is not yet clear, however, whether these reactions are equivalent to an effective anticancer response.

In individual cases, a connection between increased numbers and improved function of immunocompetent cells—in the sense of improved immunosurveillance—seems obvious (Fig. 15.**2**). However, this cannot be proved convincingly because the immune reactions to the mistletoe extract are similar in most patients within the first three months (increase in CD4$^+$ T helper/inducer lymphocytes, B cells or plasma cells producing anti-ML antibodies, and in part, also CD16$^+$/CD56$^+$

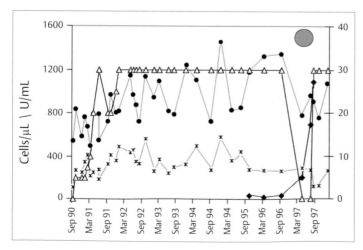

Fig. 15.2 Numbers of CD4$^+$ T helper/inducer (●) and CD16$^+$/CD56$^+$ NK- (x) as a function of the concentration of mistle-toe extract (△) (Helixor M, twice weekly, s. c. injection) applied to one of the patients (MG/f/1943) with metastasizing mammary carcinoma in the care of Professor Schietzel, Communal Hospital, Herdecke, Germany.

After discontinuation of mistletoe extract injections by the patient, the tumor marker (◆), (Ca 15-3) increased and metastases (●), which have not been growing for years, increased rapidly in size. As a result, the patient required chemotherapy and died a year later of pneumonia.

NK cells), but subsequently individual reaction patterns predominate.

The first studies carried out by our team indicate that a rapid **dose increase** should be avoided in the adjuvant treatment of cancer patients with mistletoe extract. The severe local reactions accompanying the treatment (which are, in fact, desirable in patients with metastasizing tumors) may be associated with a functional impairment of T-cell function. Although this impairment is only temporary, it can be avoided by increasing the dose slowly. The dose increase is necessary because of the formation of antibodies to mistletoe lectins. It is also not completely clear whether mistletoe extracts induce Th1-associated rather than Th2-associated immune reactions in the long term.[1]

The contradictory results on this topic can probably be traced back to different study conditions and also to clear differences in the mistletoe extracts used (8, 9, 18). The significance of the Th1/Th2 immune response for evaluating the efficacy of mistletoe therapy is unclear, particularly as one cannot exclude the possibility that there is both a mistletoe extract-induced Th2 response and, simultaneously, a Th1 response directed against the tumor.

With respect to **DNA stabilization**, it has been shown in peripheral lymphocytes that mistletoe extracts inhibit spontaneous DNA damage as well as the DNA damage caused by cyclophosphamide, an alkylating chemotherapeutic agent (8, 9). In addition, there was an improved expression of activation markers on immune cells, though it is normally suppressed by cyclophosphamide. These effects could not be achieved with defined constituents such as mistletoe lectins or viscotoxins. The protective activities were also not detected in leukemic cells, cells from amniotic fluid (i.e., cells derived from all three germ layers), or in animal experiments.

In animal experiments, simultaneous administration of **cyclophosphamide** and mistletoe extract lead to a greater decline in the number of

leukemic cells or lung metastases than chemotherapy alone (8, 9). This could mean that the immune cells were protected at both the DNA level and the functional level.

It is not clear which constituents are responsible for the protective effect, how the effects of mistletoe extracts can be optimized, and how the extract can be best applied. Nevertheless, these effects may possibly be used for alleviating the side effects of chemotherapy, either in the sense that the number and function of immunocompetent cells are less affected and/or the cells recover sooner, or that the patient's subjective condition can be improved.

- Following the injection of mistletoe extracts, distinct changes in the reactions of the immune system have been noticed (1, 8, 9, 18). In mice, Beuth and co-workers observed an increase in peritoneal macrophages, peripheral monocytes, and lymphocytes expressing the interleukin-2 receptor, and also an increase in both thymus weight and thymocyte numbers (9).

- Immune cells react to the "foreign" components of mistletoe extracts with a release of proinflammatory cytokines, in particular. Incubation of human lymphocytes, macrophages, fibroblasts, and other cells with mistletoe lectins or polysaccharides from mistletoe berries was   followed especially by the release of cytokines associated with monocytes/macrophages, namely, interleukin-1β, interleukin-6, and TNF-α (8, 9, 18). Clear interindividual differences were observed in the release of the cytokines interleukin-4 and interferon-γ after in-vitro stimulation of lymphocytes with aqueous extracts or pressed juices from mistletoes of different host trees (30).

- Like mistletoe lectins, viscotoxins also exhibit immunomodulating effects. It has been demonstrated that viscotoxins stimulate the phagocytosis of opsonized *Escherichia coli* and CD8+ T cells by human granulocytes as well as the oxidative burst induced by bacteria (32, 33). Such an improved granulocyte function could not be achieved by mistletoe lectins or by polysaccharides from mistletoe berries (34). These observations may be important for the clinical practice, especially as it was shown that a single intravenous application of a mistletoe extract prior to surgery prevented narcosis and surgical stress associated inhibition of the granulocytes' function (oxidative burst) (10). Moreover, this

---

[1] According to one of the basic postulates of tumor immunology, the Th1-associated immune reactions that lead to cellular cytotoxic immune responses (as recognized, e.g., by the presence of type 1 cytokines—interferon-γ, IL-2, and IL-12—as well as antibodies of types IgG$_1$ and IgG$_3$) are essential for an efficient anticancer response. By contrast, the humoral immune response is represented by the Th2-associated reactions involving type 2 cytokines (IL-4, IL-5, IL-10, and IL-13).

distinct route of application may be a rationale to restrict immunosuppression by surgical stress, which may accelerate the growth and metastasis of residual cancer to a minimum.

- The immunomodulating effects of mistletoe extracts are not only mediated by their cytotoxic components (mistletoe lectins and viscotoxins). Relevant effects have also been described for sugars derived from mistletoe. Rhamnogalacturonan from *Viscum album* seems to activate NK cells and monocytes/macrophages as well as stimulate the release of interferon-γ by CD4$^+$ T helper/inducer lymphocytes and the "bridge building" between CD56$^+$ NK cells and tumor cells. On the other hand, an oligosaccharide isolated from mistletoe extracts stimulated NK cytotoxicity and lead to the release of TNF-α in monocytes/macrophages (1, 8, 9, 18). The stimulation of CD4$^+$ T helper/inducer lymphocytes and the release of interleukin-6 and interferon-γ has been confirmed by incubation of human lymphocytes with polysaccharides from mistletoe berries (arabinogalactan) (33).

Clinical Studies

Immunomodulation

- Whereas mistletoe lectins did not cause T-cell proliferation by themselves, they did enhance polysaccharide-stimulated T-cell activation in some test persons, while inhibiting it in other probands (33). Pronounced interindividual differences were noticed here in the response to a constituent from mistletoe extracts—a phenomenon that might be important when evaluating the response to a mistletoe therapy, especially in the presence of pronounced local reactions. However, the clinical effects of mistletoe extracts depend to a high degree on the form of application.
- In patients with mammary carcinoma, a rise in body temperature and an increase in juvenile granulocytes, but also temporary lymphocytopenia, were observed six hours after **intravenous injection** of mistletoe extract. Within 24 hours, lymphocyte proliferation in vitro improved, the number of NK cells increased, and antibody-dependent, cell-mediated cytotoxicity in the peripheral blood increased. These ef-

fects have been attributed to the activity of the Gal-binding mistletoe lectin (ML-1) (8, 9, 18).

- Within an observation period of four to six weeks, **subcutaneous** injection of mistletoe extracts resulted in the induction of acute phase proteins, peripheral NK and T helper/inducer lymphocytes, and B or plasma cells that produced anti-ML antibodies and proinflammatory cytokines; it also caused the release of β-endorphin (8, 9, 16, 18). However, cancer patients are usually treated with mistletoe extract for several months. Short-term reactions of the immune system to the injection of "foreign" material (especially of mistletoe lectins) are therefore of secondary importance, because the injection of mistletoe extract causes the formation of anti-ML antibodies that inhibit the activity of mistletoe lectins (a fact that might be relevant especially for mistletoe extracts of relatively low ML content). After seven months of treatment with increasing doses of mistletoe extract depending on the local reactions induced, the cancer patients showed only a slight proportional increase in lymphocytes and in the number of NK cells (7), while lymphocytic subpopulations showed only a trend toward improved cell numbers.
- Likewise, in another study (35), significant changes in lymphocytic subpopulations could not be detected during an observation period of 84 weeks (though no dose increase was intended in this study).
- After **intravenous injection** of high doses of aqueous extracts, an increase in juvenile monocytes and granulocytes was observed within 24 hours (8, 9). Studies by Hajto and co-workers (for a review see ref. 8, 9, 18) confirmed such an increase in juvenile granulocytes after intravenous mistletoe extract injection.
- The **intrapleural instillation** of mistletoe extracts in patients with malignant pleural effusion lead to the elimination of tumor cells and subsequent pleurodesis in two out of three individuals (36). Significant changes in lymphocytic subpopulations in the pleural exudate could not be found here (37), but possibly a transient increase of macrophages and eosinophils in the responder group—which was not observed in nonresponders. These results indicate that the mistletoe extract-mediated pleurodesis cannot be attributed solely to mechanical stimulation and subsequent sclerosis;

rather, they suggest the stimulation of immunocompetent cells.

Quality of Life

The primary objective of medical intervention is to provide support to cancer patients and enable them to overcome their situation and to deal again in a competent way with their surroundings.

In animal experiments, it has been demonstrated convincingly that mistletoe extract injections lead to tumor remission and prolonged survival times. In the clinical application, a large number of therapeutic successes in individual cases stands against numerous studies, the majority of which are based on poor methodology and/or are no longer comparable with current therapeutic schemes (even though Grossarth-Maticek questions the meaningfulness of randomized studies)

(15). Nevertheless, some of these studies are based on good methodology and show positive results with mistletoe therapy, with the patients usually feeling better and more motivated after receiving the mistletoe extract injections (17, 18).

- Enhancement of the quality of the patient's life after injection of mistletoe extracts has been confirmed in clinical studies (11, 15, 16, 21, 39, 40, reviewed in ref. 17 and 18). Various mechanisms of action are possible, and all of the following—and others as well—may apply:
  - After injection, there is a release of mood-enhancing β-endorphins (16).
  - The patient feels "warmer" due to the cytokine-mediated mild rise in body temperature and the improved flow of blood in the skin.
  - The activated immune cells kep the tumor cells at bay and thus the patients objectively feel better.

Table 15.2 Mistletoe injection preparations for the treatment of cancer patients

Preparation (alphabetical order)	Dilution	Type of extract	Host trees	Harvest time	Plant parts
Abnoba Abnoba, Pforzheim (Germany)	1 mL: *Viscum album*, Planta tota/ Herba rec. 20, 2.0, 0.20, 0.020 mg; D6, D10, D20, D30	Pressed juice	A, Ac, Am, B, C, F, M, P, Qu	Summer and winter	Fresh leaves, shoots, and berries
Cefalektin Cefak, Kempten (Germany)	1 mL: Herb. *Visci albi* (1:10) 10 mg	Aqueous extract	Po and others	Autumn and winter	Dried leaves
Eurixor Biosyn, Fellbach (Germany)	1 mL: Herb. *Visci albi* (1:1.3) 1 mg	Aqueous extract	Po	January	Fresh leaves
Helixor Helixor, Rosenfeld (Germany)	*Viscum album*, Herba rec. (1:20) 0.01, 0.1, 1.0, 5, 10, 20, 30, 50, 100 mg	Aqueous extract	A, M, P	Summer and winter	Fresh leaves, shoots, blossoms, and berries
Iscador Weleda AG, Schwäbisch Gmünd (Germany)	*Viscum album*, Herba rec. 20, 10, 1, 0.1, 0.01, 0.001, 0.0001 mg	Aqueous fermentation	M, P, Qu, U	Summer and winter	Fresh leaves, shoots, blossoms, and berries
Iscador spezial Weleda AG, Schwäbisch Gmünd (Germany)	*Viscum album*, Herba rec. 5 mg (mistletoe lectins in M: 250 ng/mL, in Q: 375 ng/mL)	Aqueous fermentation	Qu, M	Summer and winter	Fresh leaves, shoots, blossoms, and berries
Iscucin Wala, Eckwälden (Germany)	1 mL: *Viscum album*, Planta tota (according to HAB 38)	Aqueous extract[1]	A, C, M, P, Po, Qu, S, T	Summer and winter	Dried leaves, berries, and layer
Lektinol Madaus, Cologne (Germany)	0.5 mL: Herb. *Visci albi* (1:1.1–1.5) 0.02–0.07 mg (mistletoe lectins: 30 ng/mL)	Aqueous extract	Po	January	Fresh leaves
Plenosol N Madaus, Cologne (Germany)	1 mL: Herb. *Visci albi* (1:1.3) 1 mg	Aqueous extract	Po	January	Fresh leaves and berries

Host trees: A, Abietis; Ac, Aceris; Am, Amygdali; B, Betulae; C, Crataegi; F, Fraxini; M, Mali; P, Pini; Po, Poplar; Qu, Quercus; S, Salicis; T, Tiliae; U Ulmi; [1] Fermented extracts are also available (Abietis, Mali, and Pini). (*Modified according to Büssing, 2000*)

– The mistletoe extracts provide the proverbial straws to which the patient can hang on, thus feeling less helpless in the face of unavoidable fate.
– The patients accept responsibility for themselves by performing the injections on their own.

• It has been demonstrated that the survival time of cancer patients depends significantly on their ability to deal actively with their surroundings ("self-regulation"). It is especially the patient with a high level of "self-regulation" who profits most from the treatment with mistletoe extracts (14, 15).

Summary

Is it then possible to "heal" with mistletoe therapy? Mistletoe is certainly not the cure-all wonder drug described by Pliny. The expectations of those affected and of the attending physicians may be very high here. Properly performed, adjuvant mistletoe therapy can be of valuable help in the care of cancer patients. Adequate treatment of a cancer patient must always consider the patient's individual situation and possible reactions. Fintelmann (13) emphasizes that, provided that a healing effect of mistletoe does exist, "the physician sees this effect in connection with the deeper causes of cancer and not just as a complex phytomechanism."

Any mistletoe treatment should therefore always be an integrated part of a comprehensive therapeutic concept that considers the patient in his/her overall personality. This includes, for example, also various forms of artistic therapy, meditation, rhythmic massages, as well as psychotherapeutic or pastoral care.

The significance of anthroposophical mistletoe therapy for complementary cancer treatment cannot yet be foreseen. Advances especially in different forms of application or improvements in the characterization of potencies of different mistletoe extracts (Table 15.1) may be possible for defined types of cancer. The combination with other therapies might also represent a promising approach.

References

1. Berg PA, Stein GM: Beeinflusst die Misteltherapie die Abwehr epithelialer Tumoren? Eine kritische immunologische Analyse. Deutsche Medizinische Wochenschrift. 2001; 126:339–345.
2. Büssing A, Stein GM, Pfüller U: Selective killing of CD8+ cells with a "memory" phenotype (CD62L^{lo}) by the N-acetyl-D-galactosamine-specific lectin from Viscum album L. Cell Death Diff. 1998; 5:231–240.
3. Büssing A, Wagner M, Wagner B, et al.: Induction of mitochondrial Apo 2.7 molecules and generation of reactive oxygen-intermediates in cultured lymphocytes by the toxic proteins from Viscum album L. Cancer Letters. 1999; 139:79–88.
4. Büssing A, Stein GM, Wagner M, et al.: Accidental cell death and generation of reactive oxygen intermediates in human lymphocytes induced by thionins from Viscum album L. Eur. J. Biochem. 1999; 262:79–87.
5. Büssing A, Vervecken W, Wagner M, Wagner B, Pfüller U, Schietzel M: Expression of mitochondrial Apo 2.7 molecules and caspase-3 activation in human lymphocytes treated with the ribosome-inhibiting mistletoe lectins and the cell membrane permeabilizing viscotoxins. Cytometry. 1999; 37: 131–139.
6. Büssing A, Stein GM, Pfüller U, Schietzel M: Induction of Fas ligand (CD95L) by the toxic mistletoe lectins in human lymphocytes. Anticancer Research. 1999; 19:1785–1790.
7. Büssing A, Rosenberger A, Stumpf C, Schietzel M: Entwicklung lymphozytärer Subpopulationen bei Tumorpatienten nach subkutaner Applikation von Mistelextrakten. Forschende Komplementärmedizin. 1999; 6:196–204.
8. Büssing A (ed): Mistletoe. Genus Viscum. Amsterdam, Harwood Academic Publishers, 2000.
9. Büssing A. Pharmakologische Wirkungen von Mistelextrakten. In: Fintelmann V (ed): Onkologie auf anthroposophischer Grundlage. Suttgart, Johannes M. Mayer-Verlag, 2002; chapter 3.2.4.1, p. 1–40.
10. Büssing A, Bischof M, Hatzmann W, et al.: Granulozytenfunktions-Beeinflussung durch eine einmalige perioperative Mistelextrakt-Infusion. Deutsche Zeitschrift für Onkologie 2004; 36: 148–153.
11. Dold U, Edler L, Mäurer HC, et al. (eds): Krebszusatztherapie beim fortgeschrittenen nicht-kleinzelligen Bronchialkarzinom. Stuttgart, Georg Thieme Verlag, 1991; p. 1–144.
12. Drees M, Berger DP, Dengler WA, Fiebig GH: Direct cytotoxic effect of preparations used as unconventional methods in cancer therapy in human tumour xenografts in the clonogenic assay and in nude mice. In: Arnold W, Köpf-Maier P, Micheel B (eds)

Immunodeficient animals. Models for cancer research. Contrib. Oncol. 1996; 51:115–122.

13. Fintelmann V (ed): Onkologie auf anthroposophischer Grundlage. Stuttgart, Johannes M. Mayer-Verlag, 2005.

14. Grossarth-Maticek R: Systemische Epidemiologie und präventive Verhaltensmedizin chronischer Erkrankungen. Berlin, Walter de Gruyter Verlag, 1999.

15. Grossarth-Maticek R, Kiene H, Baumgartner SM, Ziegler R: Use of Iscador, an extract of European mistletoe (*Viscum album*), in cancer treatment: prospective nonrandomized and randomized matched-pair studies nested within a cohort study. Alternative Therapies in Health and Medicine. 2001; 7:57–78.

16. Heiny BM, Beuth J: Mistletoe extract standardized for the galactoside-specific lectin (ML-1) induces β-endorphin release and immunopotentiation in breast cancer patients. Anticancer Research. 1994; 14:1339–1342.

17. Kienle GS, Berrino F, Büssing A et al.: Mistletoe in Cancer. A Systematic Review on Controlled Clinical Trials. Eur J Med Res 2003; 8: 1–11.

18. Kienle GS, Kiene H: Die Mistel in der Onkologie. Fakten und konzeptionelle Grundlagen. Schattauer, Stuttgart, 2003.

19. Kovacs E: Serum levels of IL-12 and production of IFN-gamma, IL-2 and IL-4 by peripheral blood mononuclear cells (PBMC) in cancer patients treated with *Viscum album* extract. Biomed. & Pharmacother. 2000; 54: 305–310.

20. Kuttan G, Menon LG, Kuttan R: Prevention of 20-methylcholanthrene-induced sarcoma by a mistletoe extract, Iscador. Carcinogenesis. 1996; 17: 1107–1109.

21. Lenartz D, Stoffel B, Menzel J, Beuth J: Immunoprotective activity of galactoside-specific lectin from mistletoe after tumor destructive therapy in glioma patients. Anticancer Research. 1996; 16:3799–3802.

22. Mathes H: Intraläsionale Mistelinjektionen in Lebermetastasen bei kolorektalem Karzinom und in das primäre Hepatozelluläre Karzinom (HCC) (Abstract). Der Merkurstab 50 Sonderheft, Juni 1997; S. 41.

23. Matthes H: Onkologische Misteltherapie (*Viscum album* L.) aus klinisch-anthroposophischer Sicht. In: Scheer R, Bauer R, Becker H, Berg PA, Fintelmann V (eds): Die Mistel in der Tumortherapie. Grundlagenforschung und Klinik. KVC Verlag Essen. 2001, p. 253–274.

24. Nabrotzki M, Scheffler A: Komplette Remission nach intratumoraler Misteltherapie eines Duodenum-Karziom-Rezidivs. In: Scheer R, Bauer R, Becker H, Berg PA, Fintelmann V (eds): Die Mistel in der Tumortherapie. Grundlagenforschung und Klinik. KVC Verlag Essen. 2001, p. 413–422

25. Ribéreau-Gayon H, Jung ML, Beck JP, Anton R: Effect of fetal calf serum on the cytotoxic activity of mistletoe (*Viscum album* L.) lectins in cell culture. Phytotherapy Research. 1995; 9:336–339.

26. Ribéreau-Gayon G, Jung ML, Frantz M, Anton R: Modulation of the cytotoxicity and enhancement of cytokine release induced by *Viscum album* L. extracts or mistletoe lectins. Anticancer Drugs 1997; 8 (Suppl 1), pp. 3–8.

27. Samuelsson G: Mistletoe toxins. System. Zool. 1974; 22:566–569.

28. Scheffler A, Mast H, Fischer S, Metelmann HR: Komplette Remission eines Mundhöhlenkarzinoms nach alleiniger Mistelbehandlung. In: Scheer R, Becker H, Berg PA (eds): Grundlagen der Misteltherapie. Akueller Stand der Forschung und klinische Anwendung. Stuttgart, Hippokrates Verlag. 1996; p. 453–464.

29. Stein GM, Henn W, von Laue HB, Berg PA: Modulation of cellular and humoral immune responses of tumor patients by mistletoe therapy. European Journal of Medical Research. 1998; 3:194–202.

30. Stein GM, Berg PA: Modulation of cellular and humoral immune responses during exposure of healthy individuals to an aqueous mistletoe extract. European Journal of Medical Research. 1998; 3:307–314.

31. Stein GM, von Laue HB, Henn W, Berg PA: Human anti-mistletoe lectin antibodies. In: Bardocz S, Pfüller U, Pusztai A (eds): COST 98. Effects of anti-nutrients on the nutritional value of legume diets, Vol. 5, Luxembourg: Office for Official Publications of the European Communites. 1998; p. 168–175.

32. Stein GM, Schaller G, Pfüller U, et al: Characterisation of granulocyte stimulation by thionins from European mistletoe and from wheat. Biochimica et Biophysica Acta. 1999; 1426:80–90.

33. Stein GM, Edlund U, Pfüller U, Büssing A, Schietzel M: Influence of polysaccharides from *Viscum album* L. on human lymphocytes, monocytes and granulocytes in vitro. Anticancer Research. 1999; 19:3907–3914.

34. Stein GM, Pfüller, Schietzel M: Viscotoxin-free aqueous extracts from European mistletoe (*Viscum album* L.) stimulate activity of human granulocytes. Anticancer Research. 1999;19:2925–2928.

35. Steuer-Vogt MK, Bonkowsky V, Ambrosch P et al.: The effect of an adjuvant mistletoe treatment programme in resected head and neck cancer patients: a randomised controlled clinical trial. European Journal of Cancer. 2001; 37: 23–31.

36. Stumpf C, Schietzel M: Intrapleurale Instillation eines Extraktes aus Viscum album (L.) zur Behandlung maligner Pleuraergüsse. Tumourdiagnostik und Therapie. 1994; 15:57–62.

37. Stumpf C, Büssing A: Stimulation of antitumour immunity by intrapleural instillation of a Viscum al-

bum L. extracts. Anticancer Drugs. 1997; 8 (Suppl. 1), pp. 23–26.

38. Stumpf C, Ramirez-Martinez S, Becher A, Stein GM, Büssing A, Schietzel M.: Intratumorale Mistelapplikation bei stenosierendem Rezidiv eines Cardia-Carcinoms. Erfahrungsheilkunde, Sonderausgabe August. 1997; 509–513.

39. Wetzel D, Schäfer M: Results of a randomised placebo-controlled multicentre study with PS76A2 (standardised mistletoe preparation) in patients with breast cancer receiving adjuvant chemotherapy: 3rd International Congress on Phytotherapy, Munich 2000, Phytomedicine Suppl. II, Abstr. SL66. 2000; p. 34.

40. Wolf P, Freudenberg N, Konitzer M: Analgetische und stimmungsaufhellende Wirkung bei Malignom-Patienten unter hochdosierter Viscum album Infusionstherapie Erfahrungsheilkunde. 1994; 43: 262–264.

16 Thymic Peptides

Josef Beuth

General Remarks

In 1965, Angelo Mario DiGeorge observed a congenital immune defect with pronounced T lymphocytopenia. This defect was associated with thymic hypoplasia caused by malformation of the third and fourth pharyngeal pouches due to disturbed embryonic development during the twelfth week of pregnancy (DiGeorge syndrome). It soon became clear that the thymus gland represents the key organ in the establishment and functionality of cellular immunity. Its far-reaching tasks include:
- regulation of hematopoiesis in the bone marrow
- differentiation of T lymphocytes (helper T cells developing through specific contacts with major histocompatibility complex [MHC] class II+ cells, and cytotoxic T cells developing through specific contacts with MHC class I+ cells) as well as their maturation and release
- development of immune tolerance for the body's own tissues
- secretion of thymic hormones, cytokines, and growth factors (8, 12).

Cytokines and growth factors (colony stimulating factors) control the functions of immune cells and have been recommended for diverse clinical indications. Meanwhile, the initial euphoria over their discovery has been put into perspective by the realization that a multitude of cofactors complicates a therapeutically meaningful application. Thymic peptides, thymic hormones, and thymic cytokines finally received increasing attention in the context of experimental and clinical evaluation of cytokines and growth factors. Promising biological activities and pharmacological effects of thymus peptides were described, thus leading to an increase in preclinical research.

For purposes of this discussion we distinguish between:
- total thymic extracts
- thymic peptides
- standardized thymic peptide mixtures (1, 2, 6, 8, 9, 12).

Total Thymic Extracts (Complex Mixtures)

Data on the preclinical efficacy of total thymic extracts are not available in scientific databases (e. g., MEDLINE). The multitude of published data—in nonpeer-reviewed journals, mostly published or sponsored by product manufacturers—does not prove the scientific relevance of total thymic extracts.

Thymic Peptides

Thymic peptides have properties that can restore and stimulate the immune system. It has been shown that the activity of natural killer (NK) cells against tumor cells, which is suppressed in cancer patients, can be significantly increased in vitro. In addition to this restoring or activating activity, there is evidence that thymic peptides influence the cytokine balance. It has been demonstrated experimentally that preparations of thymic peptides induce the release of interleukin-8 and monocyte chemotactic protein-1 (MCP-1), both of which act as cytokines that enhance the anticancer activity of monocytes.

Standardized Thymic Peptide Mixtures

Some effects of standardized thymus peptide mixtures have been well documented in oncology. They include:
- restoration and stimulation of immune cells in case of immunosuppression due to therapy or cancer
- increase in cell numbers and activity of T lymphocytes, NK cells, and LAK cells (lymphokine-activated killer cells)
- compensation of undesired drug effects and, especially, of tumor-destructive radiation therapy or chemotherapy
- activation of the neuroendocrine network
- enhancement of the quality of life.

Table 16.1 Total thymic extracts and relevant thymic peptides (examples)

	Molecular weight (Da[**])	Constituents
I Complex mixtures		
Total thymic extract (THX)		Proteins, peptides, amino acids
II Low molecular weight mixtures		
Thym Uvocal[*]	< 5 000	Protein-free, chromatographically
Thymoject[*]	< 10 000	standardized peptide mixtures
III Thymic fractions		
Thymic humoral factor	< 3 400	Biochemically characterized, synthetic
Thymosin fraction V	< 12 000	Biochemically characterized
IV Thymic peptides		
Thymopentin	680	Pentapeptide
Thymosin α-1	3 100	Polypeptide
Thymopoietin II	5 600	Polypeptide

[*]Pharmaceutical and biological qualities, including BSE security, certified by the BfArM (Germany). [**] DA = Daltons

Table 16.2 Experimental in-vitro and in-vivo data on the effects of standardized thymic peptide mixtures (a), thymosin α-1 (b), and thymic humoral factor (c)

In vitro	In vivo (murine models)
↑ Immunocyte activity (a, b, c)	↑ Immunocyte number/activity in peripheral blood (a, b, c)
↑ Cytokine release (a, b, c)	
↑ Proliferation, maturation, and differentiation of thymocytes (a, b, c) and bone marrow progenitor cells (b)	↑ Thymocyte proliferation (a, b, c)
	↑ Antiviral activity (b)
↑ Antiviral activity (a, b)	↑ Anticancer/antimetastatic activity (a, b, c)
	↑ Immunocyte restoration (b, c)

The following stocktaking focuses essentially on approved, clinically available, and standardized thymus peptide mixtures. These preparations meet the regulations of the German Federal Institute for Drugs and Medical Devices (BfArM) and, after adequate clinical evaluation, seem to be suitable as indication-specific measures in complementary oncology (Table 16.1).

Experimental Studies

Scientifically adequate, experimental, preclinical effects have been established for standardized thymic peptide mixtures as well as for several biochemically defined thymic peptides or fractions, such as thymosin α-1, thymic humoral factor (Table 16.2). The preclinical knowledge on individual thymic peptides has been well documented, including immunocyte modulation, stimulation, and restoration, as well as anticancer, antimetastatic, and antiviral activities.

Clinical Studies

The biological properties of defined thymic peptides or standardized thymic peptide mixtures have been well documented. On the whole, they reflect the huge therapeutic potential for oncological indications. Up to now, however, there are no clinical studies with a structure and design suitable for providing evidence.

- The ability of standardized thymic peptide extracts to reconstitute the immune system has been demonstrated repeatedly in clinical studies. In one study, for example, the low CD4/CD8 ratio in mammary carcinoma patients prior to therapy shifted to the normal range after treatment with a standardized thymic peptide mixture.
- Other authors observed an increase in CD4+ T cells and NK cells in patients with colorectal carcinoma following treatment with thymostimulin.
- In addition to these immunological activities of thymic peptides, other mechanisms have been

demonstrated that may positively affect the patient's quality of life. Thymosins are neuroactive immunotransmitters that pass information from the immune system to the central nervous system (CNS). For example, thymosin-stimulated lymphocytes produce β-endorphin, a transmitter formerly regarded as a CNS-derived neuropeptide. These substances are transmitted to the neuroendocrine system and induce physiological reactions, such as analgesia or an enhanced sense of well-being. In addition, it has been shown that thymic peptides can also influence psychological reactions, such as anxiety and depression. In animal experiments, thymopentin and its synthetic peptide analogue revealed stress-protective activities in rats. It is assumed that the anxiolytic effect of thymopentin is based on the modulation of nicotinic receptors in the CNS.

- In 42 patients with smal cell lung carcinoma, thymic peptides significantly improved the immune response (number and function of T cells) and the survival time of cancer patients when administered as an adjuvant to radiation therapy, as compared with placebo in the control group.
- New is the discovery that defined thymic peptides have a pronounced inhibitory effect on angiotensin-converting enzyme (ACE). This mechanism may prolong the half-life of neuropeptides in the brain and improve the well-being of the patient—as has already been shown for other ACE inhibitors. There is increasing

clinical evidence that standardized thymic peptides enhance the quality of life, a finding that should be taken seriously In the context of application studies in 809 cancer patients, there was a relevant improvement in the quality of life, general clinical conditions, and fitness of the patients under treatment with standardized thymus peptide mixtures.

- Currently, there are about 25 controlled studies on thymic peptide therapy as a complementary oncological treatment. A total of 1700 patients (with bronchial, mammary, colorectal, ovarian, and esophageal carcinoma as well as malignant melanoma and non-Hodgkin lymphoma) were enrolled in these studies. Only six of the controlled studies on complementary thymic peptide therapy involved more than 60 patients and thus reached the biometrically acceptable minimum number of patients required for establishing efficacy (Table 16.**3**).

A short analysis of these studies (Table 16.**3**) shows statistically significant therapeutic effects only in two studies:

- Patients with non-smal cell lung carcinoma survived significantly longer when receiving complementary thymic peptide treatment. However, this study was not published in a peer-reviewed journal and is, therefore, not acceptable as evidence for efficacy.
- Patients with colorectal carcinoma benefited from complementary thymic peptide therapy because the side effects of the standard therapy

Table 16.3 Controlled clinical studies on thymic peptide therapy

Indication	Therapy	Patients (n)	Results	Reference
Mammary carcinoma	Chemo ± TP[1]	296	↓ SE from Chemo	13
Colorectal carcinoma	Chemo ± TP[1]	211	↓ SE from Chemo* ↑ Remission rate*	11
Non-Hodgkin lymphoma	Chemo ± TP[1]	150	↑ Remission rate ↑ Survival time ↑ Immune function	5
Small cell lung carcinoma	Chemo + Rad ± TP[2]	91	↓ SE from Chemo, Rad ↑ Remission rate/period	14
Non-small cell lung carcinoma	Rad ± TP[3]	87	↑ Survival time* ↓ Relapse rate	
Mammary carcinoma	Chemo ± TP[4]	78	↑ Survival time ↑ Immune function	7

*Statistically significant as compared to the control group. Chemo, chemotherapy; Rad, radiation therapy; SE, side effects; TP, thymic peptides; [1]thymostimulin; [2]thymosin fraction V; [3]thymosin α-1; [4]thymopentin.

were significantly reduced (enhanced quality of life) and remission rates were significantly improved as well. However, this study had no placebo control group, and the enhancement of the quality of life was not necessarily due to the complementary treatment. Despite significantly improved remission rates, the survival time was reduced (though not significantly) in the group of patients receiving thymic peptide therapy.

In all other studies, therapeutic effects were observed that were not statistically relevant, and they were also scientifically irrelevant because of marginal effects, absence of placebo controls, low patient numbers, or absence of stratification.

Summary

Thymic peptide therapy is a complementary therapeutic measure and is supposed to optimize tumor-destructive standard therapies. Chromatographically standardized thymic peptide mixtures are administered as complementary oncological treatment depending on the indication (e. g., clearly demonstrated immunosuppression after tumor-destructive treatment). Documented benefits for the patient include, among others, restoration of immunocytes or T cells, prevention of infections, and enhancement of the quality of life.

Up to now, it has not been demonstrated that thymic peptide therapy can protect against relapses or metastases or that this therapy prolongs the survival time of cancer patients. Although a multitude of clinical studies on thymic peptide therapy is available, definitive statements on the behavior of relapses or metastases are not yet possible from a scientific point of view, because all studies have shortcomings and do not meet the current scientific requirements. The first studies did not conform to Good Clinical Practice (GCP) guidelines but were promising; however, definitive evidence will hopefully come from the controlled clinical studies that are currently being undertaken and that do conform to GCP.

Finally, the suggested, but scientifically unproved, activity of total thymic extracts should be addressed. Some authors suppose these to be superior to standardized thymic peptide mixtures. Total thymic extracts, like thymic peptide mixtures, are preparations containing multiple components, and the reproducibility of their pharmacological and immunological activities depends on the quality of standardization. Hence, a specification of their constituents is essential. Unless reproducible standardization of individual thymic components is guaranteed (in addition to obligatory proof of their pharmaceutical and biological qualities), such therapeutic agents should be considered obsolete in scientifically oriented medicine.

Several well-documented application studies of standardized thymic peptide mixtures (or defined thymic fractions) are available that demonstrate an effect of the therapy on both the state of immunity and the quality of life (i.e., reduction of side effects by tumor-destructive therapies). It should be emphasized, however, that application studies cannot prove efficacy. Also, the existing clinical studies on treatment with standardized thymic peptides in oncology do not allow any definitive statements regarding the behavior of relapses or metastases, or regarding the survival time of cancer patients, because all of the studies have shortcomings with regard to randomization, blinding, stratification, and/or patient numbers (4). Uncritical protagonists of treatment with total thymic extracts or thymic peptides like to dispute that a selection bias should be suspected: positive results are published, while negative ones are rejected. This certainly does not apply to all studies, but it is a fact that most of the present therapy studies have been published in journals without peer review. (3) Thus, there is an absolute need to evaluate this therapeutic approach.

Outlook

Research into the structure, activity, and mechanism of action of thymic peptides is currently vigorously pursued in the experimental and clinical fields. With the increase in knowledge about tumor biology and tumor immunology, the immunotherapeutic approaches to cancer treatment become very interesting as well. Despite many setbacks, promising data on immunotherapy have been published (e. g., with malignant melanoma). Under defined conditions (selection of therapeutically meaningful preparations and integration into the therapeutic concept), standardized thymic peptide mixtures can also contribute to the patient's well-being.

A multicenter study that meets all scientific criteria regarding the therapy with standardized thymic peptide mixtures (and carries the "A" seal of quality by the German Cancer Society) has begun (10). Within the scope of this study, a comparison is made between therapy using a standardized thymic peptide mixture combined with 5-fluorouracil and folinic acid, vs. placebo combined with 5-fluorouracil and folinic acid, in patients with UICC stage IV colorectal carcinoma (T1–4 N0–3 M1).

It is the objective of this study to demonstrate the clinical efficacy of a low molecular weight, standardized thymic peptide mixture (which is registered in Germany) in patients with metastatic colorectal carcinoma as compared with placebo. Within the scope of this study, either thymic peptide mixture or placebo is administered as an adjuvant to the internationally recognized standard treatment of metastatic colorectal carcinoma. Thus, all patients receive the consensus therapy for UICC stage IV colorectal carcinoma. The target criteria are defined as follows:
- primary: quality of life, tumor response, or remission
- secondary: age-corrected survival time, time period before progression
- frequency or intensity of undesired drug effects of chemotherapy
- changes in cell-mediated immunity.

This representative controlled study is presented here to document that complementary therapy with standardized thymic peptide mixtures—which might be replaced in future by defined (synthetic) thymic peptides (e.g., thymosin α-1 or thymic humoral factor)—may be on the right path to enter evidence-based oncology.

■ References

1. Ben-Efraim S, Keisari Y, Ophir R, Pecht M, Trainin N, Burstein Y: Immunopotentiating and immunotherapeutic effects of thymic hormones and factors with special emphasis on thymic humoral factor (THF-γ-2). Critical Rev. Immunol. 1999; 19:261–284.

2. Beuth J, Schierholz JM, Ko HL, Braun JM: Application-dependent immunomodulating and antimetastatic efficacy of thymic peptides in BALB/c-mice; In Vivo. 2001;15:403–406.

3. Cassileth BR: Thymus therapy for cancer; Eur. J. Cancer. 1997; 33:517–518.

4. Ernst E: Thymus therapy for cancer? A criteria-based, systemic review. Eur. J. Cancer. 1997; 33: 531–535.

5. Federico M, Gobbi PG, Mretti G, et al.: Effects of thymostimulin with combination chemotherapy in patients with aggressive non-Hodgkin lymphomas. Am. J. Clin. Oncol. 1995; 18:8–14.

6. Low TLK, Goldstein AL: Thymosins: structure, function and therapeutic applications. Thymus. 1984; 6:27–32.

7. Mallmann P, Krebs D: Investigations on cell-mediated immunity in patients with breast and ovarian carcinomas receiving a combination of chemotherapy and immunotherapy with thymopentin. Exp. Clin. Pharmacol. 1990; 12:333–340.

8. Maurer HR, Goldstein AL, Hager ED (eds): Thymic peptides in preclinical and clinical medicine. W. Zuckschwerdt Verlag, Munich, 1997.

9. Mayer G, Pohlmeyer K, Caliebe A, et al.: Low molecular thymic peptides stimulate human blood dendritic cells. Anticancer Res. 2000; 20:2873–2884.

10. Mayer G, Wolf F, Schmidt UJ: Erste plazebokontrollierte Doppelblindstudie mit Thymuspeptiden bei Patienten mit metastasiertem kolorektalen Karzinom in Deutschland. Z. Onkol./J. of Oncol. 1999; 31:8–13.

11. Mustacchi G, Pavesi L, Milani S: High-doses of folinic acid and fluorouracil plus or minus thymostimulin for treatment of metastatic colorectal cancer. Results of a randomized multicenter clinical trial. Anticancer Res. 1994; 14:617–620.

12. Neumeyer G (ed): Thymuspeptide zur Behandlung chronischer und maligner Erkrankungen. Karl F. Haug Verlag, Heidelberg, 1996.

13. Pavesi L: Fluorouracil with and without high-dose folinic acid plus epirubicin and cyclophosphamide (FEC) versus HDFA-FEC plus or minus thymostimulin in metastatic breast cancer. Results of a multicenter study. Eur. J. Cancer. 1993; 29:77–80.

14. Scheer HI, Shank B, Chapman R, et al.: Randomized trial of combined modality therapy with and without thymosin fraction V in treatment of small cell lung cancer. Cancer Res. 1988; 481:1663–1670.

17 Probiotic Therapy

Volker Rusch

Introduction

The objective of probiotic therapy is to optimize the body's defense mechanisms with microbiotics and autovaccines and, possibly, to replace antibiotics with probiotics.

Probiotics are increasingly becoming established as a therapeutic option in addition to antibiotics. Antibiotics and probiotics are not necessarily antagonistic. Antibiotics are still the last resort in cases of severe bacterial or parasitic infections. Positive effects of antibiotics can be maximized and negative effects on the immune system minimized by strictly controlling their application.

Probiotics are useful therapeutic tools in numerous cases of acute and, above all, chronic infections. Prerequisite for applying probiotics is the critical delimitation of life-threatening infections or imminent complications. Probiotics can reduce the negative effects of antibiotics, e.g., problems posed by resistance, and optimize their positive effects on immunological functions.

The International Study Group on New Antimicrobial Strategies (ISGNAS) defines three categories of probiotics (5, 16, 17, 21):

- **Medical probiotics:** microbial preparations (microbiotics) that contain live and/or inactivated (dead) microorganisms—including their constituents and products—and are used for therapeutic purposes. These bacterial preparations and autovaccines are used as remedies, the efficacy of which has been documented.
- **Pharmaceutical probiotics:** microbial preparations that are used as food additives. As a rule, these are products manufactured under pharmaceutical conditions; they contain lyophilized microorganisms in high concentrations and are available at pharmacies.
- **Alimentary probiotics:** microbial preparations that play a role in food fermentation or food production. Alimentary probiotics are usually dairy products, such as yogurt. Probiotic dairy products can play a useful role in nutrition. However, despite assertion to the contrary, yogurt cannot be considered a medicine.

We focus here on the use of symbiotic microorganisms in the form of medical and pharmaceutical probiotics that can control complex immune mechanisms, modulate the endogenous microflora interactively, and control metabolic processes.

Man and Microbes

Homo sapiens represents only a snapshot in evolution and will continue to evolve in the future. From the very beginning, microbes played an important role. Mutual dependencies and requirements developed, and these are reflected in complex functional areas and diverse differentiations of structural interrelationships. The term symbiosis is often used in this connection. However, the definition of **symbiosis** includes a range of partnerships, such as parasitism, neutralism, commensalism, and mutualism. In a partnership such as parasitism, only one of the partners is the beneficiary, namely the parasite, whereas the other partner is harmed by the parasite. A symbiotic association in which partners coexist without mutual interaction and without obvious advantages or disadvantages is called neutralism. Commensalism is a close association from which only one of the two partners benefits without causing harm to the other partner. A partnership in which both partners benefit from each other is called **mutualism** (mutualistic symbiosis – coexistence for mutual benefit).

Gnotobiology

Much of our knowledge on the interaction between unicellular and multicellular organisms comes from gnotobiology, the science dedicated to studying animals raised in a germ-free environment, comparing them with microflora-associated normal animals, and also studying monoflora-associated or polyflora-associated animals.

We distinguish between microflora-associated characteristics (MAC) and germ-free animal characteristics (GAC). There are essential differences between conventional, microflora-associated, and germ-free animals. Germ-free animals are not able to defend themselves effectively against infections. Their association with pathogenic microorganisms is lethal. This can be attributed to the fact that, in germ-free animals, essential components of the complex immune system are underdeveloped and function only to a limited extent or not at all. In particular, the mucosa-associated immune system is developed only to a rudimentary degree. The intestine-associated lymph tissue is particularly affected. The lymph vessels in the intestinal wall (lacteal vessels) are hardly present, or not at all. Peyer's plaques and lymph follicles are smaller

and intraepithelial T lymphocytes are severely reduced in numbers. The effectivity of immune cells is greatly decreased or does not exist at all. Serum immunoglobulin levels are extremely low.

The structure and function of all components of the defense system of multicellular organisms depend therefore directly on the microbial populations at various locations on skin and mucosa, but primarily in the entire intestinal tract. Many other factors are influenced by the presence of the microflora (Table 17.**1**).

Microbial Populations

The structures of the mucosa as interface and the colonization of this surface by symbiotic microorganisms represent a phylogenetically and ontogenetically determined functional unit and are part of the innate immune system. In stable layers of microbial populations, such as the intestinal flora, mutualistic and commensal microorganisms are in the majority. Together with the immune system, this majority keeps the minority of opportunists under surveillance and usually restricts the number of germs.

The most common intestinal microorganisms are *Bifidobacterium*, *Eubacterium*, *Lactobacillus*, and other genera that ensure the stability of the microbial populations. Elements of instability include many species of *Enterobacteriaceae*, *Pseudomonas*, and *Clostridium*. An intermediary position is taken by *Escherichia coli*, *Enterococcus*, and *Bacteroides*, which have positive as well as negative properties. The minorities in the microbial populations, however, have by far the broadest effects on the range of defensive functions (Fig. 17.**1**).

The affected functions concern the entire spectrum from innate to adaptive immunity, from nonspecific to specific immune reactions, and they control both mucosal and systemic immunity. *Bifidobacterium* and *Lactobacillus* are accepted by the host as "friendly" inhabitants and stimulate the intestine-associated lymphatic system with their predominantly nonspecific activities and functions (Fig. 17.**2**).

Microbial populations play a decisive role in health and disease. The continuous interactions between individual members of the complex microbial populations stabilize this "social community" in a dynamic equilibrium, and it is the stability

Table 17.1 Positive effects of the intestinal microflora

Establishment of a microbial barrier
- Resistance to colonization: the dominance of autochthonous microbes in intestinal biotopes and microecologic niches inhibits colonization by heterogenous germs or by invasive or toxic microorganisms (e.g., inhibition of *Candida*, *Clostridium difficile*, *Staphylococcus aureus*, and others)
- Competition for nutrients, vitamins, and other essential factors
- Acidification of the intestinal milieu (lactic acid, acetic acid)
- Production of microbicidal or microstatic substances that inhibit the growth of pathogenic germs (bacteriocins, short-chain fatty acids, hydrogen sulfide, hydrogen peroxide)
- Adhesion of friendly microbes to mucosal receptors prevents colonization by pathogenic invaders

Training of the immune system
- Development and differentiation of lymphatic organs
- Function of the immune system, especially of the mucosal immune system
- Immunoregulation (immunomodulation, immunostimulation, immunosuppression)

Intestinal motility
- Stimulation of peristalsis
- Blood supply to the intestinal mucosa

Effect on epithelia
- Proliferation of epithelial cells
- Nutritional supply of epithelial cells by short-chain fatty acids as energy source for the colon's epithelium

Vitamin production
- Vitamin K
- Vitamin B12
- Folic acid
- Nicotinamide

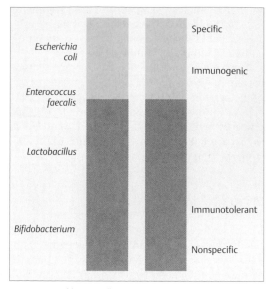

Fig. 17.**1** Profile microflora and immune system

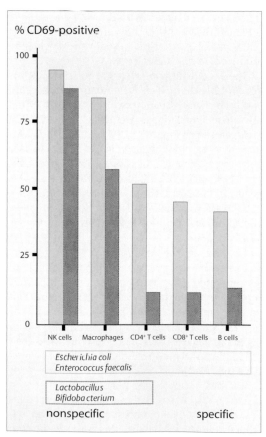

Fig. 17.**2** Immunological reaction profiles

or instability of this equilibrium that benefits or harms the human body. Normally, the coexistence of the human body with its own microflora is harmonious throughout life. Endogenous microorganisms mediate important protective functions:

– resistance to colonization: the control over colonization with endogenous, facultative pathogenic germs and heterogenous invaders
– stimulation and stabilization of epithelial integrity
– stimulation and differentiation of lymphatic organs.

Any external or internal disturbance of the well-balanced equilibrium of the unicellular microbes with the multicellular body of *Homo sapiens* has more or less severe consequences for physiological functions and health.

Pathogenic Microbes

A typical sign of the pathogenicity of microorganisms is their ability to break through the barriers of the innate defense system and to propagate in the internal milieu. In the classic case, these are natural pathogens or obligatory pathogens that are normally not members of the partnership between man and microbes, i.e., they are nonsymbionts. The adaptive immune system is responsible for dealing with the assault by such pathogens.

A microorganism can develop pathogenic properties only when it possesses genes that code for pathogenicity factors and when certain conditions lead to the expression of these genes. In the genomes of many pathogenic species of bacteria, transfer and recombination processes have established certain genetic structures that are called pathogenicity islands. These are DNA fragments that occur as genomic islands also in many nonpathogenic microbes. Their genetic codes include information for metabolic functions, secretion processes, or resistances. In terms of evolutionary biology, such genetic islands may be advantageous for microorganisms under certain conditions of selection.

Microorganisms in the environmental reservoir, as well as in symbiotic microbial populations, are constantly involved in the exchange of genes. Pieces of genetic information are continually mixed through horizontal gene transfer, and new microbial variants are thus formed.

Especially pathogenic microorganisms are subjected to intense selection pressure and, in response, have enormously increased their genetic flexibility, which is required for undergoing evolutionary processes quickly and successfully. The continual horizontal gene transfer and the existence of pathogenicity islands are indications that the evolution of pathogenicity happens in big leaps. Pathogenic microorganisms must deal with, and survive, extremely hostile environments that carry many risks. When new pathotypes can be put to the test, there are better chances for survival. As a result, new pathogens are constantly emerging. Likewise, the classic infectious agents continuously redevelop new variants that are extremely well adapted to their milieu and have a high pathogenic potential. The genetic flexibility of pathogenic microorganisms and the highly effective adaptation processes correlate also with the constant appearance of new resistances against antibiotics and, thus, demonstrate how dangerous can be the unscrupulous use of antibiotics (3).

Antibiosis

The absolutely uncritical use of antibiotics is reflected in figures of the German Institute for Medical Statistics (IMS). The use of antibiotics in Germany has more than doubled between 1987 and 1997, and it has increased by a factor of six for some indications. For example, it is interesting to note that, while the number of upper respiratory tract diseases has tripled, their treatment with antibiotics has increased by a factor of five. The trend to overprescription particularly affects children. The IMS figures for 1996 reveal that 64% of infants and children under four received antibiotics. Every fourth child was treated up to three times a year with antibiotics. In the period from 1994 to 1996, almost half of all antibiotics were prescribed to four million children with diseases of the ENT area, as compared with 76 million mostly adults with the same indication (17).

This chemotherapeutic bombardment results in a considerable ecological selection pressure. Multiple resistances have developed, and the media are full of reports on killer microbes and the end of the era of antibiotics. Meanwhile, it is becoming obvious that there has been no development of new, effective agents against microbes during the last 20 years, because it was thought that the issue of infectious diseases has been dealt with. Also vancomycin, which is used today as the last resort, is failing increasingly often. Resistant *Staphylococcus* strains have already developed even against the most recently introduced linezolid.

The **uncontrolled use of antibiotics** creates ideal selection conditions for pathogens, and the numerous new variants of these pathogens can spread easily due to global mass tourism. The dramatic increase in multiresistant pathogens could have been far less alarming, without jeopardizing the health of entire populations, if antibiotics had been used in a more controlled manner as demanded by medical microbiologists.

On the contrary, there are indications that immediate administration of antibiotics to children with otitis and tonsillitis resulted in a relapse rate after four weeks that was twice as high as in children without treatment with antibiotics (KVH aktuell 16/1996). Shifts in the composition of symbiotic microbial populations are direct consequences of the extensive use of antibiotics. Postantibiotic colitis is caused by *Clostridium difficile* and is the result of antibiotic treatment. It has also been documented that the propagation of pathogenic fungi, such as *Candida albicans*, is a result of antibiotic treatment. The significant increase in atopic disorders in industrialized countries has been correlated in recent studies with excessive hygiene, antibiotic decontamination, and lack of contact with the microbial environment. The fecal flora in atopic patients and, above all, in children exhibits considerable abnormalities; these abnormalities are evident in a significant propagation of pathogenic yeasts and enteric bacteria as well as a significant reduction in bifidobacteria and lactobacilli.

▬ Probiotic Therapy

The positive effects of certain microorganisms on the immune system and metabolism can be successfully imitated by the therapeutic application of selected bacterial strains. The most important effects of probiotic therapy are:
- immunoregulation
- improvement of metabolic functions (especially in the intestine)
- modulation of the mucosal microbial flora.

In view of the multitude of microbes that colonize the human skin and mucosa, only a small selection of germs is therapeutically important. They include primarily *Enterococcus* species, *Escherichia coli*, and lactic bacteria, such as *Bifidobacterium bifidum* or *Lactobacillus acidophilus*. Whereas *Enterococcus* and *E. coli* have primarily an effect on immunoregulation, lactic bacteria are primarily used for stabilizing the intestinal milieu. Regular intake of lactic bacteria causes acidification of the intestinal milieu. The pH value of the stool lies normally between 5.8 and 6.5, but it is often shifted to the alkaline range due to diets rich in fat and protein. This causes a reduction in the flora of lactic bacteria and leads to limitations in functions normally performed by these bacteria. Therapeutic doses help the body's own flora of lactic bacteria to stabilize and regenerate.

Microorganisms Used

Probiotic therapy uses primarily human symbiotic microorganisms. Application of human microbial species makes sense because these are already adapted to humans. Nonhuman symbiotic microorganisms, such as *Saccharomyces boulardii,* are an exception to this rule.

The majority of microbiotics are manufactured from the following microorganisms:
- *Bifidobacterium*
- *Lactobacillus*
- *Enterococcus*
- *E. coli.*

Bifidobacteria and lactobacilli restore the floral balance, regenerate the integrity of epithelial tissues, and stimulate the immune functions of the intestinal mucosa. The effects of orally applied microbiotics prepared from *Enterococcus* and *E. coli* are much more pronounced in their intensity and range than those of bifidobacteria and lactobacilli, and they cover almost all components of cellular and humoral immunity.

Autovaccines

Autovaccines are autogenous vaccines prepared from the endogenous, inactivated (dead) bacteria isolated from a patient; they are used as individualized medicine for this patient only and are optimally adapted to the patient's immune system. When type, severity, and chronicity of the disease, or a problematic course of treatment, require special intensification of the therapy, autovaccines are considered in the indication-specific treatment scheme. As compared with the sole use of microbial preparations, the addition of autovaccines can considerably enhance the intensity of immunomodulating signals and, thus, guarantee an extraordinary adaptation to individual immunological situations.

Autovaccines prepared from intestinal bacteria are of special importance because of the prominent role that the intestine-associated immune system and the intestinal microflora play in influencing the immune system. Nonpathogenic, inactivated E. coli is used for this purpose, and the autogenous vaccines are referred to as **intestinal tract autovaccines**. Other autovaccines are also a possibility (16).

Indications and Forms of Administration

Probiotic therapy has a relatively broad spectrum of indications because of its regulating effects on the immune system, metabolism, and flora (Table 17.**2**).

Different **forms of administration** are available for autovaccines. Injections are preferred because the bacterial agents are directly brought into contact with the immune system, and the effect occurs usually faster than with oral and percutaneous autovaccines. As patients have to appear in the practice twice a week for receiving the injection, patient counseling is also optimal this way. Good results can also be achieved with autovaccines that are either taken by mouth (oral autovaccine) or are rubbed in (percutaneous autovaccine). These

Table 17.2   Indications for probiotic therapy (16)
• Atopic disorders (allergic rhinitis, bronchial asthma, etc.)
• Acute, chronic, or chronic recurrent infections of respiratory tract, gastrointestinal tract, and urogenital tract
• Chronic and chronic recurrent mycoses
• Inflammatory skin diseases
• As an adjuvant measure in the treatment of rheumatic and malignant diseases

forms of application are especially important when treating children, but also adults for whom treatment by injection is not an option.

Extent and Duration

The extent and duration of probiotic therapy always depend on the respective diagnosis, severity, and chronicity of the disease as well as the age of the patient. In case of chronic respiratory infection or when treating children, it often suffices to perform the probiotic therapy exclusively with oral or percutaneous microbial preparations.

When treating disorders of the gastrointestinal tract or diseases that are often accompanied by changes in the intestinal microflora (e. g., atopy or mycosis), the **milieu-stabilizing effect of lactic bacteria** should be used as an additional treatment.

The more severe and far-reaching the disturbance of the diseased body's regulatory capacity, the more important is the concomitant use of autovaccines. If, at the start of the treatment, it is not yet clear which components are required, it is recommended that the microbial preparations are used initially only for six to eight weeks; based on the clinical development, a decision is then made whether further measures are necessary at all.

When making such a decision, **fecal diagnosis** can be helpful as well. In principle, probiotic therapy is not bound to any microbiological findings in the stool and can be carried out independently of such findings. The microbiological diagnosis—which is ideally combined with other fecal parameters (digestive remnants, inflammation markers)—may provide additional findings and clues for practical measures of complementary therapy in cases of gastrointestinal or atopic diseases as well as other difficult cases, or when the response to treatment is extremely slow.

Side Effects

The majority of patients tolerate probiotics very well. However, very high doses can cause side effects in patients with a hypersensitive disposition, like the one associated with severe atopy or inflammatory gastrointestinal diseases. Meteorism (i. e., flatulent distention of the abdomen), abdominal pain, or aggravation of the existing syndrome may indicate that the dose is too high. In such cases, the dose is reduced by a few drops, and symptoms abate within a few days.

To prevent reactions from occurring in very sensitive patients, it is recommended that treatment starts with a low dose that is then increased within the limits of good tolerance. It is not important for the success of the therapy to reach the recommended treatment doses. It makes far more sense to treat the patient with a dose adapted to his/her reactive disposition for as long as it is clinically necessary (16).

Clinical Application

The different components of the probiotic therapy make it possible to address the individual needs of the patient specifically and to vary the extent of the necessary therapeutic measures depending on type, severity, and chronicity of the disease.

- Especially in the treatment of chronic diseases, it has proved ideal to use different microbial preparations, nutrient supplements containing lactic acid bacteria, and autovaccines in **indication-specific treatment schemes**. The following approach makes it possible to control the immune system with different signals (16):
  - **Initiation.** The basic scheme of probiotic therapy for treating chronic or chronic recurrent diseases includes an initial step of fine-tuning the immune system. In this step, autolysates prepared from inactivated *E. coli* and *Enterococcus* are administered.
  - **Phase 1.** initiation is followed by administration of live *Enterococcus*. If lactic acid bacteria and autovaccines are to be applied, this is also done when starting phase 1.
  - **Phase 2.** Phase 1 is followed by administration of live *E. coli* in addition to live *Enterococcus* (Fig. 17.**3**). The concomitant use of both these bacteria is based on the fact that *Enterococcus* and *E. coli* send out different immunological signals and control the defense functions in different ways. In the end, both bacteria have a synergistic effect on the immune system and, together, they lead to an intense control of defense functions. If lactic acid bacteria and autovaccines have been used in addition to these microbial preparations, their administration may continue into phase 2 (Fig. 17.**3**).

Table 17.3 Therapeutic measures of probiotic therapy	
Basic therapy (usually *Enterococcus faecalis* and/or *E. coli*)	Microbial preparations for oral application (medical probiotics)
Intensified, individualized therapy	Additional administration of autovaccines in case of therapy resistance or a severe chronic course of the disease; also obligatory in cases of atopic allergies, urogenital infections, or chronic inflammatory intestinal diseases
Complementary therapy with lactic acid bacteria	Additional oral administration in cases of allergies, mycoses, gastrointestinal diseases or discomfort, indigestion (pharmaceutical probiotics)

- On average, the **length of treatment** for chronic diseases is around five to nine months and should be varied according to the severity and chronicity of the disease. In the end, it is always the clinical picture that decides the length of treatment. It is important here that the treatment lasts long enough to reach a stable condition. In very severe cases, this could mean that probiotic therapy has to be continued for one or two years. As a rule of thumb, the treatment period often corresponds in months to the number of years that have elapsed since the beginning of the disease.
- It is important for **compliance** to inform patients prior to therapy about the treatment period required and also about the fact that, in severe cases, improvement often comes only after months. Important prerequisites for a therapeutic success with chronically ill patients are perseverance, patience, and discipline.
- The basic scheme of application needs to be modified according to indication. For example, using a combination of inactivated *Enterococcus* and *E. coli* is of special importance in the case of allergies. On the other hand, initiation with inactivated bacteria is not essential in the treatment of acute infections.

Malignant Diseases

The improvement of immune functions ranks high in complementary oncological therapy and follow-up. Apart from this, probiotic therapy serves to stimulate metabolic functions and often also to remove treatment-induced damages, especially in the intestine. The application of microbial preparations and autovaccines should be understood primarily as adjuvant measures.

Because of the hypersensitive disposition of patients with malignancies, probiotic therapy requires a lot of tact and experience with these patients. It is therefore not recommended that one gets into probiotic therapy by treating such severe diseases. Rather, one should first gain experience and confidence in dealing with microbial preparations and autovaccines by starting with less complicated syndromes, such as chronic infections, mycoses, pollinosis, or atopic dermatitis.

- Because of the hypersensitive disposition of cancer patients, probiotic therapy should be approached with special care (Tables 17.**4** and 17.**5**).

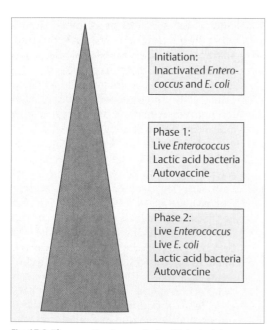

Initiation:
Inactivated *Enterococcus* and *E. coli*

Phase 1:
Live *Enterococcus*
Lactic acid bacteria
Autovaccine

Phase 2:
Live *Enterococcus*
Live *E. coli*
Lactic acid bacteria
Autovaccine

Fig. 17.**3** Therapeutic phases of microbiological therapy

Table 17.4 Therapeutic phases of probiotic therapy for malignant diseases, adults

Initiation	ProSymbioflor	Start with 2 × 1 drop and increase to 2 × 20 drops	4 weeks
Phase 1	Symbioflor 1 (+/− lactic acid bacteria) Autovaccine	2 × 20 drops	20 weeks
Phase 2	Symbioflor 2 Symbioflor 1 (+/− lactic acid bacteria) Autovaccine	Start with 2 × 1 drop and increase to 2 × 20 drops 2 × 20 drops	24 weeks

Table 17.5 Therapeutic phases of probiotic therapy for malignant diseases, children

Initiation	ProSymbioflor	Start with 2 × 1 drop and increase to 2 × 20 drops	4 weeks
Phase 1	Symbioflor 1 (+/− lactic acid bacteria) Autovaccine	2 × 20 drops	20 weeks
Phase 2	Symbioflor 2 Symbioflor 1 (+/− lactic acid bacteria) Autovaccine	Start with 1 × 1 drop and increase to 1 × 20 drops 2 × 20 drops	24 weeks

- Therapy is initiated very cautiously, beginning with only 2 × 1 drop daily.
- The dose is increased during the following days by adding one drop every day until a maximal dose of 2 × 20 drops is reached.
- After four weeks, initiation by administering inactivated bacteria is finished, and phase 1 follows with the application of live *Enterococcus*. After at least five months of phase 1 therapy, live cultures of *E. coli* are administered in addition to *Enterococcus*. Phase 2 also lasts for at least five months. The entire probiotic treatment thus covers approximately one year. In severe cases, treatment is also possible over a much longer period. The important thing is to adapt the total treatment period to the clinical necessities and to avoid premature termination of the therapy after the first signs of improvement.
- Especially when dealing with gastrointestinal cancer or when the patient suffers from intestinal discomfort, indigestion, or disturbed well-being, the addition of lactic acid bacteria is recommended when starting phase 1 of probiotic therapy.
- Autovaccines are an integral component of probiotic therapy and facilitate a very specific immunoregulation that is fine-tuned to the individual's defense situation. It is essential to start the therapy with highly diluted autovaccines. To make sure that these can be prepared in adequate dilutions, it is very important to emphasize that one is dealing with a cancer patient. This notion is relevant, even though the cancer may have occurred decades ago and the probiotic therapy is aimed at treating another disease.
- In cases of cancer, probiotic therapy should never be discontinued abruptly but always very gradually. For this purpose, the current dose is changed into a **maintenance dose** for the last six weeks of treatment. This means applying the doses of *Enterococcus* and *E. coli* in daily alternation: 1 × 20 drops of live cultures of *Enterococcus* on the first day, 1 × 20 drops of live cultures of *E. coli* on the next day, and so on, for approximately six weeks. In exceptional cases—above all, when the final discontinuation of probiotics creates problems—the maintenance dose can be continued for much longer periods, even for years, if deemed necessary.
- Since immune functions are suppressed by chemotherapy and radiation therapy, the effect of concurrent probiotic therapy is diminished. Nevertheless, the simultaneous use of probiotics during chemotherapy or radiation therapy can contribute to the general well-being of the patient.

▬ References

1. Fuller R, Heidt PJ, Rusch V, van der Waaij D (eds): Probiotics—aspects of use in opportunistic infections. Old Herborn University Seminar Monograph 8. Herborn-Dill, Herborn Litterae, 1995.
2. Habermann W, Zimmermann K, Skarabis H, Kunze R, Rusch V: Einfluss eines bakteriellen Immunstimulans (humane *Enterococcus faecalis*-Bakterien) auf die Rezidivhäufigkeit bei Patienten mit chronischer Bronchitis. Arzneimittel-Forschung/Drug Research. 2001; 51(II):931–937.
3. Hacker J, Heesemann J: Infektionsbiologie. Interaktionen zwischen Mikroorganismen und Zellen. Heidelberg, Spektrum Akademischer Verlag, 2000.
4. Hanson LÅ, Yolken R (eds): Probiotics, other nutritional factors, and intestinal microflora. Nestlé Nutrition Workshop Series, Vol 42. Philadelphia, Lippincott-Raven, 1999.
5. Heidt PJ, Midtvedt T, Rusch V, van der Waaij D (eds): Probiotics. Bacteria and bacterial fragments as immunomodulatory agents. Old Herborn University Seminar Monograph 15. Herborn-Dill, Herborn Litterae, 2002.
6. Jansen GJ: The influence of oral treatment with *Enterococcus faecalis* on the human gut microflora and on the systemic humoral immune response. Dissertation. Groningen, Rijksuniversiteit Groningen, 1994.
7. Kalinski S: Steigerung der körpereigenen Abwehr bei chronisch rezidivierender Tonsillitis. Fortschritte der Medizin. 1986; 104:843–846.
8. Kalinski S: Immunstimulation bei Infektionen der oberen Luftwege und im HNO-Bereich. Klinische Prüfung eines Streptokokken-Präparates. Therapiewoche. 1987; 37:3371–3378.
9. Kalliomaki M, Salminen S, Arvilommi H, Kero P, Koskinen P, Isolauri E: Probiotics in primary prevention of atopic disease: a randomised placebo-controlled trial. Lancet. 2001; 357:1057–1059.
10. Ottendorfer D, Zimmermann K: Mikrobiologische Therapie. Wirkung bei allergischen Erkrankungen. Forum Immunologie. Stockdorf, Forum-Medizin, 1997.
11. Panijel M, Burkard I: ProSymbioflor zur Behandlung des irritablen Kolons. Jatros Naturheilkunde 2/3, 1993.
12. Rappenhöner B, Pfeil T, Herrmann E, Rychlik R: Zur Behandlung der chronisch-obstruktiven Bronchitis mit einem Immunstimulator. Eine Kosten-Nutzen-Analyse zu Symbioflor 1. Die Medizinische Welt 3/96, 1996.
13. Rembacken J, Snelling AM, Hawkey PM, Chalmers DM, Axon ATR: Non-pathogenic *Escherichia coli* versus mesalazine for the treatment of ulcerative colitis: a randomised trial. Lancet. 1999; 354:635–639.
14. Reuter G, Klein G, Heidt PJ, Rusch V (eds): Proceedings of the Symposium on "Probiotics in Man and Animal," Berlin, 1996. Microecology and Therapy 26. Herborn-Dill, Herborn Litterae, 1997.
15. Rosenkranz W, Grundmann E: Immunmodulatorische Wirkung lebender nicht-pathogener Enterococcus faecalis-Bakterien des Menschen. Arzneimittel-Forschung/Drug Research. 1994; 44:691–695.
16. Rusch K, Rusch V: Mikrobiologische Therapie. Grundlagen und Praxis. Heidelberg, Karl F. Haug Verlag, 2001.
17. Rusch V: Bakterien–Freunde oder Feinde? Berlin, Urania, 1999.
18. Rusch V, Ottendorfer D, Zimmermann K, et al.: Results of an open, non-placebo controlled pilot study investigating the immunomodulatory potential of autovaccine. Arzneimittel-Forschung/Drug Research. 2001; 51(II): 690–697.
19. Schaffstein W, Burkhard I: Symbioflor 2-eine therapeutische Alternative zur Behandlung des irritablen Kolons. Jatros Gastroenterologie 2/4, 1993.
20. Schöllmann C, Zimmermann K: Intestinale Mikroflora und Immunsystem. Edition Materia Medica. Stockdorf, Forum-Medizin, 1997.
21. Schrezenmeir J, de Vrese M: Probiotics, prebiotics, and synbiotics—approaching a definition. American Journal of Clinical Nutrition. 2001; 73:361–364.
22. Tannock GW (ed): Probiotics. A critical review. Norfolk UK, Horizon Scientific Press, 1999.

18 Blockade of Adhesion Molecules

Joseph Beuth

Lectins and Tumor Metastasis

The discovery that human liver contains membrane-associated β-D-galactose-specific lectins has initiated new lines of thought and experimental approaches (1). Based on this finding, the organotropism of metastatic malignant tumors has been interpreted in the light of a lectin-receptor theory for the first time (2). According to this theory, the galactose residue on tumor cell membranes may be regarded as a tumor-associated cryptantigen.

This carbohydrate group could have formed secondarily during malignant transformation by losing a terminal sugar molecule (e.g., *N*-acetylneuraminic acid, NANA), or it could just be a component of a precursor substance that has not changed into a "normal" glycoconjugate. Such "precursors" are known to occur in tumor cell membranes in the form of glycoproteins as well as glycolipids. They usually are formed due to the absence or inhibition of glycosyltransferases and belong, from the serological point of view, to the human blood groups (2).

As it turned out, vertebral lectins (e.g., the liver cell receptor for asialoglycoproteins, or liver lectin) also possess mitogenic properties. It is therefore assumed that these lectins play a decisive role in the adhesion of circulating tumor cells and, through appropriate stimulation, also in their growth behavior by interacting with exposed carbohydrate structures on the tumor cells ("contact stimulation"). Paradoxically, the metastatic tumor cell, with its incomplete, membrane-associated sugar molecules—often identical with the tumor marker—is recognized by the organ-specific lectins as belonging to the organ and is therefore captured. A corresponding mechanism has been found, for example, for neuraminidase-treated serum glycoproteins and hormones, where the loss of NANA means aging (9).

The process of **metastasis** is no accident but is governed by inhibiting and promoting interactions between the tumor and its host organism. Experimental research on tumor metastasis suggests that specific changes on the tumor cell membrane (such as the appearance of incomplete carbohydrate chains as tumor markers) and on organ-specific lectins (which act as mitogenic adhesion molecules) play a decisive role for the organotropism of metastasis (3, 4). The discovery and biochemical analysis of the galactose-specific liver lectin (hepatic binding protein, HBP) finally lead to the hypothesis that a liver damaged by disease (with lectins reduced in numbers or functionally restricted) might be relatively unreceptive for metastases. If an organ (e.g., the liver) is altered through disease (such as cirrhosis, fatty liver), the organ-specific lectins no longer function; hence, they can no longer recognize and bind the sugar molecules exposed on the tumor cell membrane. As a result, metastasis can no longer occur in the classic (hematogenous, lymphogenic) manner.

Analyzing the medical histories of more than 1500 cancer patients at the Surgical University Clinic, Cologne, Germany, has confirmed the following hypothesis: in a pathologically altered liver, the organ-specific adhesion molecules (lectins) can no longer fulfill their task of clearing the serum from asialoglycoproteins and neuraminic acid-free cells (such as tumor cells with a terminal galactose in membrane-associated carbohydrate residues).

In patients with liver damage, we found a considerable increase in asialoglycoproteins in the se-

Table 18.1 Development of liver metastases in cancer patients with/without liver diseases, such as cirrhosis, chronic hepatitis, fatty liver (11)

	Cancer patient examined	Patients with liver metastases
Normal liver	1047	710 (68%)
Damaged liver	495	33 (7%)
Total number of cancer patients	1542	743 (48%)

rum and a significantly reduced incidence of metastasis of malignant tumors in the liver (Table 18.**1**) (11). These results were confirmed by a Japanese study (10), where 40 out of 250 patients with colorectal carcinoma developed liver metastases (16%) but cirrhotic liver damage was detected in none of these. In the same cohort, however, metastatic growth could not be found in patients with a pathologically altered liver.

— Experimental Blockade of Liver Lectins

After the role of organ-specific lectins (liver lectins) in glycoprotein metabolism and tumor metastases in the liver had been demonstrated by experimental and statistical studies (4), the following experiments basically focused on evidence for interactions at the molecular level between organ cells and tumor cells:

- In-vitro adhesion of human tumor cells (derived from mammary, cervical, laryngeal, bronchial carcinoma) to freshly isolated homologous hepatocytes was inhibited by means of **galactose** as well as different galactoglycoconjugates.

- Arabinogalactan (a high molecular weight, galactose-rich, vegetable polysaccharide) and galactose turned out to be the best inhibitors in these studies; they completely prevented rosette formation between hepatocytes and tumor cells. Nonspecific carbohydrates had no effect on rosette formation. Treatment of tumor cells with neuraminidase (to unmask the penultimate galactose residues of membrane glycoconjugates) resulted in increased rosette formation with hepatocytes, which was inhibited with galactoglycoconjugates. Incubation of tumor cells with galactose oxidase (for enzymatic cleavage and elimination of membrane-associated galactose residues) completely prevented rosette formation (5).

- The adhesion experiments in vitro with human tumor cells and homologous hepatocytes confirmed the galactose specificity of this intercellular recognition mechanism. In order to demonstrate also in vivo that galactoglycoconjugates block liver lectins, BALB/c mice received intravenous injections of tritium-labeled α1-acid asialoglycoprotein. The rapid elimination of asialoglycoprotein from the serum of the test animals and its rapid uptake into their liver was

much delayed by prior injection of galactose or arabinogalactan. These results suggest that the blockade of asialoglycoprotein receptors of the liver (liver lectins) by receptor-specific sugar molecules was responsible for the delayed elimination of asialoglycoprotein from the serum (3).

- The hypothesis that the **metastasis** of malignant tumors is a specific, **receptor-mediated process** and that organ-specific lectins play a role in the adhesion of disseminated tumor cells, or in the organotropism of metastasis, was confirmed for the first time in vivo by means of two murine tumor models (L-1 sarcoma in BALB/c mice; ESb lymphoma in DBA/2 mice). In these experiments, different galactose-containing glycoconjugates were used in diverse application schemes and at different treatment intervals in order to inhibit the adhesion of tumor cells to parenchymal liver cells by blocking the organ-specific liver lectins. Only the regular administration of galactose or arabinogalactan was able to inhibit occurrence of metastases in the liver in a statistically significant manner, while no effect was observed on the tumor's manifestation in other organs. Of all treatment schedules tested in a mouse model, the best results were obtained with the injection of galactose or arabinogalactan over a limited period of three days and at eight-hour intervals (with the first injection one hour prior to tumor cell inoculation). This was obviously correlated with the restricted life span of tumor cells in the vascular system, or with their destruction by mechanical or immunological mechanisms when they fail to find an adhesion molecule as anchoring site (3, 4).

- Mannan and other galactose-free substances, which have been tested in the same manner (same doses and schedules of application), did not prevent metastasis into the liver, thus impressively documenting the specificity of this process. In both tumor models, other organ systems were not affected by this glycoconjugate treatment. In particular, no additional formation of metastases was observed in any of the individuals, although appropriate tests were carried out routinely (3, 4).

- Meanwhile these results have been confirmed in another tumor model (6). Here, the hepatoma MBH 1 in C57B1/65 mice was used, which metastasizes predominantly in the liver after subcutaneous or intravenous inoculation. Liver metastasis was significantly reduced with arabinogalactan (1 mg/kg body weight; one hour prior to and then at eight-hour intervals after tumor cell inoculation, over a total period of 48 hours). However, no significant inhibitory effect was detected with an appropriate administration of galactose, which was attributed to the rapid elimination of galactose from the blood of the test animals.

▬ Clinical Studies

Based on the present experimental and clinical data, three clinical studies on the clinical efficacy of the blockade of liver lectins with galactose were carried out in patients with colorectal carcinoma and stomach cancer.

- In a prospective randomized study (7), 93 patients with **colorectal carcinoma** in the treatment group received perioperative infusions of galactose; they were compared with 100 patients in the control group. The study included patients with tumors of stages UICC (Union International Centre Cancer) I–III. The two patient cohorts were comparable with respect to age, sex, tumor stage, tumor grading, and adjuvant therapies. After an observation period of 36 months, no liver metastases were found in the treatment group containing 27 patients at stage II, while in the control group two out of 31 patients had liver metastases. At stage III, the number of patients with liver metastases was five out of 31 in the treatment group, but nine out of 44 in the control group. Late appearance of liver metastases was observed in the treatment group. There was no difference at that stage with respect to disease-free survival; however, there was an advantage in the total survival of 70% in the treatment group as compared with 50% in the control group (Table 18.**2**). This difference was not statistically significant.

- In another prospective randomized study (12), 39 patients with **colon cancer** received perioperative galactose infusions; they were compared with 37 patients in the control group who received perioperative glucose infusions. The two cohorts were comparable with respect to patient characteristics. After an observation period of 48 months, liver metastases were found in 15 patients of the control group, but only in eight patients of the treatment group (Table 18.**3**). This difference was statistically significant.

- In a third study (8), 80 patients with **stomach cancer** were randomized into a treatment group with perioperative galactose infusions and a control group with glucose infusions. The two cohorts of 40 patients each were comparable with respect to patient characteristics. After an observation period of 48 months, liver metastases were found in 15 patients of the treatment group, but in 25 patients of the control group (Table 18.**4**). This difference was statistically significant.

Table 18.2 Development of liver metastases and distant nonliver metastases in patients with colorectal carcinoma (7)

		Control group	Treatment group
Number of patients (n)		100	93
Mean observation time		36 months	36 months
Stage I $n = 60$	Location of metastases: liver other organs	$n = 25$ 1 1	$n = 35$ 2 0
Stage II $n = 58$	Location of metastases: liver other organs	$n = 31$ 2 1	$n = 27$ 0 3
Stage III $n = 75$	Location of metastases: liver other organs	$n = 44$ 9 7	$n = 31$ 5 8
Stages I–III	Liver metastases	12 (12%)	7 (7%)

Table 18.3 Development of liver metastases in patients with colon cancer. Randomized comparison between a group of patients treated perioperatively with galactose and a control group (12)

	Control group		Treatment group	
Number of patients	37		39	
Mean observation time	48 months		48 months	
Tumor stage: T1–3 N0 M0, stage II	Patients (n)	Liver metastases	Patients (n)	Liver metastases
T1 N0 M0	10	2	9	1
T2 N0 M0	6	3	7	2
T3 N0 M0	21	10	23	5
T1–T3	37	15	39	8

Table 18.4 Development of liver metastases in patients with stomach cancer. Randomized comparison between a group of patients treated perioperatively with galactose and a control group (8)

	Control group		Treatment group	
Number of patients	40		40	
Mean observation time	48 months		48 months	
Tumor stage: T1–3 N0 M0, stage II	Patients (n)	Liver metastases	Patients (n)	Liver metastases
T1 N0 M0	4	2	5	1
T2 N0 M0	7	4	8	3
T3 N0 M0	29	19	27	11
T1–T3	40	25	40	15

▬ Summary

These three clinical studies suggest that the blocking of liver lectins by galactose has a favorable effect in the sense that it reduces the incidence of liver metastases. In view of the fact that the differences were too negligible in the study by Isenberg et al (7) and that the patient numbers were too low in the studies by Warczynski et al. (12) and Kosik et al. (8), these studies cannot serve as definitive proof of the validity of the hypothesis on the prevention of liver metastasis. Together with the experimental in-vitro and in-vivo data as well as the findings with patients, however, these clinical studies indicate that the galactose specificity of tumor cell metastasis in the liver is valid in humans as well and that the intraoperative spread of tumor cells is relevant for the process of metastasis. Thus, two important premises for carrying out confirmative clinical studies have been realized.

A confirmative study according to GCP guidelines has been initiated for definitive clarification of the therapeutic rating of the liver lectin blockade by means of receptor-specific (D-galactose-terminated) glycoconjugates. The results of this study will throw light on whether this relatively nontoxic technique can indeed be added to the armamentarium of integrative oncology.

▬ References

1. Ashwell G, Moorell AG: The role of surface carbohydrates in the hepatic recognition and transport of circulating glycopeptides. Edv. Enzymol. 1974; 41: 99–128.
2. August DA, Otthow RT, Sugarbaker P: Clinical perspectives on human colorectal cancer metastasis. Cancer Metastasis Rev. 1984; 3:303–324.
3. Beuth J, Ko HL, Oette K, et al.: Inhibition of liver metastasis in mice by blocking hepatocyte lectins with arabinogalactan infusions and D-galactose. J. Cancer Res. Clin. Oncol. 1987; 113:51–55.
4. Beuth J, Ko HL, Schirrmacher V, et al.: Inhibition of liver tumor cell colonization in two animal tumor models by lectin blocking with D-galactose or arabinogalactan. Clin. Exp. Metastasis. 1988; 6:115–120.
5. Beuth J, Oette K, Uhlenbruck G: Liver lectins as receptors for tumor cells in metastasis. Lectins. 1986; 5:229–235.
6. Hagmar B, Ryd W, Skomedal H: Arabinogalactan blockade of experimental metastases to liver by

murine hepatoma. Invasion Metastasis. 1991; 11: 348–355.

7. Isenberg J, Stoffel B, Stuetzer H, et al.: Liver lectin blocking with D galactose to prevent hepatic metastases in colorectal carcinoma patients. Anticancer Res. 1997; 17:3767–3772.

8. Kosik J, Szmigielski S, Beuth J, et al.: Prevention of hepatic metastases by liver lectin blocking with D-galactose in stomach cancer patients. A prospectively randomized clinical trial. Anticancer Res. 1997; 17:1411–1415.

9. Springer GF: T and Tn, general carcinoma autoantigens. Science. 1984; 224:1198–206.

10. Uetsuji T, Yamamura M, Yamamichi K, et al.: Absence of colorectal cancer metastasis to the cirrhotic liver. Am. J. Surg. 1992; 164:176–177.

11. Uhlenbruck G, Beuth J, Weidtmann V: Liver lectins: mediators for metastasis? Experientia. 1983; 39: 1314–1315.

12. Warczynski P, Gil J, Szmigielski S, et al.: Prevention of hepatic metastases by liver lectin blocking with D-galactose in colon cancer patients. A prospectively randomized clinical trial. Anticancer Res. 1997; 17:1223–1226.

19 Tumor Vaccination and Antibody-Mediated Immunotherapy

Volker Schirrmacher

Introduction

Tumor vaccination attempts to stimulate the patient's own immune system in such a way that immune reactions against the tumor are assisted in a targeted manner. Recently, this field has again become a burning issue due to three new developments:

- new ways of identifying and isolating tumor-associated antigens (TAA)
- new cell culture methods for propagating antigen-presenting cells (APC) and tumor-reactive immunocytes
- molecular biology methods for targeted gene transfer in tumor cells or other cells.

The idea of using antitumor vaccination for the targeted destruction of tumor cells in the body is not new (14), but only recent advances in immunology and molecular biology have prepared the ground for evaluating immunotherapy in controlled studies. Various approaches aim at selective immunostimulation, though they differ considerably in concept and realization.

In contrast to viruses and bacteria, tumor-associated antigens usually lead only to weak immune defenses; this is due to the fact that the expressed tumor antigens differ only slightly from physiologically occurring antigenic cell structures (42).

This tolerance of the immune system needs to be lowered. Here, we discuss the two most promising strategies: vaccines and monoclonal antibodies (MAbs).

Tumor Vaccines and Active Specific Immunotherapy (ASI)

All forms of vaccination rely on the immune system's active cooperation and support in order to provoke a targeted immune response. This is true also for tumor vaccination, which is therefore referred to as active specific immunotherapy (ASI).

The thesis favored initially, namely, that the immune system distinguishes only between "self" and "nonself," is no longer valid today (13). Obviously, the immune system recognizes tumors and develops immune responses, although these are often inefficient (48). The recognized antigens are often classic autoantigens, which therefore also occur on normal cells of the body.

Table 19.1 provides a list of representative human tumor antigens. These include, for example, oncofetal antigens and cancer-testis antigens (CTA), which are expressed on embryonic cells or germ cells; they are suppressed in differentiated body cells but may be re-expressed in tumor cells. In addition, tumor antigens include differentiation antigens, viral antigens, and also peptide sequences derived from proteins coded for by mutated or overexpressed genes.

If a tumor cell is supposed to induce a T-cell-mediated immune reaction, a professional antigen-presenting cell (e.g., a dendritic cell) must phagocytose tumor proteins and, subsequently, present peptide fragments of the tumor antigens on its surface together with genetically determined major histocompatibility complex (MHC) molecules (55). The complex of MHC molecule and tumor peptide is then recognized by cytotoxic (CD8⁺) or helper (CD4⁺) T lymphocytes. T-cell activation can only occur when, in addition to antigen recognition, activation signals are mediated to the T cells. This activation includes their proliferation and maturation into effector cells, which are either cytotoxic or release cytokines, such as IFN-γ. Cytotoxic T cells can recognize and directly destroy the tumor cell, once the same MHC–tumor–peptide complex has been identified on the malignant cell. This complex sequence of events must be taken into account when developing a successful tumor vaccine.

Clinical Studies

Active Immunization with Intact Modified Tumor Cells

A tumor vaccine made up of intact tumor cells from the patient has the advantage that all relevant tumor proteins and peptides are present in the vac-

Table 19.1 Representative human tumor antigens

Antigen[1]	MHC restriction[2]	T-cell epitope[3] (amino-acid sequence)
Cancer-testis Antigen		
MAGE-1	HLA-A1	EADPTGHSY
NY-ESO-1	HLA-A2	QLSLLMWIT
Differentiation antigen		
Tyrosinase	HLA-A2	MLLAVLYCL
CEA	HLA-A2	YLSGANLNL
Immunoglobulin isotype (myeloma)	Individual differences	Patient-specific
Product of a mutated gene		
β-catenin	HLA-A24	SYLDSGIF
Bcr/Abl	HLA-DR4	ATGFKQSSKALQRPVAS
Product of an overexpressed gene		
HER-2/neu	HLA-A2	KIFGSLAFL
p53	HLA-A2	LLGRNSFEN
Viral antigen		
HPV-E7	HLA-A2	YMLDLQPETT

[1] All tumor antigens are derived from cellular proteins. [2] Intracellular degradation of these proteins creates the peptides listed in the right column; these peptides are associated with the HLA molecules listed here and are transported as MHC–peptide complexes to the cell surface. [3] The MHC–peptide complexes are recognized by tumor antigen-specific T cells by means of accurately fitting T-cell receptors. The sequences of the T-cell epitopes are shown in amino-acid code.

cine and that the molecular characterization of their structures is not required (41, 53, 60). To increase the efficiency and immunogenicity of the tumor cells, they can be transfected ex vivo, for example, with cytokine gene sequences (21). After proper selection, the genetically modified tumor cells will secrete the desired cytokines aimed at enhancing the body's immune response. The difficulty is to achieve a sufficiently high transfection rate with tumor cells (1), a problem that can be solved by using new vector constructs that are usually based on adenoviruses or retroviruses (73), but also by using so-called virus-like particles (VLP) (39).

The Newcastle disease virus (NDV), an avian paramyxovirus, has the following special features:
– tumor-selective replication (52)
– induction of proinflammatory cytokines and chemokines (70)
– mediation of costimulatory signals for T cells (62)
– oncolytic effects (45)
– high degree of safety (no DNA integration, no risk of viral spread or infection)
– high tolerance and few side effects (36).

In the future, this virus can also be used for the purpose of gene therapy, because lately it has been produced by recombinant technology (43, 47).

Thus, NDV represents an interesting alternative in tumor gene therapy. It has been used in Heidelberg, Germany, since 1986 for infecting tumor cells in order to enhance their tumor immunogenicity (19, 25, 50, 51, 68). The virus-modified autologous tumor vaccine, called ATV-NDV, is being produced in a special laboratory from tumor tissue freshly obtained from the patient and then used postoperatively as an adjuvant therapy for the prevention of metastasis: (2)

• In a study involving 18 patients with **renal cell carcinoma** and eight patients with **prostatic carcinoma**, tumor cells were obtained during surgery and transfected with a retroviral vector coding for GM-CSF (37). After irradiating these tumor cells, they were applied subcutaneously to the patients at four-week intervals. The side effects were minor (mild fever, chills, pain in the limbs, and itching). One of the renal cell carcinoma patients showed regression of pulmonary metastases for seven months. None of the patients in the group with prostatic carcinoma responded to the treatment. The biggest problem in these studies was to harvest and propagate sufficient amounts of autologous tumor cells.

• In a second study, which involved 17 patients with **metastatic renal cell carcinoma** (30) and with a positive cutaneous reaction to recall antigens, the primary tumor was first removed. Cell hybrids were then created within 12 hours from autologous tumor cells and allogeneic dendritic cells by means of electrofusion. At intervals of six weeks, the patients received at least two subcutaneous injections into the region of the inguinal lymph nodes. In case of a clinical response after 12 weeks, a booster vaccination followed every three months. No major side effects were observed. Eleven out of 17 patients treated developed positive skin reactions (delayed type hypersensitivity, DTH) as a sign of a specific immune response following the exposure to tumor cells. Seven patients (41%) responded to the therapy, with four complete remissions (23%), two partial remissions (12%), and one mixed response (6%). The problem of this study was with the size and selection of the patient cohort. Thus, "spontaneous" remissions of metastases after removal of the primary tumor have been observed in nonselected patients in up to 10% of the individuals (32). Whether the better result of this study can be attributed solely to the selection of immunocompetent patients or whether the vaccine therapy had contributed to the result, must be clarified in larger case–control studies without preselected patients.

- Long-term survival advantages were observed in an earlier study on **metastatic renal cell carcinoma** in which we participated (44). This study included 40 patients with advanced renal cell carcinoma, each of whom had distant metastases in at least one organ at the time of surgery. Following nephrectomy, active immunization with intact, NDV-modified autologous tumor cells was performed by multiple vaccinations. In addition to immunization with the tumor vaccine ATV-NDV, the patients received low-dose recombinant interleukin-2 and interferon-α in three two-week cycles. In 40 patients evaluated, the following observations were made:
  - five complete remissions (CR)
  - six partial remissions (PR)
    12 individuals with stable disease (SD; median 25 months)
  - 17 tumor progressions
  - median survival time of CR and PR patients: more than four years
  - median survival time of SD patients: 31 months.

Twenty-three (57.5%) of the 40 patients with CR, PR, or SD seemed to gain a survival benefit from this adjuvant treatment as compared with the progressive patients or with a historical reference group (44).

- **Melanoma**: For several years now, David Berd and co-workers in Philadelphia, USA, have evaluated a dinitrophenyl-modified autologous tumor vaccine. For 62 patients with stage III melanoma and lymphadenectomy, who were treated postoperatively with this vaccine, the five-year survival rate was 58% (7). The results of earlier studies on clinical tumor vaccination against malignant melanoma have been summarized in 1995 (53).

- After fusion with a tumor cell, an antigen-presenting cell is thought to present a major portion of the tumor antigens on its surface and, hence, should efficiently stimulate the immune system (59). This idea led to a clinical study involving 16 patients with **metastatic melanoma** of an advanced stage (65). These patients received three subcutaneous vaccinations with at least 3×10^7 tumor cells at two sites that were located as far away from the tumor as possible. The treatment was well tolerated and never reached level II of the World Health Organization scale of side effects. Two patients developed local vitiligo as a sign of induction or expansion of melanocyte-specific T cells. The mean survival time of 16.1 months was clearly better that the six months historically expected for such patients.

- In the case of primary **mammary carcinoma**, we can look back on long-term experience with postoperative adjuvant therapy using active specific immunization with the autologous tumor vaccine ATV-NDV: In a phase II study involving 62 patients, there were indications for a clear improvement in the five-year survival rate by approximately 30% when using the most favorable application (2, 54). The number of tumor cells and their vitality were decisive for the quality and effectiveness of this virus-modified autologous tumor vaccine (2).

- In another study on vaccination, 38 patients with primary **colorectal carcinoma** (Dukes stage C) were postoperatively treated with the autologous tumor vaccine ATV-NDV. As was the case with the mammary carcinoma study, patients treated with the most favorable live cell vaccine obviously gained a long-term survival benefit as compared with those treated with a less favorable vaccine or those receiving no postoperative immunotherapy at all (40, 50).

- In a prospective randomized phase III study on active specific immunotherapy, 254 patients with **colon cancer** received a BCG-modified autologous live cell vaccine. In patients with stage II (Dukes Stage 132/133) and stage III (Dukes Stage C) colon cancer, this lead to a reduction of recurrences by 43 % and of deaths by 32 % (*P* < 0.01) (67).

Active Immunization with Peptides and Heat Shock Proteins

Whereas the tumor-associated antigens in the tumor vaccines do not undergo further characterization prior to application, the situation is different for vaccination with TAA peptides. Only used here are antigenic proteins or peptide fragments of known amino-acid sequence, against which specific CD4$^+$ and/or CD8$^+$ T-cell responses have been demonstrated in vitro in the respective MHC context (20). However, it is very costly to define the immunogenic peptide domains of a tumor protein and to restrict the immune response to only the one or a few peptide domains that are usually limited to a few human leukocyte antigen (HLA) molecules.

To activate the immune system, the peptides must be presented on antigen-presenting cells in the context of MHC. This can be achieved by direct injection of peptides into the skin or into the region of draining lymph nodes, where they are then taken up by antigen-presenting cells (such as dendritic cells), processed, and presented to the immune system on their cell surface. Another approach is to treat dendritic cells ex vivo (4). For this purpose, precursors of dendritic cells are isolated from the patient, loaded with peptides, and reinfused into the patient once the cells have matured. To enhance the immune response, substances that support this stimulation (e.g., cytokines) are almost always administered together with the dendritic cells, independently of the procedure chosen.

Direct administration of peptides is the approach most frequently used, because it is both technically simple and safe for the patient. Many tumor antigens have been identified in malignant melanoma, which is why this tumor is still the prototype for many immunotherapeutic strategies.

Instead of individually defined tumor peptides, certain **heat shock proteins** (HSP) can be obtained from tumor cells and used for tumor immunotherapy (4). Heat shock proteins are natural chaperones of peptides and represent the total peptide composition of the cell. Heat shock protein–peptide complexes are particularly immunogenic and have shown therapeutic effects in preclinical studies with animal tumors (8). First clinical studies have already started.

Most of the data obtained so far are derived from melanocyte differentiation antigens, such as Melan-A/MART-1, gp100, or also tyrosinase (69). In the phase I/II studies performed, no side effects worth mentioning were observed after peptide vaccination. Half of the patients treated developed peptide-specific skin reactions or in-vitro reactions. There were isolated cases where the core of the tumor was reduced in size, but no significant tumor regression or prolonged survival was observed. The use of differentiation antigens as a vaccination substance turned out to be problematic because of the genetic instability of the tumor cells. Under the selection pressure of the vaccination and the immune response generated thereby, the tumor cells partly lost expression of the differentiation antigens used as the target structure (26). Apart from the pigment loss seen in local vitiligo, the tumor continued to grow independently of the immune response induced. The more recently used tumor antigens with stable expression—especially those from the group of cancer-testis antigens, such as NY-ESO-1—may represent an alternative (27).

Ex-Vivo Loading of Dendritic Cells

In principle, standardizing the administration of peptides in vivo is problematic. The peptide must reach the local lymph node in sufficient amounts and within a certain time frame in order to induce an immune response rather than blocking it (74). Therefore, the loading of professional antigen-presenting cells in the lymph node plays a decisive role:

- The first attempts of a more efficient ex-vivo loading of dendritic cells (DC) with tumor antigens were again undertaken with **malignant melanoma**. The dendritic cells of 16 patients were isolated, expanded in the presence of granulocyte–macrophage colony stimulating factor (GM-CSF) and interleukin-4 (IL-4), and then loaded with tumor peptides (tyrosinase, gp100, Melan-A/MART-1) or tumor lysate (38). Vaccination was well tolerated. Eleven of the 16 patients developed a positive skin reaction after renewed exposure to the antigen or tumor lysate. Five patients showed also a clinical response, with two complete (15%) and three partial remissions (19%). A reduction in tumor size was observed in various organs, e.g., skin, soft tissue, lungs, and also pancreas. Immunohistochemical analysis of vaccine-infiltrating lymphocytes in a similar therapeutic approach revealed a dominance of CD8+ T cells in nine out of 17 patients (9). In three out of five patients evaluated, the specificity of these lymphocytes for the tumor lysate of the patient has been demonstrated. However, neither the infiltration with CD8+ T cells nor their specificity can be unambiguously assigned to the vaccination procedure, because no tumor biopsies were examined prior to therapy.

- Also **prostate cancer** has been treated with peptide-loaded dendritic cells (49, 63). This usually involved the use of HLA-A2-specific peptides of the prostate-specific membrane antigen (PSMA). In a first phase I study involving 51 patients with hormone-refractory metastatic prostate cancer, the excellent tolerance of this approach was confirmed once again. On average, the PSA level dropped after treatment. In a subsequent phase I/II study, 74 patients with advanced prostate cancer were treated at six-week intervals with six intravenous DC applications (approximately 2×10^7 peptide-loaded DC per intravenous application). The response rate was 25–30%. The duration of the response correlated positively with the number of dendritic cells applied.

Instead of dendritic cells, Epstein–Barr virus-transformed, spontaneous lymphoblastoid cell lines (LCL) from cancer patients can also be used as antigen-presenting cells (29). A study on vaccination with mutated p21 ras peptides and autologous LCL involving healthy donors and a single patient with pancreatic tumor revealed adequate and specific activation of the immune system. As the disease of the patient was very advanced, a response of the tumor to the treatment was not to be expected and was also not observed.

▬ Monoclonal Antibodies and Passive Immunotherapy

In contrast to the vaccination strategies just described, passive immunotherapy with MAbs does not require the immune system's active cooperation and support in order to provoke a specific immune response against the tumor cells. Within the scope of passive immunotherapy, monoclonal antibodies are supposed to find and destroy specific tumor cells in the patient. After binding to the tumor cells, the antibodies show their activity in different ways:
- blockade of signal transduction pathways (e.g., inhibition of proliferation stimuli)
- local initiation of complement cascade (complement-dependent cytotoxicity, CDC)
- recruitment of effector cells (antibody-dependent cellular cytotoxicity, ADCC) (11, 22, 55).

In 1982, a patient with non-Hodgkin lymphoma was the first to experience a complete remission after receiving individually produced monoclonal anti-idiotype antibody (34). In spite of numerous studies on the treatment of other tumors, these therapeutic attempts have remained unsuccessful. Special problems were created by the high costs and also by the regular appearance of blocking antibodies (human antimouse antibodies, HAMAs) after repeated applications. At the beginning of the 1990s, only the murine anti-CD3 antibody (Muromonab CD3), designed to treat acute rejection reactions following organ transplantation, was successful (72). It was only through the development of recombinant antibodies—as chimeric or humanized antibodies—that repetitive treatment cycles became possible in the mid-1990s. Improved manufacturing procedures also allowed for cost-effective production of the amounts required (18). Today, antibody-based therapeutics make up 25% of the new products now studied in early clinical research. So far, the American health authorities (FDA) have approved nine antibodies with different indications (Table 19.**2**), and more than 70 antibodies are being tested in phase I/II studies.

A major problem is insufficient accessibility of the target antigen. In several studies involving patients with colorectal carcinoma, specific accumulation of the antibody in the tumor area or in regions of metastases was detected after intravenous administration (71). After biopsy or resection of the tumor, however, it was found that the anti-

Table 19.2 Monoclonal antibodies approved by the Food and Drug Administration (FDA)

Antibody	Trade name	Target antigen	Indication
Muromomab	OKT3	CD3 (T cells)	Transplant rejection
Basiliximab	Simulect	CD25 (T cells)	Transplant rejection
Daclizumab	Zenapax	CD25 (T cells)	Transplant rejection
Infliximab	Remicade	TNF-α (soluble)	Rheumatoid arthritis, Crohn disease
Pavilizumab	Synagis	RSV	Respiratory syncytial virus
Abciximab	ReoPro	GP IIa/IIIb (thrombocytes)	Coronary revascularization
Rituximab	Mabthera	CD20 (B cells)	Follicular B-cell non-Hodgkin lymphoma
Trastuzumab	Herceptin	HER-2/neu	Metastatic mammary carcinoma
Gemtuzumab ozogamicin	Mylotarg	CD33	Recurrent acute myeloid leukemia

bodies were distributed unevenly, accumulating predominantly in the marginal regions. Obviously, central tumor parts are not reached by conventional antibody constructs due to tumor necrosis, uneven antigen distribution, and increased interstitial tissue pressure. Here, a solution to the problem may be the use of smaller antibody molecules with altered binding properties or also antibody conjugates in which the antibody serve as a vehicle to achieve specific accumulation of cytotoxic substances (chemotherapeutic agents, radionucleotides) in the tumor (24, 64).

Clinical Studies

Herceptin: A Prototype for Antibody Therapy of Solid Tumors

With respect to solid tumors, therapeutic success has been reported especially in cases of breast cancer. Trastuzumab (Herceptin) is a humanized monoclonal antibody that has recently been approved also in Europe for treating metastatic mammary carcinoma overexpressing the HER-2/neu oncogene.

HER-2/neu is a growth factor receptor tyrosine kinase that is overexpressed in 25–30% of all mammary carcinomas as well as in some other tumors and is associated with decreased survival. It is the target structure for the monoclonal antibody:

- In women with metastatic **mammary carcinoma**, who had undergone several cycles of chemotherapy and still showed overexpression of HER-2 in the tumor tissue, antibody mono-

therapy resulted in objective remission (CR and PR) in 15% of the patients for eight months on average (12). As compared with pure chemotherapy, the combination of Herceptin with doxorubicin/cyclophosphamide or with paclitaxel (Taxol) resulted in an impressive increase in remission rates from 42% to 65%, or from 25% to 57%, respectively, and the progression-free interval was prolonged by two to four months (57). However, especially under combination therapy with anthracyclin/doxorubicin—one of the most effective classes of cytostatic substances for mammary carcinoma—the cardiotoxic side effects increased. Hence, the problem of the most favorable combination is still unsolved.

Monoclonal Antibody C225

The chimeric C225 MAb recognizes the epidermal growth factor receptor (EGFR), which is overexpressed in many epithelial tumors; it is therefore another important representative of the group of growth factor receptor-binding monoclonal antibodies (33). In phase I/II studies involving patients with various types of tumors (head and neck, bronchial, renal, prostate, ovarian, pancreas, breast, or bladder cancer), C225 proved to be well tolerated and rarely induced inhibiting antibodies (5.2%). Like Herceptin, it seemed to act synergistically when used in combination with chemotherapy or radiation therapy and also with new therapeutic concepts, such as inhibitors of angiogenesis (6, 10).

- In a small pilot study involving 12 patients with head-and-neck cancer, the combination of C225 (starting dose: 100, 400, or 500 mg/m²; 250 mg/ m² weekly as maintenance dose for six weeks) with cisplatin (100 mg/m²) achieved a distinct clinical response in six out of nine patients evaluated, with a 22% rate of complete remission (56). These results need to be confirmed in phase III studies.

With both **Herceptin** and **C225**, the target antigens are not tumor-specific antigens, and their ubiquitous expression patterns also on nonneoplastic epithelial cells seems to be, at first glance, counterproductive to wide clinical application. The reason why they are effective lies probably in the interaction of the antibody with the respective receptor, namely, in blocking the physiological interaction of the growth factor with its receptor in case of the C225 antibody or in altering receptor-dependent signal transduction in case of Herceptin (17, 58). Thus Herceptin, as well as C225, affects the proliferation of tumor cells by binding to the growth factor receptor and directly inducing apoptosis (cell death). In addition, Herceptin blocks the cellular DNA repair mechanism, which explains the synergism of chemotherapy and antibody therapy (5). Further research thus focuses on the isolation and characterization of new antibodies that can block receptor–ligand interactions that are important for the homeostasis of cells.

Antibody Conjugates
Carefully chosen radionuclides can kill tumor cells across a distance of several cell diameters. This allows it to also reach antigen-negative tumor cells. The poor penetration of antibodies in solid tumors can thus be counterbalanced, at least in part. So far, however, the response rates of solid tumors to therapy with antibody–radionuclide conjugates have not been impressive (with more than 700 patients involved in over 40 studies) (16, 28).

Only individual cases of this therapy have been reported for melanoma, neuroblastoma, ENT tumors, and medullary thyroid carcinoma as well as renal, prostate, breast, and bronchial cancer.

Nevertheless, the following approaches attempt to increase the effectiveness of the treatment:
• dose escalation with autologous stem cell transplantation, e.g., in the case of gastrointestinal tumors (61) and mammary carcinoma (46)
• use of humanized carrier monoclonal antibody with the potential for repeated application (15)

• combination with whole body hyperthermia (35).

Outlook

In recent years, technical developments have provided new impulses to tumor vaccination as well as monoclonal antibody therapy. They include new methods for identifying human tumor antigens by serological expression cloning (SEREX) (48), an improved understanding for antigen processing and presentation by antigen-processing cells (23), and better reagents for determination and follow-up of the immune response induced in the patients (3). Nevertheless, immunotherapeutic treatment of tumors is still in its infancy. In recent years, advances in tumor immunology and molecular biology have broadened our understanding of the complex interactions between the immune system and tumor cells and have provided us with new reagents for tumor therapy. Recombinant monoclonal antibodies are increasingly being introduced in the clinical practice and have, in part, already been approved for treating certain hemoblastoses and solid tumors.

The biggest impulse for innovation is expected to come from new antibody constructs and from the coupling of antibodies to cytotoxic substances. In contrast to antibody therapies, the vaccination strategies for treating solid tumors are not yet fully accepted. However, individual observations and the results of small studies are encouraging.

The discovery of numerous new human tumor antigens and a new understanding of the process of antigen uptake and presentation have lead to a revival of vaccination strategies, the therapeutic importance of which cannot yet be determined.

References

1. Agha-Mohammadi S, Lotze MT: Immunomodulation of cancer: potential use of selectively replicating agents. J. Clin. Invest. 2000; 105:1173–1176.
2. Ahlert T, Sauerbrei W, Bastert G, et al.: Tumor cell number and viability as quality and efficacy parameters of autologous virus modified cancer vaccines. J. Clin. Oncol. 1997; 15:1354–1366.
3. Altman J, Moss PAH, Goulder P, et al.: Direct visualization and phenotypic analysis of virus-specific T lymphocytes in HIV-infected individuals. Science. 1996; 274:94–96.

4. Baar J: Clinical applications of dendritic cell cancer vaccines. Oncologist. 1999; 4:140–144.

5. Baselga J, Norton L, Albanell J, Kim YM, Mendelsohn J: Recombinant humanized anti-HER2 antibody (Herceptin) enhances the antitumor activity of paclitaxel and doxorubicin against HER2/neu overexpressing human breast cancer xenografts. Cancer Res. 1998; 58:2825–2831.

6. Baselga J, Pfister D, Cooper MR, et al.: Phase I studies of anti-epidermal growth factor receptor chimeric antibody C225 alone and in combination with cisplatin. J. Clin. Oncol. 2000; 18:904–914.

7. Berd D, Maguire HC, McCue P, Mastrangelo MJ: Treatment of metastatic melanoma with an autologous tumor-cell vaccine: Clinical and immunological results in 64 patients. J. Clin. Oncol. 1990; 8:1858–1867.

8. Blachere NE, Li Z, Chandawarkar RY, et al.: Heat shock protein-peptide complexes, reconstituted in vitro, elicit peptide-specific cytotoxic T lymphocytes response and tumor immunity. J. Exp. Med. 1997; 186:1315–1322.

9. Chakraborty NG, Sporn JR, Tortora AF, et al.: Immunization with a tumor-cell-lysate-loaded autologous-antigen-presenting-cell-based vaccine in melanoma. Cancer Immunol. Immunother. 1998; 47:58–64.

10. Ciardiello F, Bianco R, Damiano V, et al.: Antiangiogenic and antitumor activity of anti-epidermal growth factor receptor C225 monoclonal antibody in combination with vascular endothelial growth factor antisense oligonucleotide in human GEO colon cancer cells. Clin. Cancer Res. 2000; 6:3739–3747.

11. Clynes RA, Towers TL, Presta LG, Ravetch JV: Inhibitory Fc receptors modulate in vivo cytoxicity against tumor targets. Nat. Med. 2000; 6:443–446.

12. Cobleigh MA, Vogel CL, Tripathy D, et al.: Efficacy and safety of Herceptin™ (humanized anti-HER2 antibody) as a single agent in 222 women with HER2 overexpression who relapsed following chemotherapy for metastatic breast cancer. Proc. Amer. Soc. Clin. Oncol. 1998; 17:97a.

13. Cohen IR: Discrimination and dialogue in the immune system. Sem. Immunol. 2000; 12:215–219.

14. Coley W: The treatment of inoperable sarcoma by bacterial toxins (the mixed toxins of the *Streptococcus erysipelas* and the *Bacillus prodigius*). London: John Bale & Sons Publishers. 1909; 1–48.

15. De Bree R, Roos JC, Plaizier MA, et al.: Selection of monoclonal antibody E48 IgG or U36 IgG for adjuvant radioimmunotherapy in head and neck cancer patients. Br. J. Cancer. 1997; 75:1049–1060.

16. De Nardo GL, O'Donnell RT, Kroger LA, et al.: Strategies for developing effective radioimmunotherapy for solid tumors. Clin. Cancer Res. 1999; 5:3219–3223.

17. Diardiello F, Damiano V, Bianco R, et al.: Antitumor activity of combined blockade of epidermal growth factor receptor and protein kinase A. J. Nat. Cancer Inst. 1996; 88:1770–1776.

18. Dillman RO: Antibodies as cytotoxic therapy. J. Clin. Oncol. 1994; 12:1497–1515.

19. Ertel C, Millar NS, Emmerson PT, et al.: Viral hemagglutinin augments peptide specific cytotoxic T-cell responses. Eur. J. Immunol. 1993; 23:2592–2596.

20. Falk K, Rotzschke O, Rammensee HG: Cellular peptide composition governed by major histocompatibility complex class I molecules. Nature. 1990; 348:248–251.

21. Fearon ER, Pardoll DM, Itaya T, et al.: Interleukin-2 production by tumor cells bypasses T helper function in the generation of an antitumor response. Cell. 1990; 60:97–403.

22. Flieger D, Renoth S, Beier I, Sauerbruch T, Schmidt-Wolf I: Mechanism of cytotoxicity induced by chimeric mouse human monoclonal antibody IDEC-C2B8 in CD20-expressing lymphoma cell lines. Cell Immunol. 2000; 204:55–63.

23. Germain RN: T-cell signaling: the importance of receptor clustering. Curr. Biol. 1997; 7:640–644.

24. Goldenberg M: The role of radiolabeled antibodies in the treatment of non-Hodgkin's lymphoma: the coming of age of radioimmunotherapy. Crit. Rev. Oncol. Hematol. 2001; 39:195–201.

25. Heicappell R, Schirrmacher V, von Hoegen P, et al.: Prevention of metastatic spread by postoperative immunotherapy with virally modified autologous tumor cells. Int. J. Cancer. 1986; 37:569–577.

26. Herr W, Wolfel T, Heike M, Meyer zum Buschenfelde KH, Knuth A: Frequency analysis of tumor-reactive cytotoxic T lymphocytes in peripheral blood of a melanoma patient vaccinated with autologous tumor cells. Cancer Immunol. Immunother. 1994; 39:93–99.

27. Jäger E, Nagata Y, Gnjatic S, et al.: Monitoring CD8 T cell responses to NY-ESO-1: correlation of humoral and cellular immune responses. Proc. Nat. Acad. Sci., 2000; 97:4760–4765.

28. Kairemo KJA: Radioimmunotherapy of solid cancers. Acta Oncol. 1996; 35:343–355.

29. Kubuschok B, Cochlovius C, Jung W, et al.: Gene-modified spontaneous Epstein-Barr-virus transformed lymphoblastoid cell lines as autologous cancer vaccine: p21 ras oncogene as a model. Cancer Gene Ther. 2000; 7:1231–1249.

30. Kugler A, Stuhler G, Walden P, et al.: Regression of human metastatic renal cell carcinoma after vaccination with tumor cell-dendritic cell hybrids. Nat. Med. J. 2000; 6:332–336.

31. Lindner M, Schirrmacher V: Tumor cell-dendritic cell fusion for cancer immunotherapy: comparison of therapeutic efficiency of polyethylene-glycol versus electro-fusion protocols. Europ. J. Clin. Invest. 2002; 32:207–217.

32. Lokich J: Spontaneous regression of metastatic renal cancer. Case report and literature review. Am. J. Clin. Oncol. 1997; 20:416–418.

33. Mendelsohn J, Baselga J: The EGF receptor family as targets for cancer therapy. Oncogene. 2000; 19:6550–6565.

34. Miller RA: Treatment of B-cell lymphoma with monoclonal anti-idiotype antibody. N. Engl. J. Med. 1982; 306:517–522.

35. Mittal BB, Zimmer MA, Sathiaseelan V, et al.: Phase I/II trial of combined 131I anti-CEA monoclonal antibody and hyperthermia in patients with advanced colorectal adenocarcinoma. Cancer. 1996; 78: 1861–1870.

36. Nelson NJ: Scientific interest in Newcastle disease virus is reviving. J. Nat. Cancer Inst. 1999; 91:1708–1710.

37. Nelson WG, Simons JW, Mikhak B, et al.: Cancer cells engineered to secrete granulocyte-macrophage colony-stimulating factor using ex vivo gene transfer as vaccines for the treatment of genitourinary malignancies. Cancer Chemother. Pharmacol. 2000; 46 (Suppl.):67–72.

38. Nestle FO, Alijagic S, Gilliet M, et al. : Vaccination of melanoma patients with peptide-or tumor lysate-pulsed dendritic cells. Nat. Med. 1998; 4:328–332.

39. Nieland JD, Da Silva DM, Velders MP, et al.: Chimeric papillomavirus virus-like particles induce a murine self-antigen-specific protective and therapeutic antitumor immune response. J. Cell. Biochem. 1999; 73:145–152.

40. Ockert D, Schirrmacher V, Beck N, et al.: Newcastle disease virus infected intact autologous tumor cell vaccine for adjuvant active specific immunotherapy of resected colorectal carcinoma. Clin. Cancer Res. 1996; 2:21–28.

41. Offringa R, van der Burg SH, Ossendorp F, Toes RE, Melief CJ: Design and evaluation of antigen-specific vaccination strategies against cancer. Curr. Opin. Immunol. 2000; 12:576–582.

42. Overwijk WW, Lee DS, Surman DR, et al.: Vaccination with a recombinant vaccinia virus encoding a "self" antigen induces autoimmune vitiligo and tumor cell destruction in mice: Requirement for CD4+ T lymphocytes. Proc. Nat. Acad. Sci., 1999; 96(6):2982–2987.

43. Peeters BPH, de Leeuw OS, Koch G, Gielkens ALJ: Rescue of Newcastle disease virus from cloned cDNA: Evidence that cleavability of the fusion protein is a major determinant for virulence. J. Virol. 1999; 73:5001–5009.

44. Pomer S, Schirrmacher V, Thiele R, et al.: Tumor response and 4 year survival data of patients with advanced renal cell carcinoma treated with autologous tumor vaccine and subcutaneous r-IL-2 and IFN-alpha 2b. Int. J. Oncol. 6: 947–954, 1995.

45. Reichard KW, Lorence RM, Cascino CJ, et al.: Newcastle disease virus selectively kills human tumor cells. J. Surg. Res. 1992; 52:448–453.

46. Richman CM, DeNardo SJ, O'Grady LF, De Nardo GL: Radioimmunotherapy for breast cancer using escalating fractionated doses of 131I-labeled chimeric L6 antibody with peripheral blood progenitor cell transfusions. Cancer Res. 1995; 55 (Suppl. 23): 5916s–5920s.

47. Römer-Oberdörfer A, Mundt E, Mebatsion T, Buchholz UJ, Mettenleiter TC: Generation of recombinant lentogenic Newcastle Disease Virus from cDNA. J. Gen. Virol. 1999; 80:2987–2995.

48. Sahin U, Türeci Ö, Pfreundschuh M: Serological identification of human tumor antigens. Cur. Opin. Immunol. 1997; 9: 709–716.

49. Salgaller ML, Thurnher M, Bartsch G, Boynton AL, Murphy GP: Report from the International Union Against Cancer (UICC) Tumor Biology Committee: UICC workshop on the use of dendritic cells in cancer clinical trials. Cancer. 1999; 86:2674–2683.

50. Schirrmacher V, Ahlert T, Pröbstle T, et al.: Immunization with virus-modified tumor cells. Semin. Oncol. 1998; 25:677–696.

51. Schirrmacher V, Griesbach A, Zangemeister U: γ-Irradiated viable tumor cells as whole cell vaccines can stimulate in situ syngeneic anti-tumor CTL and DTH reactivity while tumor cell lysates elicit only DTH reactivity. Vaccine Res. 1994; 3:31–48.

52. Schirrmacher V, Haas C, Bonifer R, et al.: Human tumor cell modification by virus infection: An efficient and safe way to produce cancer vaccine with pleiotropic immune stimulatory properties when using Newcastle Disease Virus. Gene Ther. 1999; 6:63–73.

53. Schirrmacher V: Immuntherapie maligner Tumoren unter besonderer Berücksichtigung der aktiv-spezifischen Immuntherapie. In: Zeller WJ, zur Hausen H (ed.): Onkologie; Grundlagen, Diagnostik, Therapie, Entwicklungen. Ecomed, Landsberg/Lech, 1–17, 1995.

54. Schirrmacher V: Tumor vaccines–new therapeutic approaches against cancer. Euro-Biotech, Special Edition. Verlag Büro f. Publizistik GmbH. p. 64–66, 2001.

55. Shan D, Ledbetter JA, Press OW: Signaling events involved in anti-CD20-induced apoptosis of malignant human B cells. Cancer Immunol. Immunother. 2000; 48:673–683.

56. Shin DM, Donato NJ, Perez-Soler R, et al.: Epidermal growth factor receptor-targeted therapy with C225

and cisplatin in patients with head and neck cancer. Clin. Cancer Res. 2001; 7:1204–1213.

57. Slamon DJ, Leyland-Jones B, Shak S, et al.: Use of chemotherapy plus a monoclonal antibody against HER2 for metastatic breast cancer that over-expresses HER2. N. Engl. J. Med. 2001; 344:783–792.

58. Sliwkowski MX, Logren JA, Lewis GD, Hotaling TE, Fendly BM, Fox JA: Nonclinical studies addressing the mechanism of action of trastuzumab (Herceptin). Semin. Oncol. 1999; 26 (Suppl. 12):60–70.

59. Stuhler G, Walden P: Recruitment of helper T cells for induction of tumor rejection by cytolytic T lymphocytes. Cancer Immunol. Immunother. 1994; 39: 342–345.

60. Sun Y, Paschen A, Schadendorf D: Cell-based vaccination against melanoma—background, preliminary results and perspective. J. Mol. Med. 1999; 77:593–608.

61. Tempero M, Leichner P, Dalrymple G, et al.: High-dose therapy with iodine-131-labeled monoclonal antibody CC49 in patients with gastrointestinal cancers: a phase I trial. J. Clin. Oncol. 1997; 15: 1518–1528.

62. Termeer CC, Schirrmacher V, Bröcker EB, Becker JC: Newcastle-Disease-Virus infection induces a B7-1/ B7-2 independent T-cell-costimulatory activity in human melanoma cells. Cancer Gene Therap. 2000; 7(2):316–323.

63. Tjoa BA, Simmons SJ, Bowes VA, et al.: Evaluation of phase I/II clinical trials in prostate cancer with dendritic cells and PSMA peptides. Prostate. 1998; 36: 39–44.

64. Tolcher AW, Sugarman S, Gelmon KA et al.: Randomized phase II study of BR96-doxorubicin conjugate in patients with metastatic breast cancer. J. Clin. Oncol. 1999; 17:478–484.

65. Trefzer U, Weingart G, Chen Y, et al.: Hybrid cell vaccination for cancer immune therapy: first clinical trial with metastatic melanoma. Int. J. Cancer. 2000; 85:618–626.

66. Trowsdale J: Genomic structure and function in the MHC. Trends Genet. 1993; 9:117–122.

67. Vermorken JB, Claessen AM, van Tinteren H, et al.: Active specific immunotherapy for stage II and stage III human colon cancer: a randomized trial. Lancet. 1999; 353:345–350.

68. Von Hoegen P, Weber E, Schirrmacher V: Modification of tumor cells by a low dose of Newcastle disease virus: Augmentation of the tumor-specific T cell response in the absence of an anti-viral response. Eur. J. Immunol. 1988; 18:1159–1166.

69. Wang F, Bade E, Kuniyoshi C, et al: Phase I trial of a MART-1 peptide vaccine with incomplete Freund's adjuvant for resected high-risk melanoma. Clin. Cancer Res. 1999; 5:2756–2765.

70. Washburn B, Schirrmacher V: Human tumor cell infection by Newcastle disease virus leads to up-regulation of HLA and cell adhesion molecules and to induction of interferons, chemokines and finally apoptosis. Int. J. Oncol. 2002; 21:85–93.

71. Welt S, Divgi CR, Real FX, et al.: Quantitative analysis of antibody localization in human metastatic colon cancer: a phase I study of monoclonal antibody A33, J. Clin. Oncol. 1990; 8:1894–1906.

72. Wilde MI, Goa KL, Muromonab CD: A reappraisal of its pharmacology and use as prophylaxis of solid organ transplant rejection. Drugs. 1996; 51:865–894.

73. Wildner O, Blaese RM, Morris JC: Therapy of colon cancer with oncolytic adenovirus is enhanced by the addition of herpes simplex virus-thymidine kinase. Cancer Res. 1999; 59:410–413.

74. Zinkernagel RM: Localization, dose and time of antigens determine immune reactivity. Sem. Immunol. 2000; 12:163–171.

20 Hyperthermia

E. Dieter Hager

General Remarks

There are two types of heat application: **active hyperthermia**, which provokes fever episodes by means of pyrogen administration, and **passive hyperthermia**, which raises the temperature of tissues or body fluids by various physical means.

The classic, pyrogen-induced **fever therapy** with target temperatures between 39–40 °C results in enhanced migration of leukocytes and monocytes from the peripheral blood into the tissues and also improves chemotaxis and activates phagocytosis. In addition, it activates metabolic processes, enhances the blood supply, and potentiates the effects of some cytostatic agents.

Passive hyperthermia (Tables 20.**1** and 20.**2**) has different results depending on the range of temperatures:

- **Moderate hyperthermia** has immunological effects similar to fever; it also increases membrane permeability and alters the blood supply within the tumor tissue. Synergistic effects with certain cytostatic agents in vitro and in vivo have been reported.
- **Extreme hyperthermia** has direct cytostatic and cytotoxic effects, especially within the tumor tissue, and produces synergistic effects with cytostatic agents.

In principle, hyperthermia can be applied to all solid malignant tumors. Temperatures above approximately 42 °C have cytostatic or cytotoxic effects on cells in general. In malignant tissues, however, heat seems to be cytotoxic already at lower temperatures because of the altered microenvironment. Damages to membranes of the endoplasmic reticulum, to the cytoskeleton, and to the mitotic spindle are induced already at temperatures in the range of 41–42 °C. In addition, hyperthermia causes the induction of apoptosis.

During passive hyperthermia, the tumor tissue is warmed up by means of external energy sources. The temperature range differs depending on the type of application:

- 39–40 °C for moderate whole body hyperthermia
- 41–42 °C for extreme whole body hyperthermia
- 42–43 °C for superficial or deep hyperthermia
- 46–58 °C for transurethral hyperthermia.

Hyperthermia must be distinguished from **thermoablative methods**. These procedures induce coagulation necrosis at temperatures of above 90 °C. They are usually performed with interstitial techniques, but also with ultrasound and alternating magnetic fields.

The **thermosensitivity** of tumors depends on internal cellular factors and on the cellular environment (e. g., energy deficit, or low pO_2 and low pH). At low pH and low oxygen saturation, cells are more sensitive to higher temperatures. This might explain why malignant tissues are more sensitive to heat than healthy tissues with a normal blood supply. In addition to specific conditions of physical absorption and the altered microenvironment, the tumor's blood vessels are probably less capable of thermoregulation. This creates higher tempera-

Table 20.1 Subdivision of hyperthermia according to temperature ranges	
37.5–38.5 °C	Subclinical hyperthermia
38.5–40.5 °C	Moderate hyperthermia
40.5–41.5 °C	Intermediary hyperthermia
41.5–43.0 °C	Extreme hyperthermia
> 43.0 °C	Thermotherapy

Table 20.2 Mechanisms of action of hyperthermia
• Cytostatic/cytotoxic effects through metabolic changes and denaturation of molecular structures (e. g, enzymes)
• Induction of apoptosis through heat and through hyperacidity caused by metabolites that are not sufficiently eliminated by the blood stream
• Inhibition of cellular repair mechanisms
• Increased permeability of cell membranes for chemotherapeutic agents
• Synergistic effects with radiation therapy and chemotherapy (additive and potentiating)
• Nonspecific immunostimulation and, possibly, induction of a specific immune response mediated by HSP-TAA
• Alleviation of pain by blocking pain receptors

tures within the tumor and stimulates some of the tumor cells to produce **heat shock proteins** (HSP). These proteins are then expressed on the cell membrane together with tumor-associated antigens (HSP-TAA), thus increasing the cell's antigenicity and inducing additional local immunoreactions that contribute to the destruction of the tumor cells (10, 14, 16). Depending on the temperature and duration of treatment, there may also be some regional overheating with increased blood flow in the healthy tissue surrounding the tumor, thus causing a reduction in the tumor's blood supply.

Unlike the thermoablative procedures, however, hyperthermia on its own does not kill all tumor cells, and its biological effects are usually reversible. In general, other therapies should be used simultaneously in order to achieve complete tumor regression. Hyperthermia is therefore usually combined with chemotherapy, radiation therapy, and/or immunotherapy (e. g., mistletoe extracts, tumor vaccines, or antibodies), not least because of its additive and potentiating effects together with classic cytostatic agents and modern immunotherapeutics. The increase in cytotoxicity caused by hyperthermia is due, in part, to an increased influx of the cytostatic agent into the cells and, in part, to an increased cellular metabolism, thus reducing the resistance to chemotherapy.

Hyperthermia Combined with Radiation Therapy or Chemotherapy

The main problem with the sole application of high temperatures as cancer therapy lies in the technical area, i. e., in reaching sufficiently high and homogenous temperatures in tumors of well-vascularized organs or of deep location, and also in the prevention of so-called hot spots in healthy tissues.

In addition to having direct cytotoxic effects on the tumor tissue and making the tumor tissue more sensitive to chemotherapy or radiation therapy (e. g., by increasing membrane permeability), high temperatures also increase the cytotoxic effects of cytostatic agents and ionizing radiation. Hence, it makes sense to combine these methods. There are also clinical indications that the resistance to chemotherapy can be overcome by heat. The combined therapies may be performed simultaneously, or sequentially at defined alternating intervals.

The **cytotoxic effects** of hyperthermia are essentially based on molecular and metabolic changes in the cells. Due to the breakdown of molecular structures, the cells become more sensitive to heat not only during mitosis but also during S phase. This might explain the better response rate when radiation therapy and hyperthermia are combined—in addition to the changes in metabolic processes and blood supply—because cells in S phase and mitosis are certainly resistant to radiation. However, they are also especially thermosensitive. Another explanation for the potentiating effect of this combination therapy might be a thermal inhibition of the repair processes following radiation-induced DNA damage. In addition, hyperthermia is first of all effective in hypoxic areas, whereas radiation is more effective in oxygen-rich areas.

The sensitizing effect of hyperthermia on chemotherapy depends on the type of the cytostatic agent and on the temperature. The improved blood supply resulting from the initial hyperthermia in tumor and surrounding tissue may lead to an increased permeability of cell membranes, thus increasing the concentration of the cytostatic within the tumor. However, there are also known temperature-dependent changes in the intracellular biotransformation of various cytostatics (e. g., gemcitabine, capecitabine). Alkylating agents, platinum complexes, and anthracyclines (such as doxorubicin) are currently regarded as the ideal cytostatic agents in combination with hyperthermia (17). However, for most antimetabolites (such as vinca alkaloids and taxines), there are so far no indications of synergistic effects. Supplementary effects may also be expected from the fact that vascularized tumor regions are more accessible to cytostatic chemotherapy, whereas less vascularized hypoxic areas respond better to hyperthermia.

▬ Generation of Hyperthermia

The best effects for cancer therapy are achieved at temperatures above 41.5 °C. In order to reach the temperature required in the target region, various technically expensive procedures have been developed in recent years (Table 20.**3**). It is only through these procedures that the clinical application of hyperthermia has become possible. Today,

Table 20.3 Subdivision of hyperthermia according to size and location of the overheated body area

Hyperthermia procedure	Size and location of tumor
Local hyperthermia (LHT) [or superficial hyperthermia (SHT)]	Superficial skin tumors or metastases
Interstitial hyperthermia (IHT)	Direct overheating of tumors by implantation of applicators
Regional hyperthermia (RHT) [or deep hyperthermia (DHT)]	Deep location of organ tumors or metastases
Perfusion hyperthermia (PHT)	Hollow organs or extremities with disseminated metastases
Whole body hyperthermia (WBHT)	Generalized metastases
Interstitial thermotherapy (ITT)	Locally targeted tumor therapy (e. g., prostate cancer, ENT tumors, liver metastases)

Table 20.4 Subdivision of hyperthermia according to energy sources

Hyperthermia procedure	Energy source
Superficial hyperthermia (SHT)	Infrared A[1], short waves/microwaves
Deep hyperthermia (DHT)	Short waves/decimetric waves, ultrasound
Perfusion hyperthermia[2] (PHT)	Heat convection, extracorporal heat exchange
Whole body hyperthermia (WBHT)	Infrared A, extracorporal heat exchange
Interstitial thermotherapy (ITT)	Antennas, ferromagnetic particles
Magnetic fluid hyperthermia (MFH)	Magnetite, magnetic alternating field

[1]Water-filtered irradiation with infrared A; [2]intracavitary perfusion or perfusion of extremities

hyperthermia is mainly generated by infrared radiation, radio waves, microwaves, ultrasonic waves, or alternating magnetic fields (Table 20.**4**):

- **Infrared radiation** Infrared A (IRA) radiation is generally used because it penetrates better into the tissue. In order to prevent skin burns resulting from intense absorption of some of the IRA radiation by water molecules in the uppermost layers of the skin, water-filtered infrared A (wIRA) radiation is sometimes applied. The most important fields of IRA application are superficial hyperthermia (e. g., Hydrosun irradiator) and whole body hyperthermia (e. g., IRATHERM 2000; Heckel hyperthermia bed).
- **Radio waves** Radio frequency hyperthermia (RF-HT) is usually used for tumors in deeper locations, because short waves penetrate better into the tissue (5–10 cm) than waves of higher frequencies. Depending on the frequency, energy transmission occurs by means of capacitive or radiative applicators. Radio waves that are used frequently for therapeutic purposes operate in the range of 8–27 MHz. By selecting certain frequencies and, thereby, determining the

interactions between the electromagnetic field and cellular structures, it may be possible to achieve also direct cytostatic (nonthermal) effects. For example, the dielectric constant is approximately 10–30 times higher in tumors than in healthy tissues (6), and the electric conductivity in tumors is up to 100 times higher (11), which may be important especially when applying short waves.

- **Decimetric waves** Some devices for deep hyperthermia operate in the frequency range of 400–912 MHz. By using several radiative applicators, the temperature can be selectively increased to a predetermined range by phase shift. However, the higher the frequency, the lower the penetrating power, thus resulting in increased heterogeneity of temperature distribution (hot spots).
- **Microwaves** The frequencies used in microwave hyperthermia (MW-HT) are in the GHz range, and their penetrating power is low. Microwaves are a possibility especially for local hyperthermia. With some of these methods there is an increased risk that nonspecific cou-

pling and heterogeneous field distribution induce hot spots, which may cause damage to healthy tissues as well.

- **Magnetic field** Magnetic field hyperthermia (MF-HT) uses the implantation or infusion of ferrimagnetic or ferromagnetic particles. Depending on the size of these particles (nano particles, microspheres), they can accumulate in the tumor so that selective overheating can be achieved within the tumor (e. g., magnetic fluid hyperthermia, MFH). Energy can be transmitted onto the implanted magnetic particles by externally applying alternating magnetic fields (hysteresis), which finally leads to selective overheating.

▬ Clinical Application

Local Hyperthermia

The aim of local hyperthermia is to transmit thermal energy into the tumor while avoiding the healthy tissue as much as possible. Noninvasive approaches are only possible for superficial tumors by means of infrared radiation, laser light, or ultrasonic waves (Fig. 20.1). The combination of photosensitizing substances with point-source laser therapy or water-filtered infrared radiation is promising for small, superficial malignant skin alterations. Superficially spreading recurrences can be treated by methods using flexible applicators (e. g., spiral microstrip antennas). There are findings of phase I and phase II clinical trials on the treatment of superficial tumors by radiation therapy combined with hyperthermia (18).

Selective, homogeneous overheating within a tumor is hardly possible because the well-vascularized, proliferating peripheral parts and oxygen-deficient, partially necrotic, central parts of the tumor lie next to each other. Efforts are therefore aimed at achieving a sufficiently homogeneous transmission of energy and, thus, even heat distribution within the tumor by intravenous or intratumoral application of ferromagnetic particles (thermal seeds) as the pharmacological agent. These particles are then heated by means of alternating magnetic fields. A largely homogeneous temperature distribution can also be achieved with invasive therapy (interstitial hyperthermia), e. g., by inserting ferromagnetic wires or rods (thermal rods).

Indications
Local hyperthermia is applied to superficial tumors, such as skin tumors, chest wall cancer, or its recurrences, and individual cervical lymph node metastases. Magnetic particles are used primarily for metastases in the liver, lungs, and brain (e. g., SIR-Spheres, Sirtex Medical Inc., USA). The size of the treatment area and the penetrative power depend decisively on the method used and on the size of the applicator.

Regional Hyperthermia

Regional hyperthermia with radio waves or decimetric waves is the noninvasive, percutaneous transmission of energy to larger areas, e. g., in the region of the small pelvis. The various methods used are:

- radiative hyperthermia by means of antennas; these are distributed in a ring around the patient and can be individually controlled by phase shift in order to radiate energy selectively into an area (e. g., SIGMA-60 applicator with eight pairs of antennas; BSD Medical Corporation, USA)
- capacitive hyperthermia by means of plate electrodes that generate an electromagnetic field in the short wave range, thus producing a target temperature in the tumor that ranges between 42–43 °C (e. g., OncoTherm, Hungary; Synchrotherm, Switzerland/Italy).

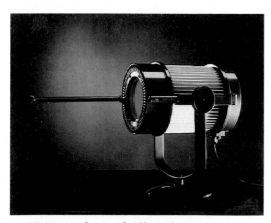

Fig. 20.1 Device for superficial hyperthermia.

Regional hyperthermia is costly and requires thorough quality assurance. The distributions achieved for field and temperature are limited by the electric interphase at bones, air, or fat and are therefore not homogeneous. This heterogeneity is enhanced by the variable blood supply in tumors.

Indications

In oncotherapy, regional hyperthermia is a comparatively gentle procedure and is used when local invasive methods are not possible, or when the tumor has disseminated into the region. It is applied to larger areas, such as the pelvic region, the abdominal region, the thighs, or other body parts of up to 30–40 cm expansion. Regional hyperthermia is used in combination with radiation therapy or chemotherapy for **mammary carcinoma metastases**, tumors in the throat and neck region, or **bone metastases**. It is preferably combined with chemotherapy and/or radiation therapy and biological immunotherapy. A comparative phase II clinical study shows that hyperthermia combined with radiation therapy leads to an improved three-year survival rate from 27 % to 57 % in patients with locally advanced cervical carcinoma (22, 23). Tumors located in the liver, lungs, pancreas, and brain may be treated additionally with short waves.

Side Effects

- During treatment, the energy-transmitting antenna or electrode is cooled in a cooling loop to prevent **burns** of the skin. Mild erythema is rare and disappears rapidly. Subcutaneous paresthesia, caused by the development of heat in deep regions, also regresses after treatment.
- Scars are poorly vascularized, and their temperature regulation is disturbed; these areas must therefore be protected properly.
- Patients under powerful **pain management** fail to judge heat accurately, and this may lead to burns of the skin.
- Several hours or days after hyperthermia treatment, there may be mild **fever episodes** as a result of increased cell death.
- If the patients carry implanted foreign bodies, such as **pacemakers** or joint replacements, burns may occur because of unwanted overheating. Warning: disturbance of the electronics of pacemakers cannot be excluded. In such cases, the manufacturers need to be consulted prior to application of hyperthermia.

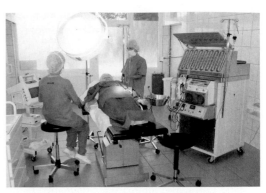

Fig. 20.2 Device for perfusion hyperthermia.

Hyperthermic Perfusion

Here, cavities (abdomen, bladder, pleura) or extremities are perfused with warm (42–43 °C) physiological solution or blood in combination with cytostatics or cytokines. This is done by extracorporal warming of the blood or fluid (Fig. 20.**2**). We distinguish between intracavitary hyperthermic perfusion and extremity perfusion.

Intracavitary Hyperthermic Perfusion (ICHP)

The physiological fluid in cavities—such as the abdomen (intraperitoneal hyperthermic perfusion, IPHP), the bladder (intravesical hyperthermic perfusion, IVHP), or the pleura (intrapleural hyperthermic perfusion, IPLHP)—is warmed up by extracorporal heat exchange.

IPHP was developed primarily for the treatment of metastases in the abdomen or bladder (12, 20). The abdomen is perfused with a warm (up to 50 °C) cytostatic-containing fluid, whereby intraperitoneal temperatures of 41–43 °C are achieved. This makes it possible to reach metastases or primary tumors that are distributed between pelvis and diaphragm. The treatment can be helpful if abdominal lymph nodes are affected by cancer of the colon, stomach, or pelvic organs, as well as in cases of ascites.

These procedures are performed in combination with cytostatic agents. Intraperitoneal instillation of cytostatics in combination with ICHP offers the following advantages:

- a 20 to 1000 times higher concentration of the cytostatic agent in the region of the tumor than in the plasma

- prolonged period of action, thereby affecting more cells undergoing division
- simultaneous overheating has an additive or potentiating effect on some cytostatic agents
- reduced resistance to chemotherapy
- induction of immunological reactions, especially those mediated by hyperthermia-induced heat shock proteins in combination with tumor-associated antigens (HSP-TAA).

This method can also be used perioperatively, e. g., after cytoreductive therapy in the case of peritoneal carcinomatoses resulting from ovarian or stomach cancer.

Perfusion of Extremities

Regional hyperthermic perfusion of an extremity is an effective treatment for sarcoma and malignant melanoma located in a limb (19). This treatment is carried out with the intention of facilitating organ-preserving surgery. The blood supply to the extremity carrying the tumor is separated from the main blood flow, and the blood is warmed up by extracorporal circulation. This form of hyperthermia is usually done in combination with cytostatic agents or cytokines (e. g., TNF-α).

Indications

- Important indications for intraperitoneal hyperthermic perfusion chemotherapy (IPHC) are **peritoneal carcinomatoses** with or without ascites (e. g., metastases from ovarian, stomach, or colon cancer (5), and also sarcoma and pseudomyxoma peritonei). This method is not effective (and should not be used) for large solid tumors when the diffusion distance is too large (tumor diameter > 3 cm) or in cases of extensive adhesions, because the cavity must be sufficiently perfused and the tumor sufficiently immersed.
- By using IPHC, high remission rates can be achieved even in cases of systemic chemotherapy resistance. A direct effect of heat on the tumor's resistance to cytostatics may play a role, in addition to increased membrane permeability. Because of delayed absorption of the cytostatics from the cavities, concentrations in the peripheral blood are low, and systemic side effects are therefore relatively minor.
- IPHC may also represent a promising adjuvant therapy for gastrointestinal tumors (first of all, **stomach cancer**) and ovarian tumors because metastases of these tumors often spread intraperitoneally.
- Apart from the peritoneum, the primary organ affected by **metastases** is usually the liver. Micrometastases (< 2 mm) are supplied with blood through the portal circulation in the same way as the stroma of the liver. This is the same path taken by drugs after intraperitoneal instillation and substantial absorption by the visceral peritoneum (approximately 70 %).
- Likewise, intravesical hyperthermic perfusion chemotherapy (IVHC) may be successfully used for the treatment of **recurrent bladder carcinoma**. Mitomycin and also epirubicin and mitoxantron are usually employed for superficial bladder cancer. As shown in a preliminary clinical study (4), the rate of recurrences can be significantly reduced and chemotherapy resistance overcome, thus avoiding cystectomy. When using this method as a neoadjuvant treatment, the rate of complete remission was 65 % (5) and the rate of recurrences was significantly lower than with conventional therapies.
- So far, treatment of **malignant pleural effusion** by means of intrapleural hyperthermic perfusion chemotherapy (IPLHC) did not achieve better results than pleurodesis. In the attempts undertaken thus far, the cooling effects caused by respiration and circulation were probably to blame for the failure to reach temperatures high enough to ensure a synergistic effect with cytostatic agents.

Transurethral Hyperthermia

By using hyperthermia, benign and malignant tumors of the prostate can be treated with lower risks than those associated with surgery performed for incontinence or impotence. A catheter containing an emitter of decimetric waves or microwaves is inserted into the urethra in such a way that it comes to lie close to the prostate. This way, the tissue can be locally overheated to above 48 °C (**thermotherapy**). For the treatment of prostate cancer, however, the implantation of thermal rods or thermal seeds has proved effective. This type of hyperthermia is successfully used in combination with percutaneous and interstitial radiation therapy and is indicated especially when surgery is not an option.

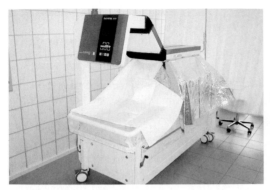

Fig. 20.3 IRATHERM 2000 device

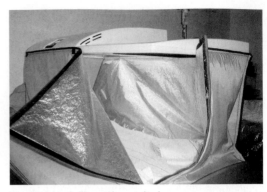

Fig. 20.4 Heckel hyperthermia bed

Whole Body Hyperthermia

In clinical studies, some techniques of whole body hyperthermia (WBHT or WBH) have become increasingly effective for the treatment of expanded systemic malignant tumors (1, 13, 15, 21). Raising the body temperature safely to 42 °C and acceptable levels of toxicity were used as criteria. The devices currently in use operate primarily with infrared radiation:

- Enthermics RHS-2001 (Enthermics Medical Systems, Menomonee Falls, Wisconsin, USA)
- IRATHERM 2000 (Fig. 20.**3**; Von Ardenne Institute of Applied Medical Research, Dresden, Germany)
- Heckel hyperthermia bed (Fig. 20.**4**; Heckel Medizintechnik, Esslingen, Germany)
- WBH 2000 (HOT OncoTherm, Budapest, Hungary).

When combined with cytostatic agents, the previously well-tried method of extracorporal overheating as well as overheating in a bath or by microwaves resulted in undesirable toxic effects that were not proportional to the therapeutic success (e.g., extreme overheating of organs, poor controllability). In recent years, overheating by means of water-filtered infrared irradiation has therefore gained acceptance in clinical studies. Extreme extracorporal whole body hyperthermia may have a place in the treatment of viral diseases (hepatitis C virus, HCV; human immunodeficiency virus, HIV).

For the purpose of whole body hyperthermia, the entire body is overheated to core body temperatures of 41.5–42 °C (**extreme hyperthermia**). The treatment phase lasts 60 minutes. Whole body hyperthermia is usually performed in combination with cytostatic agents, thus taking advantage of a synergistic effect of the systemic temperature rise and the synchronized administration of cytostatics. During treatment, the patient receives general anesthesia or deep sedation (analgosedation). The warm-up phase and the cooling phase last one to two hours each.

Recent studies in experimental animals (9, 12, 20) indicated that moderate overheating (39–40 °C for four to six hours) in combination with cytostatics may possibly yield response rates that are comparable to those of extreme hyperthermia (41.0–42.5 °C for one hour) but are associated with less medical and technical expenses and fewer complications.

According to these studies, a target temperature of 39–40 °C (**moderate hyperthermia**) for four to six hours seems to have a satisfactory potentiating effect on cytostatic agents while being much better tolerated by the patient. Overheating in a warming bed that is completely isolated by a surrounding aluminum foil (Heckel hyperthermia bed, Fig. 20.**4**) is less expensive. Moderate hyperthermia often replaces or supports fever therapy by warming the body up to 40 °C, with the overheating time lasting four to six hours.

Phase II/III clinical trials on the **combination of whole body hyperthermia with cytostatics** suggest that such a therapy might be an alternative to high-dose chemotherapy, as it is associated with greater tolerance (13, 15, 21), lower long-term toxicity, and much lower overall expenses. This alone should be all the more reason to use a therapeutic method that has relatively few side effects (Table

20.**7**) as compared with high-dose chemotherapy, even though the mechanism of action is not completely clear and the method still needs to be improved technically. Especially for patients with advanced stages of cancer, any method that improves the patient's quality of life should be preferred in the context of palliative care.

Indications

- Whole body hyperthermia is indicated in cases of generalized cancer with metastases in several regions of the body. However, it may also be used for regionally circumscribed neoplasms.
- In case of long-term or repeated hyperthermia, temperatures of 40 °C and above are already sufficient to ensure the induction of heat shock proteins in the tumor tissue, thus eliciting an enhanced immunological reaction against the tumor.
- In phase II/III clinical trials, much higher response rates were achieved in some cases and a higher rate of survival in others when hyperthermia was combined with chemotherapy and/or radiation therapy for carcinoma in the abdomen, pelvis, and extremities.
- The treatment seems to be especially effective for advanced ovarian cancer, breast cancer, melanoma recurrences, and lymphoma (6), and also for sarcoma (8).
- First clinical studies involving tumors or metastases located in bone, liver, lungs, and pancreas showed that the sole application of hyperthermia over relatively long periods can lead to a steady state with clearly improved findings or

even partial (and in rare cases, complete) remission (2, 3).

Selection of Patients

Prior to hyperthermia treatment, patients must undergo a thorough medical and cardiological examination (Tables 20.**5** and 20.**6**). This is especially important for extreme whole body hyperthermia.

- Electrocardiograms (ECGs) and ergometry.
- Spirometry.
- Serochemical determination of heart enzymes and electrolytes, if applicable.
- Measurement of oxygen tension (pO_2).
- Coagulation status.
- Arterial hypertension and diabetes mellitus must be brought under control prior to treatment.
- If a brain tumor is suspected, cerebral computed tomography or magnetic resonance imaging is recommended prior to treatment.
- Warning: lymphedema may be enhanced during treatment with whole body hyperthermia. It may help to let the compression bandage in place during treatment. There is an increased risk of pressure ulceration in previously irradiated regions. Here, an especially thorough monitoring is required as well as covering the area with a terry towel during treatment.
- If general anesthesia is planned, it is obligatory to have a consultation with an anesthesiologist once all findings of the examination are available.

Table 20.5 Inclusion criteria for extreme whole body hyperthermia
• General health according to ECOG (WHO): 0, 1, 2; life expectancy > 12 weeks
• Renal function: clearance > 60 mL/min, if potentially nephrotoxic substances are applied (e. g., platinum complexes, ifosfamide)
• Cardiac function: ejection fraction > 60 %, no detection of relevant arrhythmia and high-degree heart block
• Pulmonary function: vital capacity > 50 %, FEV1 > 50 %, diffusion capacity > 50 %
• Normal ergometry or myocardial scintigraphy under stress
• Manifestations of a tumor detected by imaging procedures
• Possibility of regular, long-term follow-up

Table 20.6 Contraindications for extreme whole body hyperthermia
• Severe arrhythmia, angina pectoris, history of myocardial infarction
• State after stroke
• Thrombosis or thrombophlebitis
• Poor general health
• Cerebral edema or intracranial pressure, e. g., in patients with brain tumors and/or brain metastases (relative contraindication) or preoperative irradiation of the brain > 40 Gy
• Bone marrow insufficiency
• Partial or total respiratory insufficiency
• Hyperthyroid state (relative contraindication, symptomatic)
• Grave disease
• Risk of fractures due to osteolysis
• Polyneuropathies
• Diseases of the CNS

Table 20.7 Side effects of whole body hyperthermia

- Burns to the skin (by infrared irradiation) especially in the region of scars and on extremities after hyperthermic perfusion
- Drop in blood pressure
- Supraventricular tachycardia
- Herpes
- Increased levels of liver enzymes
- Possibly 1–2 days of exhaustion
- Transient leukopenia

- Adequate prehydration with 2–3 L of complete electrolyte solution is required, especially when administering nephrotoxic substances.
- For positioning the patient, all rules apply that are in place for general anesthesia.
- In case of analgosedation, facilities for intubation and resuscitation must be available. It is recommended that an intensive care unit is used where the patient can be monitored for at least six hours after the treatment.
- Analgosedation must be performed by a physician with experience in intensive care medicine
- Continuous monitoring of the temperatures and the control of energy input by the attending staff must be ensured.

Performing Moderate Whole Body Hyperthermia
- Treatment is carried out under intensive monitoring:
  - ECG monitoring
  - oximetry monitoring
  - control of pulse and blood pressure
  - continuous rectal monitoring of the core body temperature.
- Treatment lasts a total of about 4 hours (including warm-up phase, treatment phase, and cooling phase).
- Dressed in light cotton pajamas, the patient reclines in the tentlike hyperthermia cubicle, or in a device operating with water-filtered infrared radiation, and receives an intravenous access with physiological infusion solution and also the leads for various monitoring devices.
- The head of the patient is best positioned outside the cubicle, allowing the patient to listen to a relaxation or meditation tape via Walkman, if so desired.
- The patient may inhale oxygen by means of an oxygen mask (e.g., 4 L/min; recommended pO_2 > 90 %).

- Once all preparations are complete, the cubicle is closed. The infrared irradiators either emit water-filtered radiation, or they are arranged in such a way that they emit a widely scattered, diffuse radiation. If thoroughly monitored, the risk of burns is extremely low.
- During the subsequent period of 45–90 minutes, the patient is continuously warmed up, aiming at a target temperature of 39–40 °C.
- Without sedation or anesthesia, patients find whole body hyperthermia very exhausting. Especially the escalation of heat is often difficult to tolerate. However, if patients are well cared for, e.g., by providing drinks, wiping off sweat, and distracting them through discussion (psychotherapeutic intervention) or relaxing music, the treatment can usually be carried out without problems.
- In cases of known claustrophobic tendency, problems with accepting the treatment may arise; they, too, can be kept under control through individual care and sedation.
- Experience has shown that, once the irradiators are turned off, the body continues to warm up spontaneously by approx. 0.5 °C, thus reaching a core body temperature of 40.0–40.5 °C.
- Hyperthermia cubicles equipped with reflective foil diminish the reactive drop in temperature caused by sweating and surface cooling.
- The sweating induced in the patient should be compensated by administering Ringer infusion solution. The infusion solution is warmed up to approximately 40 °C in order to achieve optimal distribution of heat in the body.
- Once the high temperature phase is reached, the heat irradiators are turned off and the patient is wrapped into foils. This way, the temperature can be kept at a constant level for several hours.
- In some cases, patients describe a renewed spontaneous rise in temperature to approximately 39 °C, occurring about six to eight hours after completion of the treatment and subsiding without further measures after one to three hours.

— Hyperthermia Centers

Hyperthermia is predominantly performed at various cancer centers in the context of clinical studies involving selected groups of patients and, in the case of children, at the pediatric clinics of the universities of Tübingen and Düsseldorf, Germany.

Specialist Associations
- Interdisciplinary Study Group on Hyperthermia, Heidelberg, Germany; Tel: +49 (69) 630096-0

Websites
- http://www.uni-essen.de/strahlentherapie/strahlenphysik/deutsch/hyperth.html
- http://www.m-ww.de/enzyklopedie/diagnosen_therapien/hyperthermie.html

Books, Reviews, and Guidelines
- Kosaka M, et al.: Thermotherapy for Neoplasia, Inflammation and Pain: Berlin, Springer-Verlag, 2000.
- Urano M, et al.: Chemopotentiation by Hyperthermia, Utrecht, VSP BV, 1994.
- Seegenschmidt MH, et al.: Thermoradiotherapy and Thermochemotherapy. Berlin, Springer-Verlag, vols. 1, 2, 1995.
- Interdisziplinäre Arbeitsgruppe Hyperthermie: Leitlinien zur Durchführung der Ganzkörperhyperthermie, Nov. 29, 2001.
- Hager ED: Komplementäre Onkologie, Forum Medizin-Verlag, Gräfelfing 1996.
- Hager ED: Formen der Hyperthermie und klinische Ergebnisse. J. Oncol. 1997; 29 (3): 78–83.
- Bakshandeh A, et al.: Year 2000 guidelines for clinical practice of whole body hyperthermia combined with cytotoxic drugs. J. Oncol. Pharm. Practice. 1999; 5:131–134.
- Gauthery M, et al.: Biological Basis of Oncologic Thermotherapy. Berlin, Springer-Verlag, vols. 1–4, 1990.
- Wust P, et al.: Feasibility and analysis of thermal parameters for the whole-body-hyperthermia system Iratherm 2000. Int. J. Hyperthermia. 2000; 16:235–339.

▃ References

1. Dauterstedt W, et al.: IRA-Therm–eine neuartige InfrarotA-Hyperthermierichtung. Z. Klin. Med. 1987; 42:953–957.
2. Hager ED, et al.: Loco-regional deep hyperthermia with RF in patients with liver metastases from colorectal cancer. International Congress Hyperthermia in Clinical Oncology. Venice, May 28–30, 1998.
3. Hager ED, et al.: Multimodal treatment of patients with advanced pancreatic cancer in combination with locoregional hyperthermia. Southern Medical Journal. 1996; p. 145.
4. Hager ED, et al.: Prevention of cystectomy of recurrent bladder carcinoma by intravesical hyperthermic perfusion chemotherapy IVHP. Anticancer Res. 1998; 18:4876.
5. Hager ED, Dziambor H, Höhmann D, Mühe N, Strama H: Intraperitoneal hyperthermic perfusion chemotherapy of patients with chemotherapy-resistant peritoneal disseminated ovarian cancer. Int. J. Gynecol. Cancer. 2001; 11:57–63.
6. Hager ED: Komplementäre Onkologie. Gräfeling, Forum Medizin Verlag, 1996, p. 164–180.
7. Heckel M: Ganzkörper-Hyperthermie und Fiebertherapie–Grundlagen und Praxis. Stuttgart, Hippokrates Verlag, 1990
8. Issels RD, et al.: Ifosfamide plus etoposide combined with regional hyperthermia in patients with locally advanced sarcomas: a phase II study. J. Clin. Onc. 1980; 8:1818–1829.
9. Matsuda H, Strebel FR, Kaneko T et al. Long duration-mild whole hyperthermia of up to 12 hours in rats: feasibility, and efficacy on primary tumour and axillary lymph node metastases of a mammary adenocarcinoma: implications for adjuvant therapy. Int. J. Hyperthermia 1997; 13:89–98.
10. Multhoff G, et al.: A stress-inducible 72 Da heat shock protein (HSP 72) is expressed on the cell surface on human tumor cells, but not on normal cells. Int. J. Cancer. 1995; 61:272–279.
11. Nordenström B: Biologically closed electric circuits. Nordic Medical Publications, 1983.
12. Repasky EA, Tims E, Pritchard M, Burd R: Characterization of mild whole-body hyperthermia protocols using human breast, ovarian and colon tumors grown in severe combined immunodeficient mice. Infect. Dis. Obstet. Gynecol. 1999; 7:91–97.
13. Robins HI, et al: A new technological approach to radiant heat whole body hyperthermia. Cancer Letters. 1994; 79:137–145.
14. Srivastava PK: Peptide-binding heat shock proteins in the endoplasmic reticulum: role in immune response to cancer and in antigen presentation. Adv. Cancer Res. 1993; 62:153–177.
15. Steinhausen D, et al.: Evaluation of systemic tolerance of 42 °C infrared-A whole-body hyperthermia in combination with hyperglycemia and hyperoxemia. Strahlentherapie und Onkologie. 1994; 170:322–334.
16. Udono H, Srivastava PK: Heat shock protein 70-associated peptides elicit specific cancer immunity. J. Exp. Med 1993; 178: 1391–1396.
17. Urano M: Chemopotentation by Hyperthermia; Utrecht, VSP, 1994.

18. Vernon CC, Hand JW, Field SB et al.: Radiotherapy with or without hyperthermia in the treatment of superficial localized breast cancer: results from five randomized controlled trials. Int. J. Rad. Oncol. Biol. Phys. 1996; 35:731–744.

19. Wagenbach S, et al.: Die regionale hypertherme Extremitätenperfusion zur Therapie des malignen Melanoms. Ärztebl. Rheinl.-Pfalz. 1995; p. 173–177.

20. Wang XY, Ostberg JR, Repasky EA: Effect of fever-like whole-body hyperthermia on lymphocyte spectrin distribution, protein kinase C activity and uropod formation. J. Immunol. 1999; 162: 3378–3387.

21. Wiedemann GJ, et al.: Klinische Studien zur Kombination von Ifosfamid, Carboplatin und Etoposid ICE mit Ganzkörperhyperthermie. Med. Klin. 1996; 91:279–283.

22. van der Zee J, Gonzalez DG, van Rhoon GC, van Dijk JDP, van Putten WLJ: Comparison of radiotherapy alone with radiotherapy plus hyperthermia in locally advanced pelvic tumours: a prospective, randomised multicentre trial. Lancet. 2000; 355:1119.

23. van der Zee J, Gonzalez DG: The Dutch Deep Hyperthermia Trial: results in cervical cancer. Int. J. Hyperthermia. 2002; 18:1–12.

21 Applied Complementary Oncology

Josef Beuth

Anal carcinoma

Standard therapy	Efficacy-tested complementary measures	Extended complementary measures
Preoperative measures	• Nutrition • Psycho-oncology • Sodium selenite (100–200 µg/day) • Immunotherapy (depending on the indication)**	• Balanced vitamins and trace elements
Surgery	• Sodium selenite (300–1000 µg/day)	
Adjuvant therapy, or chemotherapy and radiation	• Sodium selenite (300–1000 µg/day) • Proteolytic enzymes* (4–9 tablets/day) • Nutrition • Sports • Psycho-oncology	• Restorative naturopathic measures • Balanced vitamins and trace elements • Probiotic therapy
Follow-up	• Nutrition • Sports • Psycho-oncology	• Restorative naturopathic measures • Balanced vitamins and trace elements • Probiotic therapy • Proteolytic enzymes* (4–9 tablets/day)
	• **Immunotherapy**** – mistletoe therapy	• **Immunotherapy**** – (thymic) peptide therapy – hyperthermia

*see p. 270; **see p. 270

Bronchial carcinoma (small cell or non-small cell lung cancer)

Standard therapy	Efficacy-tested complementary measures	Extended complementary measures
Preoperative measures	• Nutrition • Psycho-oncology • Sodium selenite (100–200 µg/day) • Immunotherapy (depending on the indication)**	• Balanced vitamins and trace elements
Surgery	• Sodium selenite (300–1000 µg/day)	
Adjuvant therapy, or chemotherapy and radiation	• Sodium selenite (300–1000 µg/day) • Proteolytic enzymes* (4–9 tablets/day) • Nutrition • Sports • Psycho-oncology	• Restorative naturopathic measures • Balanced vitamins and trace elements • Probiotic therapy
Follow-up	• Nutrition • Sports • Psycho-oncology	• Restorative naturopathic measures • Balanced vitamins and trace elements • Probiotic therapy • Proteolytic enzymes* (4–9 tablets/day)
	• **Immunotherapy**** – mistletoe therapy	• **Immunotherapy**** – (thymic) peptide therapy – hyperthermia

*see p. 270; **see p. 270

Cervical carcinoma

Standard therapy	Efficacy-tested complementary measures	Extended complementary measures
Preoperative measures	• Nutrition • Psycho-oncology • Sodium selenite (100–200 µg/day) • Immunotherapy (depending on the indication)**	• Balanced vitamins and trace elements
Surgery	• Sodium selenite (300–1000 µg/day)	
Adjuvant therapy, or chemotherapy and radiation	• Sodium selenite (300–1000 µg/day) • Proteolytic enzymes* (4–9 tablets/day) • Nutrition • Sports • Psycho-oncology	• Restorative naturopathic measures • Balanced vitamins and trace elements • Probiotic therapy
Follow-up	• Nutrition • Sports • Psycho-oncology	• Restorative naturopathic measures • Balanced vitamins and trace elements • Probiotic therapy • Proteolytic enzymes* (4–9 tablets/day)
	• **Immunotherapy** – mistletoe therapy	• **Immunotherapy** – (thymic) peptide therapy – hyperthermia

*see p. 270; **see p. 270

Colorectal carcinoma

Standard therapy	Efficacy-tested complementary measures	Extended complementary measures
Preoperative measures	• Nutrition • Psycho-oncology • Sodium selenite (100–200 µg/day) • Immunotherapy (depending on the indication)**	• Balanced vitamins and trace elements
Surgery	• Sodium selenite (300–1000 µg/day)	• **Blockade of adhesion molecules**
Adjuvant therapy, or chemotherapy and radiation	• Sodium selenite (300–1000 µg/day) • Proteolytic enzymes* (4–9 tablets/day) • Nutrition • Sports • Psycho-oncology	• Restorative naturopathic measures • Balanced vitamins and trace elements • Probiotic therapy • **Mistletoe therapy**
Follow-up	• Nutrition • Sports • Psycho-oncology	• Restorative naturopathic measures • Balanced vitamins and trace elements • Probiotic therapy • Proteolytic enzymes* (4–9 tablets/day)

	• **Immunotherapy**
	  – mistletoe therapy
		• **Immunotherapy**
		  – (thymic) peptide therapy
		  – hyperthermia

*see p. 270; **see p. 270

Endometrial carcinoma

Standard therapy	Efficacy-tested complementary measures	Extended complementary measures
Preoperative measures	• Nutrition • Psycho-oncology • Sodium selenite (100–200 µg/day) • Immunotherapy (depending on the indication)**	• Balanced vitamins and trace elements
Surgery	• Sodium selenite (300–1000 µg/day)	
Adjuvant therapy, or chemotherapy and radiation	• Sodium selenite (300–1000 µg/day) • Proteolytic enzymes* (4–9 tablets/day) • Nutrition • Sports • Psycho-oncology	• Restorative naturopathic measures • Balanced vitamins and trace elements • Probiotic therapy
Follow-up	• Nutrition • Sports • Psycho-oncology	• Restorative naturopathic measures • Balanced vitamins and trace elements • Probiotic therapy • Proteolytic enzymes* (4–9 tablets/day)

	• **Immunotherapy****
	  – mistletoe therapy
		• **Immunotherapy****
		  – (thymic) peptide therapy
		  – hyperthermia

*see p. 270; **see p. 270

Esophageal carcinoma

Standard therapy	Efficacy-tested complementary measures	Extended complementary measures
Preoperative measures	• Nutrition • Psycho-oncology • Sodium selenite (100–200 µg/day) • Immunotherapy (depending on the indication)**	• Balanced vitamins and trace elements
Surgery	• Sodium selenite (300–1000 µg/day)	
Adjuvant therapy, or chemotherapy and radiation	• Sodium selenite (300–1000 µg/day) • Proteolytic enzymes* (4–9 tablets/day) • Nutrition • Sports • Psycho-oncology	• Restorative naturopathic measures • Balanced vitamins and trace elements • Probiotic therapy
Follow-up	• Nutrition • Sports • Psycho-oncology	• Restorative naturopathic measures • Balanced vitamins and trace elements • Probiotic therapy • Proteolytic enzymes* (4–9 tablets/day)
	• **Immunotherapy**** – mistletoe therapy	• **Immunotherapy**** – (thymic) peptide therapy – hyperthermia

*see p. 270; **see p. 270

Gallbladder carcinoma, bile duct carcinoma

Standard therapy	Efficacy-tested complementary measures	Extended complementary measures
Preoperative measures	• Nutrition • Psycho-oncology • Sodium selenite (100–200 µg/day) • Immunotherapy (depending on the indication)**	• Balanced vitamins and trace elements
Surgery	• Sodium selenite (300–1000 µg/day)	
Adjuvant therapy, or chemotherapy and radiation	• Sodium selenite (300–1000 µg/day) • Proteolytic enzymes* (4–9 tablets/day) • Nutrition • Sports • Psycho-oncology	• Restorative naturopathic measures • Balanced vitamins and trace elements • Probiotic therapy
Follow-up	• Nutrition • Sports • Psycho-oncology	• Restorative naturopathic measures • Balanced vitamins and trace elements • Probiotic therapy • Proteolytic enzymes* (4–9 tablets/day)
	• **Immunotherapy**** – mistletoe therapy	• **Immunotherapy**** – (thymic) peptide therapy – hyperthermia

*see p. 270; **see p. 270

Head and Neck carcinoma

Standard therapy	Efficacy-tested complementary measures	Extended complementary measures
Preoperative measures	• Nutrition • Psycho-oncology • Sodium selenite (100–200 µg/day) • Immunotherapy (depending on the indication)**	• Balanced vitamins and trace elements
Surgery	• Sodium selenite (300–1000 µg/day)	
Adjuvant therapy, or chemotherapy and radiation	• Sodium selenite (300–1000 µg/day) • Proteolytic enzymes* (4–9 tablets/day) • Nutrition • Sports • Psycho-oncology	• Restorative naturopathic measures • Balanced vitamins and trace elements • Probiotic therapy • Incense (3 × 800–1200 mg/day)
Follow-up	• Nutrition • Sports • Psycho-oncology	• Restorative naturopathic measures • Balanced vitamins and trace elements • Probiotic therapy • Proteolytic enzymes* (4–9 tablets/day)

	• **Immunotherapy****
	  – mistletoe therapy
		• **Immunotherapy****
		  – (thymic) peptide therapy
		  – hyperthermia

*see p. 270; **see p. 270

Hepatocellular carcinoma

Standard therapy	Efficacy-tested complementary measures	Extended complementary measures
Preoperative measures	• Nutrition • Psycho-oncology • Sodium selenite (100–200 µg/day) • Immunotherapy (depending on the indication)**	• Balanced vitamins and trace elements
Surgery	• Sodium selenite (300–1000 µg/day)	
Adjuvant therapy, or chemotherapy and radiation	• Sodium selenite (300–1000 µg/day) • Proteolytic enzymes* (4–9 tablets/day) • Nutrition • Sports • Psycho-oncology	• Restorative naturopathic measures • Balanced vitamins and trace elements • Probiotic therapy
Follow-up	• Nutrition • Sports • Psycho-oncology	• Restorative naturopathic measures • Balanced vitamins and trace elements • Probiotic therapy • Proteolytic enzymes* (4–9 tablets/day)
	• **Immunotherapy** – mistletoe therapy	• **Immunotherapy** – (thymic) peptide therapy – hyperthermia

*see p. 270; **see p. 270

Malignant melanoma

Standard therapy	Efficacy-tested complementary measures	Extended complementary measures
Preoperative measures	• Nutrition • Psycho-oncology • Sodium selenite (100–200 μg/day) • Immunotherapy (depending on the indication)**	• Balanced vitamins and trace elements
Surgery	• Sodium selenite (300–1000 μg/day)	
Adjuvant therapy, or chemotherapy and radiation	• Sodium selenite (300–1000 μg/day) • Proteolytic enzymes* (4–9 tablets/day) • Nutrition • Sports • Psycho-oncology	• Restorative naturopathic measures • Balanced vitamins and trace elements • Probiotic therapy • **Hyperthermia** • **Vaccination with tumor cells or peptide antigens** • **Dendritic cell therapy**
Follow-up	• Nutrition • Sports • Psycho-oncology	• Restorative naturopathic measures • Balanced vitamins and trace elements • Probiotic therapy • Proteolytic enzymes* (4–9 tablets/day)
	• **Immunotherapy**** – mistletoe therapy	• **Immunotherapy**** – (thymic) peptide therapy – hyperthermia

*see p. 270; **see p. 270

Malignant mesothelioma

Standard therapy	Efficacy-tested complementary measures	Extended complementary measures
Preoperative measures	• Nutrition • Psycho-oncology • Sodium selenite (100–200 µg/day) • Immunotherapy (depending on the indication)**	• Balanced vitamins and trace elements
Surgery	• Sodium selenite (300–1000 µg/day)	
Adjuvant therapy, or chemotherapy and radiation	• Sodium selenite (300–1000 µg/day) • Proteolytic enzymes* (4–9 tablets/day) • Nutrition • Sports • Psycho-oncology	• Restorative naturopathic measures • **Hyperthermia** • Balanced vitamins and trace elements • Probiotic therapy
Follow-up	• Nutrition • Sports • Psycho-oncology	• Restorative naturopathic measures • Balanced vitamins and trace elements • Probiotic therapy • Proteolytic enzymes* (4–9 tablets/day)
	• **Immunotherapy**** – mistletoe therapy	• **Immunotherapy**** – (thymic) peptide therapy – hyperthermia

*see p. 270; **see p. 270

Mammary carcinoma

Standard therapy	Efficacy-tested complementary measures	Extended complementary measures
Preoperative measures	• Nutrition • Psycho-oncology • Sodium selenite (100–200 µg/day) • Proteolytic enzymes* (4–9 tablets/day)	• Balanced vitamins and trace elements
Surgery	• Sodium selenite (300–1000 µg/day)	
Adjuvant therapy, or chemotherapy and radiation	• Sodium selenite (300–1000 µg/day) • Proteolytic enzymes* (4–9 tablets/day) • Mistletoe therapy • Nutrition • Sports • Psycho-oncology	• Restorative naturopathic measures • Balanced vitamins and trace elements • Vaccination with tumor cells or peptide antigens • Dendritic cell therapy
Follow-up	• Nutrition • Sports • Psycho-oncology	• Restorative naturopathic measures • Balanced vitamins and trace elements • Probiotic therapy • Proteolytic enzymes* (4–9 tablets/day)

	• **Immunotherapy****
	  – mistletoe therapy
		• **Immunotherapy****
		  – (thymic) peptide therapy
		  – hyperthermia

*see p. 270; **see p. 270

Ovarian carcinoma

Standard therapy	Efficacy-tested complementary measures	Extended complementary measures
Preoperative measures	• Nutrition • Psycho-oncology • Sodium selenite (100–200 µg/day) • Immunotherapy (depending on the indication)**	• Balanced vitamins and trace elements
Surgery	• Sodium selenite (300–1000 µg/day)	
Adjuvant therapy, or chemotherapy and radiation	• Sodium selenite (300–1000 µg/day) • Proteolytic enzymes* (4–9 tablets/day) • Nutrition • Sports • Psycho-oncology	• Restorative naturopathic measures • Balanced vitamins and trace elements • Probiotic therapy • Vaccination with tumor cells or peptide antigens • Dendritic cell therapy
Follow-up	• Nutrition • Sports • Psycho-oncology	• Restorative naturopathic measures • Balanced vitamins and trace elements • Probiotic therapy • Proteolytic enzymes* (4–9 tablets/day)
	• **Immunotherapy**** – mistletoe therapy	• **Immunotherapy**** – (thymic) peptide therapy – hyperthermia

*see p. 270; **see p. 270

Pancreas carcinoma

Standard therapy	Efficacy-tested complementary measures	Extended complementary measures
Preoperative measures	• Nutrition • Psycho-oncology • Sodium selenite (100–200 µg/day) • Immunotherapy (depending on the indication)**	• Balanced vitamins and trace elements
Surgery	• Sodium selenite (300–1000 µg/day)	
Adjuvant therapy, or chemotherapy and radiation	• Sodium selenite (300–1000 µg/day) • Proteolytic enzymes* (4–9 tablets/day) • Nutrition • Sports • Psycho-oncology	• Restorative naturopathic measures • Balanced vitamins and trace elements • Probiotic therapy
Follow-up	• Nutrition • Sports • Psycho-oncology	• Restorative naturopathic measures • Balanced vitamins and trace elements • Probiotic therapy • Proteolytic enzymes* (4–9 tablets/day)

	• **Immunotherapy**
	  – mistletoe therapy
		• **Immunotherapy**
		  – (thymic) peptide therapy
		  – hyperthermia

*see p. 270; **see p. 270

Penis carcinoma

Standard therapy	Efficacy-tested complementary measures	Extended complementary measures
Preoperative measures	• Nutrition • Psycho-oncology • Sodium selenite (100–200 µg/day) • Immunotherapy (depending on the indication)**	• Balanced vitamins and trace elements
Surgery	• Sodium selenite (300–1000 µg/day)	
Adjuvant therapy, or chemotherapy and radiation	• Sodium selenite (300–1000 µg/day) • Proteolytic enzymes* (4–9 tablets/day) • Nutrition • Sports • Psycho-oncology	• Restorative naturopathic measures • Balanced vitamins and trace elements • Probiotic therapy
Follow-up	• Nutrition • Sports • Psycho-oncology	• Restorative naturopathic measures • Balanced vitamins and trace elements • Probiotic therapy • Proteolytic enzymes* (4–9 tablets/day)
	• **Immunotherapy** – mistletoe therapy	• **Immunotherapy** – (thymic) peptide therapy – hyperthermia

*see p. 270; **see p. 270

Prostate carcinoma

Standard therapy	Efficacy-tested complementary measures	Extended complementary measures
Preoperative measures	• Nutrition • Psycho-oncology • Sodium selenite (100–200 µg/day) • Immunotherapy (depending on the indication)**	• Balanced vitamins and trace elements
Surgery	• Sodium selenite (300–1000 µg/day)	
Adjuvant therapy, or chemotherapy and radiation	• Sodium selenite (300–1000 µg/day) • Proteolytic enzymes* (4–9 tablets/day) • Nutrition • Sports • Psycho-oncology	• Restorative naturopathic measures • Balanced vitamins and trace elements • Probiotic therapy • Hyperthermia
Follow-up	• Nutrition • Sports • Psycho-oncology	• Restorative naturopathic measures • Balanced vitamins and trace elements • Probiotic therapy • Proteolytic enzymes* (4–9 tablets/day)

	• **Immunotherapy****
	  – mistletoe therapy
		• **Immunotherapy****
		  – (thymic) peptide therapy
		  – hyperthermia

*see p. 270; **see p. 270

Renal cell carcinoma

Standard therapy	Efficacy-tested complementary measures	Extended complementary measures
Preoperative measures	• Nutrition • Psycho-oncology • Sodium selenite (100–200 µg/day) • Immunotherapy (depending on the indication)**	• Balanced vitamins and trace elements
Surgery	• Sodium selenite (300–1000 µg/day)	
Adjuvant therapy, or chemotherapy and radiation	• Sodium selenite (300–1000 µg/day) • Proteolytic enzymes* (4–9 tablets/day) • Nutrition • Sports • Psycho-oncology	• Restorative naturopathic measures • Balanced vitamins and trace elements • Probiotic therapy • **Vaccination with tumor cells or peptide antigens** • **Dendritic cell therapy**
Follow-up	• Nutrition • Sports • Psycho-oncology	• Restorative naturopathic measures • Balanced vitamins and trace elements • Probiotic therapy • Proteolytic enzymes* (4–9 tablets/day)
	• **Immunotherapy**** – mistletoe therapy	• **Immunotherapy**** – (thymic) peptide therapy – hyperthermia

*see p. 270; **see p. 270

Sarcoma (osteosarcoma, Ewing sarcoma, soft tissue sarcoma)

Standard therapy	Efficacy-tested complementary measures	Extended complementary measures
Preoperative measures	• Nutrition • Psycho-oncology • Sodium selenite (100–200 µg/day) • Immunotherapy (depending on the indication)**	• Balanced vitamins and trace elements
Surgery	• Sodium selenite (300–1000 µg/day)	
Adjuvant therapy, or chemotherapy and radiation	• Sodium selenite (300–1000 µg/day) • Proteolytic enzymes* (4–9 tablets/day) • Nutrition • Sports • Psycho-oncology	• Restorative naturopathic measures • Balanced vitamins and trace elements • Probiotic therapy • **Hyperthermia**
Follow-up	• Nutrition • Sports • Psycho-oncology	• Restorative naturopathic measures • Balanced vitamins and trace elements • Probiotic therapy • Proteolytic enzymes* (4–9 tablets/day)
	• **Immunotherapy**** – mistletoe therapy	• **Immunotherapy**** – (thymic) peptide therapy – hyperthermia

*see p. 270; **see p. 270

Stomach carcinoma

Standard therapy	Efficacy-tested complementary measures	Extended complementary measures
Preoperative measures	• Nutrition • Psycho-oncology • Sodium selenite (100–200 µg/day) • Immunotherapy (depending on the indication)**	• Balanced vitamins and trace elements
Surgery	• Sodium selenite (300–1000 µg/day) • **Blockade of adhesion molecules**	
Adjuvant therapy, or chemotherapy and radiation	• Sodium selenite (300–1000 µg/day) • Proteolytic enzymes* (4–9 tablets/day) • Nutrition • Sports • Psycho-oncology	• Restorative naturopathic measures • Balanced vitamins and trace elements • Probiotic therapy • **Mistletoe therapy**
Follow-up	• Nutrition • Sports • Psycho-oncology	• Restorative naturopathic measures • Balanced vitamins and trace elements • Probiotic therapy • Proteolytic enzymes* (4–9 tablets/day)
	• **Immunotherapy**** – mistletoe therapy	• **Immunotherapy**** – (thymic) peptide therapy – hyperthermia

*see p. 270; **see p. 270

Testicular tumors (seminoma, nonseminoma)

Standard therapy	Efficacy-tested complementary measures	Extended complementary measures
Preoperative measures	• Nutrition • Psycho-oncology • Sodium selenite (100–200 µg/day) • Immunotherapy (depending on the indication)**	• Balanced vitamins and trace elements
Surgery	• Sodium selenite (300–1000 µg/day)	
Adjuvant therapy, or chemotherapy and radiation	• Sodium selenite (300–1000 µg/day) • Proteolytic enzymes* (4–9 tablets/day) • Nutrition • Sports • Psycho-oncology	• Restorative naturopathic measures • Balanced vitamins and trace elements • Probiotic therapy
Follow-up	• Nutrition • Sports • Psycho-oncology	• Restorative naturopathic measures • Balanced vitamins and trace elements • Probiotic therapy • Proteolytic enzymes* (4–9 tablets/day)
	• **Immunotherapy** – mistletoe therapy	• **Immunotherapy** – (thymic) peptide therapy – hyperthermia

*see p. 270; **see p. 270

Thyroid carcinoma

Standard therapy	Efficacy-tested complementary measures	Extended complementary measures
Preoperative measures	• Nutrition • Psycho-oncology • Sodium selenite (100–200 µg/day) • Immunotherapy (depending on the indication)**	• Balanced vitamins and trace elements
Surgery	• Sodium selenite (300–1000 µg/day)	
Adjuvant therapy, or chemotherapy and radiation	• Sodium selenite (300–1000 µg/day) • Proteolytic enzymes* (4–9 tablets/day) • Nutrition • Sports • Psycho-oncology	• Restorative naturopathic measures • Balanced vitamins and trace elements • Probiotic therapy
Follow-up	• Nutrition • Sports • Psycho-oncology	• Restorative naturopathic measures • Balanced vitamins and trace elements • Probiotic therapy • Proteolytic enzymes* (4–9 tablets/day)
	• **Immunotherapy** – mistletoe therapy	• **Immunotherapy** – (thymic) peptide therapy – hyperthermia

*see p. 270; **see p. 270

Tumors of the central nervous system (glioma)

Standard therapy	Efficacy-tested complementary measures	Extended complementary measures
Preoperative measures	• Nutrition • Psycho-oncology • Sodium selenite (100–200 µg/day) • Immunotherapy (depending on the indication)**	• Balanced vitamins and trace elements
Surgery	• Sodium selenite (300–1000 µg/day)	
Adjuvant therapy, or chemotherapy and radiation	• Sodium selenite (300–1000 µg/day) • Proteolytic enzymes* (4–9 tablets/day) • Nutrition • Sports • Psycho-oncology	• Restorative naturopathic measures • Balanced vitamins and trace elements • Probiotic therapy • Incense (3 × 800–1200 mg/day) • Mistletoe therapy
Follow-up	• Nutrition • Sports • Psycho-oncology	• Restorative naturopathic measures • Balanced vitamins and trace elements • Probiotic therapy • Proteolytic enzymes* (4–9 tablets/day)
	• **Immunotherapy**** – mistletoe therapy	• **Immunotherapy**** – (thymic) peptide therapy – hyperthermia

*see p. 270; **see p. 270

Urinary bladder carcinoma

Standard therapy	Efficacy-tested complementary measures	Extended complementary measures
Preoperative measures	• Nutrition • Psycho-oncology • Sodium selenite (100–200 µg/day) • Immunotherapy (depending on the indication)**	• Balanced vitamins and trace elements
Surgery	• Sodium selenite (300–1000 µg/day)	
Adjuvant therapy, or chemotherapy and radiation	• **Instillation of keyhole limpet hemocyanin** • Sodium selenite (300–1000 µg/day) • Proteolytic enzymes* (4–9 tablets/day) • Nutrition • Sports • Psycho-oncology	• Restorative naturopathic measures • Balanced vitamins and trace elements • Probiotic therapy
Follow-up	• Nutrition • Sports • Psycho-oncology	• Restorative naturopathic measures • Balanced vitamins and trace elements • Probiotic therapy • Proteolytic enzymes* (4–9 tablets/day)
	• **Immunotherapy** ** – mistletoe therapy	• **Immunotherapy** ** – (thymic) peptide therapy – hyperthermia

*see p. 270; **see p. 270

Carcinoma of vagina and vulva

Standard therapy	Efficacy-tested complementary measures	Extended complementary measures
Preoperative measures	• Nutrition • Psycho-oncology • Sodium selenite (100–200 µg/day) • Immunotherapy (depending on the indication)**	• Balanced vitamins and trace elements
Surgery	• Sodium selenite (300–1000 µg/day)	
Adjuvant therapy, or chemotherapy and radiation	• Sodium selenite (300–1000 µg/day) • Proteolytic enzymes* (4–9 tablets/day) • Nutrition • Sports • Psycho-oncology	• Restorative naturopathic measures • Balanced vitamins and trace elements • Probiotic therapy
Follow-up	• Nutrition • Sports • Psycho-oncology	• Restorative naturopathic measures • Balanced vitamins and trace elements • Probiotic therapy • Proteolytic enzymes* (4–9 tablets/day)
	• **Immunotherapy**** – mistletoe therapy	• **Immunotherapy**** – (thymic) peptide therapy – hyperthermia

* Standardized proteolytic enzyme mixtures consisting of papain, trypsin, chymotrypsin, and/or bromelain.

** Depending on the immune status, which is determined at six to 12 weeks after finishing the standard therapy and also when indicated. The following parameters are to be analyzed: Numbers of leukocytes in the peripheral blood, granulocytes, monocytes, lymphocytes (B cells, T cells, T helper cells, T suppresser cells, cytotoxic T cells), natural killer (NK) cells, and T-cell activity expressed as the number of IL-2 receptor-positive cells.

Extended complementary measures need further study-based evaluation concerning safety and efficacy.

22 Advances in Oncology—From Research to Application

Kurt S. Zänker

Introduction

The modern scientific propositions, which still seem to be valid today, go back to Galileo, Bacon, Descartes, and others (11). The validity of knowledge depended on its implementation in both material and technique. Descartes, in particular, maintained that detailed mechanistic findings regarding the pathogenesis of diseases would certainly lead to appropriate therapies. This view has been more successful than the competing theories of natural philosophers in solving the scientific problems of the seventeenth century, and the continuous successes in medicine have obviously proved that this interpretation is correct.

At first glance, this view is undergoing a revival in molecular medicine: artificial joints and cultured organs, electrically coupled pacemakers, implantable drug pumps, and gene probes–they all remind us a bit of the artistic mechanical clocks, musical boxes, and waterworks that Descartes was so enthusiastic about.

Opposed to this monocausal, mechanistic view of the world is another type of medicine that tries to understand the human being as the sum of all somatic, emotional, and social attributes. In oncology, the two different therapeutic approaches have been vigorously competing with one another, with the treatment strategies being molded by the model idea on which they are based.

The disease "cancer" is considered an accelerated proliferation of cells no longer governed by the growth controls of the organ. The development of new drugs able to interfere with this increased cellular growth was therefore a correct and consequent approach. It was successful primarily with early childhood tumors and tumors derived from the hemopoietic organs. The success rates were far lower with solid tumors, especially in adults.

The past 50 years have been the heyday of the monocausal model (7), with the anticancer strategy consisting of surgery, radiotherapy, and chemotherapy. Therapeutic approaches not directly based on cytostasis were no longer considered. The existing medicine was founded on the undisputed basic sciences of physics and chemistry and has now elevated itself to the status of an applied science.

Something has changed, however, because treatment results in oncology have stagnated and the prayer wheel-like prophecies of a therapeutic breakthrough have not materialized. It has even been demonstrated that there was a slow but steady increase in both cancer morbidity and cancer mortality between 1950 and 1982, despite all campaigns and clinical trials (2). A follow-up study for the period of 1970 to 1994 arrived at the following impressive, unambiguous, but often criticized conclusion: "The war against cancer is far from over. Observed changes in mortality due to cancer primarily reflect changing incidence or early detection. The effect of new treatments for cancer on mortality has been largely disappointing. The most prominent approach to the control of cancer is a national commitment to prevention, with a concomitant rebalancing of the focus and funding of research" (3).

A change in paradigm took place in basic research, and cellular and molecular biology replaced pure chemistry and physics as the central sciences. It was only the sum of all findings on carcinogenesis that finally triggered a shift in thinking from a single-minded view to a more complex approach (10). Tumor growth was now more than just the uncontrolled growth of neoplastic cells. The numerous sequential genetic alterations over decades, an outwitted immune system, an adequate vascularization, and a conversion of the normal process of cellular aging are just some of the factors involved in the complex code of carcinogenesis.

Now, it is important that the achievements made so far are not abandoned and that new approaches are combined with the tried and tested strategies against cancer. Effective protocols of chemotherapy and/or radiotherapy must not be questioned only because certain circles in the scientific community might have emotional or conceptual reservations. Old and new forms of therapy should be explored together for the benefit of the patient. Here, complementary oncology can make a considerable contribution, provided a well-founded theory is put forward.

New Approaches

High-Dose Chemotherapy

There is a direct relationship between the dose of chemotherapy and the extent to which tumor cells are killed, though the data given as evidence are mainly derived from experiments with cultured cells. Based on these in-vitro data, a curative reduction in tumor cells would require a five to eight times higher dose than is actually used in clinical protocols. However, such an increase in dose usually results in a complete collapse of the hematopoietic system so that particularly the defenses against infections are no longer guaranteed. In most cases, the hematopoietic system can only be reconstituted by costly **autologous bone marrow transplantation**. For this purpose, hematopoietic stem cells are harvested by multiple iliac crest punctures prior to chemotherapy. These cells, together with growth factors, are reinfused into the patient after chemotherapy in order to restore immunocompetence.

A less invasive procedure involves the preparation of hematopoietic progenitor cells from peripheral blood (CD34+ cells) by means of cell separators. In order to increase the number of these stem cells in the peripheral blood, mobilizing chemotherapy followed by growth factors is carried out immediately before the collection of cells. This form of high-dose chemotherapy during the reconstitution of important parts of the hematopoietic system is promising in case of the following indications:

– lymphogranulomatosis
– highly malignant non-Hodgkin lymphoma during the first chemotherapy-sensitive recurrence
– plasmacytoma with good remission after conventional chemotherapy
– small cell bronchial carcinoma (limited success)
– ovarian carcinoma (limited success).

Clinical studies still need to back up the value of this therapeutic modality for various other tumors.

Unfortunately, high-dose chemotherapy is also an example of how complex developments toward efficiency control can escape supervision by the scientific community. A South African clinical study claimed to have demonstrated surprisingly good results in case of advanced mammary carcinoma. However, the results of this study could not be reproduced at the international level. During an international investigation of the data, it became conspicuous that many data were not correctly collected, negative findings were suppressed, and patient protocols were even faked. This deliberate deception of oncological experts must be regarded as a very serious violation of scientific rules, because the women received a therapy that had no life-prolonging advantage but brought on considerable side effects and, hence, treatment-induced suffering.

Treatment Optimization Studies

The therapeutic results achieved by chemotherapy and/or radiotherapy must not be given up. However, the clinical efficacy of these protocols needs to be improved in so-called treatment optimization studies. For this purpose, existing protocols of proved efficacy are complemented by substances that may help with:

– overcoming chemoresistance
– enhancing the effect of cytostatic agents
– increasing the response rate
– prolonging the survival time
– reducing side effects.

Substances used in addition to the established protocols must not interfere in terms of pharmacokinetics and pharmacodynamics with the chemotherapeutic agents and should have no, or only minor, side effects of their own.

Third generation modulators that help **overcome chemoresistance** are already available. These are modified calcium antagonists of the verapamil type. In general, however, we still have to be content with keeping the ability of tumor cells to detoxify and repair during chemotherapy as low as possible. It is therefore a doubtful practice—because undocumented—to administer cell-protecting preparations of high antioxidant potential simultaneously with chemotherapy and/or radiotherapy, for many cytostatic agents as well as radiation act by producing highly reactive radicals that destroy cellular DNA.

Another way of optimizing conventional therapies is the targeted administration of **food supplements**. In a prospective clinical study, women with mammary carcinoma consumed every day a mixture of soy bean, honey, and low-fat milk in addition to receiving treatment according to a chemotherapy/radiation protocol involving anthracycline. This adjuvant treatment significantly improved the quality of life parameters (nausea, vomiting) as well as functional parameters (lowest point of leukocytes and thrombocytes).

Cancer Treatment Based on Target Structures

The idea of attacking cancer selectively was first conceived by two scientists, von Behring and Ehrlich. Their description of cancer was based mainly on the specific differences between tumor cells and normal body cells. Today, we can indeed identify distinctive molecular features of the cell surface that represent tumor-specific or tumor-associated markers. It is possible to produce monoclonal antibodies that recognize and block these surface molecules. The specific binding of antibodies then interrupts the signal transduction cascade leading to cell proliferation, migration, and metastasis.

Rituximab—An Antibody to CD20
CD20 is a transmembrane protein of normal and malignant B lymphocytes. It is required for B-cell differentiation and is expressed on over 90 % of B-cell non-Hodgkin lymphoma. The chimeric monoclonal antibody to CD20, rituximab (Rituxan), contains some mouse but mostly human amino acid sequences. The variable part of the antibody binds to the CD20 antigen, and the Fc fragment initiates complement-mediated and antibody-dependent cellular cytotoxicity (6).

Patients with indolent non-Hodgkin lymphoma that relapsed after initial chemotherapy received monotherapy with rituximab. The remission rate was almost 50 % and the duration of remission was 13 months on average. A second cycle of therapy after renewed progression was similarly effective (8).

Trastuzumab—An Antibody to ErbB-2
Trastuzumab (Herceptin) is a humanized monoclonal antibody directed against erbB-2 (also called HER-2/neu, HER2), a member of the family of epithelial growth factor receptors (EGFR). ErbB-2 is a heterodimerization partner of EGFR and, as such, a receptor for the EGF/TGF-α family of mitogens and involved in ligand-mediated signal transduction. The intracellular domain of this transmembrane protein exhibits tyrosine kinase activity, which triggers the signal transduction cascade for proliferation and migration once the ligand binds to the cell surface (4).

Trastuzumab recognizes and binds to the erbB-2 antigen, which is overexpressed on mammary carcinoma cells by up to 30 %. The mechanism of cytotoxicity is still unclear, but antibody-dependent cellular cytotoxicity is suspected.

In women with erbB-2-overexpressing mammary carcinoma, monotherapy at the metastatic state after pretreatment with chemotherapy resulted in a remission rate of 15 %. The remission rate increased to 25 % if no chemotherapy had been carried out before. In combination with paclitaxel (Taxol), a response rate of 42 % was achieved in patients with recurrent breast cancer after adjuvant chemotherapy with anthracycline, as compared with 17 % for paclitaxel alone. Prolongation of the progression-free period from three months to almost seven months and improvement of the quality of life has been documented (6).

Imatinib—An Inhibitor of Abl Tyrosine Kinase
Imatinib mesylate (Glivec/Gleevec) is a 2-phenylamino-pyridine derivative that selectively inhibits the Abl tyrosine kinase (14). It has been approved in both Europe and the United States for patients with interferon-resistant chronic myeloid leukemia (CML). Its mechanism of action is based on the fact that malignant cell clones of CML, which express the Brc/Abl oncogene, are constitutively dependent on the activity of the Abl enzyme, whereas normal myeloid cells are only facultatively dependent. This explains why this drug is well tolerated clinically. In one study, almost all patients (up to 100 %) responded with a reduction in the number of tumor cells when they were in a blast crisis (14).

The three drugs described above have been approved for treatment of the cancer types indicated. A negative example is edrecolomab (Panorex), a monoclonal antibody directed against the 17-1A antigen on the cell surface of epithelial cells. This epitope is found at high densities on the surface of adenocarcinoma cells of the colon and rectum. It was first believed that the adjuvant administration of edrecolomab would result in a lower rate of recurrences in patients with colorectal carcinoma after complete resection at UICC (International Union against Cancer) stage III (Dukes stage C) than in patients without adjuvant treatment with edrecolomab, upon which it was temporarily approved in Europe for these indications. In the meantime, other substances already available on the market (5-fluorouracil and levamisole) proved more effective with regard to lowering the rate of recurrences and/or metastasis. Several studies subsequently demonstrated that adjuvant treatment with edrecolomab is inferior, and this monoclonal antibody has therefore been removed from the market (6).

Monoclonal antibodies have been approved based on the improvement of surrogate markers. It remains to be seen in further studies whether antibody therapy has also a positive effect on patient survival time.

Inhibition of Angiogenesis

Solid tumors can only reach a certain size if blood vessels grow from the surrounding tissue into the tumor and provide it with oxygen and nutrients. Up to a certain thickness of the border zone, conglomerates of tumor cells are supplied with oxygen and nutrients through diffusion. In addition, tumor cells can tolerate a lack of oxygen easier than normal cells (anaerobic respiration). Nevertheless, once the tumor tissue assumes a certain architecture, tumor angiogenesis is obligatory for the growth of a nodular tumor.

Experimental results have been encouraging. Several substances inhibit **tumor vascularization** and, hence, also tumor growth: endogenous proteins and peptides [such as thrombospondin, angiostatin, endostatin, interleukin-6 (IL-6), platelet factor 4] as well as tissue inhibitors of metalloproteinases (TIMP). Mutations of the endothelial cell receptor required for angiogenesis have a similar effect. Some of the endogenous angiogenesis inhibitors are subject to positive control by p53, interferon (14), or IL-12. Mutations in the *p53* gene favor the vascularization of tumors and are often found in various types of tumors. There is also evidence that angiotensin-converting enzyme (ACE) inhibitors interfere with tumor growth by means of antiangiogenic mechanisms.

Thalidomide has been rediscovered because the malformations caused in the embryo probably resulted from a restriction of angiogenesis. In addition, cytostatic agents, such as **paclitaxel**, have a direct antiangiogenic effect.

It has been shown in mice that vaccination with DNA coding for the p185 erbB-2 protein and subsequent release of interferon can suppress the development of mammary carcinoma in 90% of the vaccinated mice as compared with an untreated control group. This was mainly due to a reduction in microvascular architecture.

Based on these observations, inhibition of angiogenesis has rapidly entered the clinical phases of testing. The angiogenic target structures are well defined experimentally, but there is no clear evidence of clinical efficacy in patients. It cannot be deduced from these findings that the size (volume) of a primary tumor is directly proportional to its metastatic potential. Small nodular tumor structures without connections to blood vessels carry the same risk for metastasis as do well-vascularized larger tumors. This might explain why clinical studies on the inhibition of neoangiogenesis in tumors have been disappointing so far and why we do not hear anything about a prospective clinical use these days. Many clinical studies have been terminated prematurely because of lack of efficacy (e.g., studies on batimastat, marimastat, metastat). Here, we have to go back to the drawing board, namely, to laboratory and animal experiments.

Many years of research are therefore still necessary before we can answer the question of whether clinically relevant results may be achieved with the theoretically fascinating concept of antiangiogenesis. There are indeed some case reports that should be taken seriously. They indicate that an interruption of blood supply (e.g., to liver metastases) by means of catheter technique and bolus obstruction of afferent and efferent blood vessels can result in a reduction of tumor volume or also in the remission of such tumors. It remains an open question whether this will prolong the survival time, because there are no well-documented studies.

Invasive blocking of the blood supply is currently indicated in cases where other methods—such as surgical removal of metastases, radiotherapy, or also chemotherapy—can only be used with little hope for success but with a considerable risk of side effects and restrictions of the quality of life.

Gene Therapy: Prospects

Gene therapy is the transfer of genes into cells in the hope that these will then express proteins with therapeutic effects. A stabile transfer to eukaryotic cells is often difficult to achieve. The cells usually process the new genetic material only temporarily, and the transferred gene is removed from the cell after an undefined number of cell divisions. Somatic gene therapy therefore requires suitable vectors that integrate the desired cDNA specifically into tumor cells so that the therapeutic protein will be expressed in sufficiently high numbers of copies.

The theoretic objectives of gene transfer used as a form of cancer treatment include:
- to increase the immunogenicity of tumor cells
- to block immune escape mechanisms
- to increase the anticancer activity of immune effector cells
- to protect normal tissues from the side effects of chemotherapy
- to introduce suicide genes into the tumor cells
- to suppress the activity of oncogenes
- to enhance the expression of wild-type tumor suppressor genes in tumor cells
- to suppress angiogenesis within the tumor.

Prerequisite for using this form of treatment is a detailed knowledge about the functions of proteins in normal and malignant cells in order to ensure the stable transfer of these functions by means of cDNA.

In most attempts of gene transfer, the natural regulatory element of the gene is not co-transmitted. Instead, viral promoters or enhancing sequences are coupled with the desired cDNA. Especially retroviral genomes are used as carriers.

The target cells must divide in order to ensure the successful transfer of new genetic material. Adenoviral vectors are often used because they can be effectively employed as carriers and can infect cells that do not divide. They align themselves at a specific region of chromosome 19 and remain outside the genome until the next cell division.

The search is now on for carriers that act as cDNA vectors without having to integrate into the genome of the cell. The desired protein can thus be expressed outside the genome. Preliminary in-vitro experiments with such vectors have been promising. It is still too early to tell whether these vectors will become clinically relevant.

The scenario of gene therapy is currently still too varied and confusing. The greatest chances of success in gene therapy may exist for monogenic diseases. Cancerous diseases, however, are multigenic aberrations; in the best of cases, gene therapy will only represent part of a comprehensive therapeutic concept in oncology. The scientific and ethical aspects of gene therapy are well known. What we now need is dealing with them in a foresighted way, both at the scientific and clinical levels, to avoid that the promising approaches are prematurely abandoned because the public and the patients have built up expectations that cannot be met in the daily clinical routine (1).

As in the case of therapy through antiangiogenesis, there have been deaths during clinical studies involving gene therapy. The authorities have therefore stopped many ongoing treatments until the safety of the patients can be ensured with regard to the vectors used. In addition, the clinical successes achieved with gene therapy were only marginal. None of the strategies used on their own is currently able to replace the corresponding standard treatments for cancer. At present, gene therapy can only be regarded as part of a multimodal therapeutic strategy.

Differentiation Inducers

Carcinogenesis is a process of cellular dedifferentiation. During embryogenesis, cells differentiate into certain cell types and assume certain organ-specific features while abandoning others (gene silencing). When developing into tumor cells, epithelial cells reassume characteristics that they exhibited earlier during embryogenesis and organogenesis. These biological properties are expressed in various ways:
- change in proliferative behavior
- expression of different proteins, e.g., carcinoembryonic antigen (CEA)
- induction of cell migration
- altered course of cellular aging and death.

This is not surprising as all genes are preserved during embryogenesis and organogenesis, and only the extent of their activity is regulated differently. Experimental studies indicate that the dedifferentiation of cells can be reversed and that this is accompanied by the loss of their proliferative capacity.

A good clinical example is the induction of differentiation caused by the chromosomal translocation t(15;17) and the resulting fusion of the retinoid receptor gene with the so-called PML gene that is associated with **promyelocytic leukemia (PML)**. Treatment with **all-*trans*-retinoic acid (ATRA)** leads to maturation of dedifferentiated cell populations, and most patients with this form of acute, nonlymphatic leukemia go into remission. However, intensive chemotherapy must follow as a further treatment because resistance to ATRA may develop secondarily. The mechanism is not yet understood.

Another indication for retinoids as differentiation inducers is **leukoplakia** of the oral cavity. It has been established that this precancerous state can be reversed by administration of **isotretinoin** (13-*cis*-retinoic acid). Empirical reports on topical administration of 13-*cis*-retinoic acid and interferon-α to atypical cells of the cervix, including **in situ cervical carcinoma**, have shown that the combination of these two substances can achieve redifferentiation of the neoplastically altered cervical epithelium.

Several other differentiation inducers, such as 1,25-dihydroxyvitamin D3, tiazofurin, cyclic AMP, hexamethylene bisacetamide (HMBA), and acetylcysteine, are still under preclinical testing and in early phases of clinical trials. They, too, will most likely be integrated into a multimodal treatment scheme only as part of a therapy.

Phytoestrogens, Polyphenols, and Nutrition

The connections between cancer and nutrition are complex and are further complicated by the fact that the biology of cancer is still very little understood. It is therefore not easy to develop sufficiently safe research instruments at the epidemiological, molecular-epidemiological, and (sub-)cellular levels, in order to find new approaches to therapy in this large field.

It is currently undisputed that a diet containing a high portion of fresh vegetables and fruits, green tea, and soy bean extracts considerably reduces the risk of developing epithelial tumors. It is therefore little surprising that nutritional scientist try more than ever before to extract preventive substances from tea and various types of vegetables and fruits so that these may be of-

fered in the form of pure preparations or monopreparations.

It has been postulated that, in addition to cancer-producing substances (carcinogens), nature also provides anticarcinogenic substances that ensure the survival of unicellular and multicellular organisms in an environment containing an abundance of carcinogenic compounds. For example, plants cannot escape strong ultraviolet (UV) radiation, and it is impossible for a plant to predict whether its growth location will have high UV radiation. Short-wave UV light damages the genetic material, and these damages may cause the plant to die. In order to absorb short-wave UV light, plants have developed **secondary plant metabolites** that either absorb this light or immediately capture free radicals resulting from the transfer of electrons. As long as these plants—predominantly leafy greens and tropical fruits—are part of the human food chain, humans are provided with natural anticarcinogens. The general rule that two handfuls of vegetables and fruits (in the three colors of a traffic light) should be a component of our daily food does not exist without good reason.

A considerable cancer-preventing effect has been attributed to **green tea** (5, 9). It contains **epigallocatechin gallate (EGCG)**. This suppresses carcinogenesis not only by means of its antioxidant characteristics, but also by inducing phase I and phase II enzymes for the modulation and excretion of carcinogens, as well as by possibly inducing apoptosis and by modulating oncogene expression. EGCG blocks the receptors for EGF, PDGF, and FGF and thus inhibits the growth-promoting signal transduction into the cell. EGCG and other polyphenols of tea, e.g., theaflavin-3-3′ digallate, block the inducible nitric oxide synthase (iNOS) by reducing the activity of transcription factor NF-κB.

Many research groups are examining various flavonoids contained in **soybean** for cancer-preventing properties: genistein, daidzein, quercetin, kaempferol, luteolin, and apigenin. These compounds are also known as **phytoestrogens** because they have weak estrogen activity. They inhibit the growth and motility of malignant cells derived from mammary, colon, and prostate carcinomas. Phytoestrogens primarily interfere with signal transduction by inhibiting tyrosine kinases and thus have an effect on proliferation, differentiation, and migration.

Curcumin, mimosine, and resveratrol are naturally occurring anticarcinogens because they inhibit the proliferation and migration of tumor cells. **Curcumin** is a phytopolyphenol that is a natural yellow food pigment as well as a spice used primarily in Indian curry. **Mimosine** is a plant amino acid found in the vitamin-rich leaves and seeds of *Mimosa pudica* (Central and South America, Asia, and Oceania). **Resveratrol** is a polyphenol produced in large quantities in red grapes.

In the future, special attention may be given to **inositol hexaphosphate (IP6), γ-oryzanol**, and other compounds of rice that are similar to the compounds of soy bean. They inhibit the neoplastic transformation of cells in various animal models.

The currently available nutritional supplements derived from green tea and soy bean, as well as borage oil and vitamin E, possess the biological characteristics of the individual substances mentioned above. They are supposed to reduce the risk of metastasis and to enhance the activity of the immune system in chronic diseases and especially in cancer.

As long as controversial nutritional supplements are marketed together with scientifically established background information and are produced under strict quality control, it makes sense to use them as food supplements.

Many secondary plant metabolites are already referred to as the vitamins of the twenty-first century. As their effects are dose dependent, it is essential that consumers are well informed about the benefits and risks of these nutritional supplements.

A prospective clinical study involving 8552 individuals in Japan showed that drinking 10 cups of green tea daily (as compared with three cups daily) increased the mean age at which people developed cancer by 6.2 years in women and by 3.2 years in men (9). As not everybody can drink 10 cups of green tea daily, it makes sense to consume an equivalent amount of active ingredients in the form of green tea extract.

Cancer Prevention

The rapidly accumulating results of research in molecular medicine will guide individual tumor diagnostics to individual tumor therapies in the near future. Molecular target structures identified in a patient's tumor sample will then become the target structures for therapeutic approaches. Un-

fortunately, the principal problem will be that the gap between molecular target structures and possible forms of treatment continues to widen.

We are learning to characterize many tumor targets, but the development and approval of target-specific anticancer drugs will severely trail behind if the currently established procedures for drug approval are kept in place. Study end points, such as morbidity and survival time, are being temporarily replaced by so-called surrogate parameters in order to speed up the approval of new active principles.

Nevertheless, it will remain absolutely essential to continue testing the efficacy of a drug with respect to the three prominent patient-based parameters: morbidity, quality of life, and survival time. It is never the individual tumor cell with all its aberrations of molecular biology that presents itself to the oncologist. It is always the cancer patient who hopes to receive medical, social, and psychological help through individualized treatment that can prolong the survival time and increase the quality of life.

An important and frequently discussed question is whether cancer is a curable or preventable disease (12). Whatever the answer to this question may be, cancer prevention certainly plays a far greater role than it did during the last 50 years (13). The three pillars of cancer prevention are: primary, secondary, and tertiary prevention.

Primary prevention is precaution, which can be practiced both epidemiologically and individually and should ensure that malignant diseases do not develop. It includes nutrition, avoidance of well-defined physical and habitual risk factors (e.g., smoking, alcohol abuse, exposure to intense sunlight) and, possibly, also vaccinations. In the future, vaccinations against hepatitis B virus and against human papillomavirus will reduce the incidence of primary liver cell carcinoma and cervical carcinoma, respectively.

Secondary prevention is the screening with all available instrumental and biochemical tools, including imaging procedures. It is used to detect cancer in the entire population and/or in certain risk groups as early as possible and to treat it successfully with conventional therapy.

All arguments about the value of screening procedures, such as those for mammary or colorectal carcinoma, have been considered at the academic level. The results of future studies should demonstrate the individual value of screening methods for those examined, or the economic gain achieved by saving treatment costs or averting early retirement. Based on these results, the entire community will have to make decisions regarding public heath care.

Tertiary prevention typically includes perioperative or postoperative adjuvant chemotherapy, radiotherapy, and hormone therapy. It addresses those patients for which it was possible to show histologically that the tumor had been completely removed from the healthy tissue. Apart from this, there is no evidence that would justify diagnosing a progressive cancer with the current diagnostic possibilities. Nevertheless, measures should be taken to reduce considerably the risk of recurrences and/or metastasis. Here, too, several unanswered questions remain: Who profits from such a therapy? Who is overtreated by such a therapy? Moreover, which parameters can measure the success of an adjuvant therapy?

It has been shown by case reports and preliminary clinical results that 1,2-benzopyrone and its 7-OH derivative (umbelliferone) reduce the risk of metastasis by means of inhibiting oncogene expression, proliferation, and migration. The substances themselves have no toxicity worth mentioning and can therefore be combined with other active principles (e. g., hormone therapy) and used in outpatient clinics.

▬ Comorbidity

Until 2030, the population pyramid in Germany will change in such a way that the proportion of old people will increase from 15 % to 25 %. This will result in an increase in cancer by 50 % if the age-dependent incidence remains constant. Already now, over 50 % of cancer patients are more than 65 years old at the time of diagnosis, and over 60 % of cancer deaths occur in this age group. Hence, there is an urgent need for geriatric oncology (6).

Because of the age distribution, comorbidity will play a more prominent role in the caring for cancer patients. The percentage of diagnoses of hypertension, cardiovascular diseases, and arthritis or arthropathy in tumor patients of age 55 and over, is between 35–43 %. About 10 % of cancer patients are diabetics or have glucose intolerance. It will therefore be necessary in the near future to have therapeutic procedures at hand for such comorbidities, i. e., treatments that neither interfere

with the pharmacokinetics or pharmacodynamics of cancer therapies nor reduce the quality of life even further.

Adequate nutrition will play a major role especially with respect to metabolic diseases. It certainly makes sense here to choose, upon the advice of a physician or after consulting a pharmacist, suitable nutritional supplements, the ingredients of which have been clinically tested for their physiological curative effects but do not have the characteristics of a medicine. Recently, a nutritional supplement derived from plants (a phytonutrient) has been introduced that delays the transport of monosaccharides and disaccharides from the intestinal epithelium into the blood vessels, thus slowing down the rise in blood glucose after a meal. Case reports have shown that this does reduce the Hb A1c value to below 6.5 %. Such preparations are of high value particularly for cancer patients, because clinically tested nutritional supplements must not be toxic but should possess physiological effectiveness as distinct from pharmacological efficacy.

▬ Outlook

In this new century, oncological research and therapy will have to follow a double path. Prevention must receive the same attention as therapy, which is often ineffective. Within prevention, the early detection of malignant cell transformation (which will then lead to early treatment) will have to be promoted more vigorously. It is important to realize that the size of a tumor is no indication of its tendency to spread. Very small aggregates of malignant cells do have metastatic capacity, whereas tumors of more than 2 cm in diameter often have not yet formed any clinically detectable metastases.

The essential question in cancer research is: why does a benign, sessile cell assume a malignant, invasively migrating phenotype? If we were able to answer this question adequately, the problem of solid tumor development in adults would have long been solved satisfactorily, for a primary tumor that is detected early (and therefore treated) is not the principal cause of suffering and, ultimately, death.

We hope that molecular medicine will be able to identify the genotype of potentially metastatic cells. Combined therapeutic approaches are therefore required which supplement each other or, better yet, enhance each other in their benefits for the patient. It is understood that all treatments in complementary oncology must be subjected to critical methodical testing.

▬ References

1. Assmann G, Brandt B, Zänker KS: Research in gene diagnostics of cancer disease. Preface: Joint Meeting and Laboratory Course, Research in "Gene Diagnostics and Cancer Disease," Gene 1995; 159:ix–x.
2. Bailar III JC, Smith EM: Progress against Cancer? New Engl. J. Med. 1986; 314:1226–1232.
3. Bailar III JC, Gornik HL: Cancer undefeated. New Engl. J. Med. 1997; 336:1569–1574.
4. Brandt B, Roetger A, Dittmar T, et al.: C-erbB2/EGFR as dominant heterodimerization partners determine a mitogenic phenotype in human breast cancer cells. FASEB J. 1999; 13:1939–1949.
5. Fujiki HJ: Two stages of cancer prevention with green tea. J. Cancer Res. Clin. Oncol. 1999; 125:589–597.
6. Höffken K (ed.), Kolb G, Wedding U: Geriatrische Onkologie. Berlin, Springer-Verlag 2002.
7. Lerner M. Choices in Healing—Integrating the Best of Conventional and Complementary Approaches to Cancer. Cambridge, MA, The MIT Press, 1994.
8. McLaughlin P, Grillo-Lopez AJ: Rituximab chimeric anti-CD20 monoclonal antibody therapy for relapsed indolent lymphoma: half of patients respond to a four-dose treatment program. J Clin Oncol. 1998; 16:2825–2833.
9. Nakachi K, Matsuyama S, Miyake S: Preventive effects of drinking green tea on cancer and cardio-vascular disease: Epidemiological evidences for multiple targeting prevention. BioFactors. 2000; 13:49–54.
10. Zänker KS: Die Suche nach Stofflichkeit und Begrifflichkeit in der Vermittlung von Leib und Seele –Unterwegs zu einem anderen Medizinkonzept. In: Herkunft, Krise und Wandlung der modernen Medizin. Kulturgeschichtliche, wissenschaftsphilosophische und anthropologische Aspekte. Berliner Studien zur Wissenschaftsphilosophie und Humanontogenetik, (Wessel KF, ed.), Kleine Verlag, Bielefeld, vol. 3. 1994; 3:124–134.
11. Zänker KS: Zellkommunikation und die Theorie morphischer Felder. In: Rupert Sheldrake in der Diskussion. Das Wagnis einer neuen Wissenschaft des Lebens. (Dürr HP, Gottwald FT, eds) Bern, Scherz-Verlag, 1997; 60–77.
12. Zänker KS: Klinische Interventionsstudien zur Chemoprävention – Vom Rationale zu Ergbnissen, Der Onkologe. 1998; 4:716–722.
13. Zänker KS: Ohne die Chemoprävention wird die Onkologie im nächsten Jahrhundert schuldhaft versagen. Von der molekularen Prävention zur klinischen Anwendung. Nova Acta Leopoldina NF 78. 1998; 305:21–34.
14. Zänker KS, Tominaga S, Mihich E, Gao YT: International Symposium on Molecular Basis for Cancer Chemo- and Immunoprevention, Shanghai, China. J Cancer Res Clin Oncol. 2002; 128: 288–293.

Index

Page numbers suffixed by "t" refer to tables;
page numbers suffixed by "f" refer to figures.